At the Epicentre: Hong Kong and the SARS Outbreak

What was really happening as Hong Kong struggled with SARS? In *At the Epicentre*, the story of those extraordinary weeks unfolds with all its drama — personal, national and international, political, medical and scientific.

The authors give us the whole picture: from a day-by-day calendar of events to the experiences of a SARS-sufferer; from the heroic efforts of the medical staff in the hospitals to the work of the pioneering global network of laboratories that the World Health Organisation (WHO) created; from the amazing shift to openness of the Chinese authorities to a detailed study of how the global media covered the story.

It is a story of individuals, of Dr Gregory Cheng recounting how it felt to have SARS, of the concentrated and intense work of Professor Malik Peiris as he struggled to identify the virus, of Dr David Heyman of the WHO as he dealt with intense political pressures yet moved the international effort along at high speed.

The impact of SARS on Hong Kong was enormous and far-reaching. *At the Epicentre* explores the economic consequences, the way the community responded, and what might be the long-term political implications for Hong Kong, for China and for the international community. The authors are rigorous but fair in their criticisms, recognizing that what seems clear now was not always so in the heat of the battle. But most important are the lessons they draw from the events and experiences for the next time, for the authors all recognize that SARS is just the first global epidemic of the new century.

"Having the opportunity to help write and put this book together represents the culmination of a very special personal experience. It was a personal journey where I met many caring and energetic people who all wanted to help Hong Kong. Today, the most vivid and heart-warming memories are those of working with people from all walks of life and sharing each other's fears and joys. I am also aware of the pain and grief that SARS has left in our community. Each illness and each death affected many people. In considering the positive lessons, we must not forget that there were losses that were irreparable." — Christine Loh

AT THE
EPICENTRE

Disclaimer

Civic Exchange is a non-profit organisation that helps improve policy and decision-making through research and analysis. This is a collaborative report and the views expressed do not necessarily represent the opinions of Civic Exchange.

AT THE EPICENTRE

HONG KONG AND THE SARS OUTBREAK

Edited by Christine Loh
and Civic Exchange

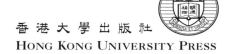

香港大學出版社
HONG KONG UNIVERSITY PRESS

Hong Kong University Press
14/F Hing Wai Centre
7 Tin Wan Praya Road
Aberdeen
Hong Kong

ISBN 962 209 683 2 (Hardback)
ISBN 962 209 684 0 (Paperback)

Secure On-line Ordering
http://www.hkupress.org

British Library Cataloguing-in-Publication Data
A catalogue record for this book is available
from the British Library.

Cover design by Jeffrey du'Vallier d'Aragon Aranita
Printed and bound by United League Graphic & Printing Co. Ltd., in Hong Kong, China

CONTENTS

PREFACE

Christine Loh

...SARS can and must be contained — pushed back out of its new human host. One by one, the many puzzling features of this new disease are being unmasked. One by one, the most severe outbreaks in the initial waves of infection are being brought under control. Recommended measures — case detection, isolation and infection control, and contact tracing and follow-up surveillance — are working. With this reassurance, the image of populations unmasked because of fear, the public face of SARS, can now begin to fade.

— The World Health Organisation (WHO)

20 May 2003

S ARS' place in history is assured. It was the first severe new disease to emerge in the twenty-first century. As such, it provided a warning of what could happen in a globally interconnected world where infectious diseases have the capacity to spread rapidly along international air travel routes. Within a period of days, SARS spread from mainland China via Hong Kong to many cities around the world. In the initial stages of the outbreak, doctors did not even know what to call the disease, much less how it should be treated. The symptoms were like those of common pneumonia but the disease was clearly more virulent. For want of a better term, doctors began referring to it as a form of "atypical pneumonia."

Fortunately, SARS was not the global pandemic that communicable disease experts had feared it would be. Despite its ability to spread via air travel, the disease was relatively inefficient in human-to-human transmission. Had it been more efficient, the world would have been in much bigger trouble. But SARS gave us a sense of what "the real thing" — a full global pandemic — could be like. Many experts fear that SARS could re-emerge as early as the winter of 2003, albeit on a less severe scale. However, new and more deadly diseases could also be lurking and the world needs to prepare for a worst-case scenario — for the emergence of an unknown disease that is efficient in human-to-human transmission. Dr. Henk Bekedam of the World Health Organisation (WHO) has warned that it is not enough to be 100% ready for infectious diseases, the authorities "need to be 300% ready." A sobering thought indeed.

So far, with the exception of HIV/AIDS, few of the new diseases that have emerged during the past several decades have presented a major threat in terms of global public health, which may be why the authorities in developed countries have become somewhat complacent about communicable diseases. Avian flu, Nipah virus, West Nile fever and the Ebola virus are worrying but to date, the impact of these diseases has been regional rather than international. However, health experts were alarmed by certain characteristics of SARS as a disease, particularly its common and non-specific symptoms and its ten-day incubation period — a period long enough to allow carriers who seemed healthy to spread SARS locally and internationally via air travel.

In the future, the outbreaks of greatest concern will be those that occur in transportation hubs, such as Hong Kong, or in densely populated areas, such as south China, because such outbreaks could affect a large number of people, which would in turn make treatment and control much more challenging. Hence, the WHO regards every country with an international airport, or bordering an area where there is an outbreak, as a high-risk area in terms of transmissible diseases. For those of us who live in the south China neighbourhood, SARS brought home to us the fact that our region has a history of being the world's incubator for new diseases. In a global world, this presents special responsibilities for regional authorities as well as citizens in terms of disease prevention and control.

The worldwide response to SARS was also atypical. Events happened quickly. Healthcare professionals had to face enormous personal risks in fighting the disease on the frontline. Scientists around the world collaborated to an unprecedented degree to find out what they could about SARS as the first step in discovering a cure. Need has been the mother of a number of useful inventions, such as the contact tracing system developed in Hong Kong. SARS also touched almost every other aspect of personal and community life in affected areas. Ministers and officials lost their jobs. Many businesses suffered. Ordinary people were forced to reassess their priorities. Communities had to find useful ways of coping with panic while continuing to fight the disease.

*   *   *

This book opens with a **Calendar of Events** compiled by William Chiu and Veronica Galbraith, two researchers at Civic Exchange, which shows key local and international events between November 2002 and September 2003. As this timeline illustrates, the pace of the SARS outbreak was breathtaking and overwhelming, particularly for communities dealing with the disease. The Calendar provides a useful reference for readers and sets the stage for Chapter 1, **Unmasking SARS: Voices from the Epicentre**, written by seasoned reporters Alexandra Seno and Alejandro Reyes. This chapter describes the looming SARS crisis by piecing together different narratives to give a sense of how SARS affected the lives of individuals in Hong Kong.

    I am grateful to Dr. Moira Chan, a well-respected respiratory health specialist, for contributing Chapter 2. **At the Frontline: The Medical Challenge** traces the progression of the disease from its emergence in mid-November 2002 in Guangdong Province, China, to its transmission to Hong Kong in February 2003, from where it was exported via air travel to Singapore, Vietnam, Toronto and other international cities. In each of the affected areas, the pattern of infection was the same. The disease first took root in hospital settings when healthcare workers were unknowingly exposed to the infectious agent. Hospital staff then spread the disease to the community. Chapter 3 is the personal story of a distinguished doctor who himself became a SARS patient. Gregory Cheng's **Healing Myself: Diary of a SARS Patient and Doctor** recounts his personal experience of SARS on a day-by-day basis. His insights as both a doctor and a patient contribute to our understanding of the disease and its impact on human lives. Dr. Chan and I co-wrote Chapter 4, **The New Coronavirus: In Search of the Culprit**, which describes the role of scientists from Hong Kong and around the world in learning more about the new disease and summarises what we know about the virus to date.

    In addition to the immediate medical challenge, SARS also presented a major public health challenge for Hong Kong. Public health scholars Gabriel Leung, Anthony Hedley, Edith Lau and Tai-Hing Lam co-wrote Chapter 5, **The Public Health Viewpoint**, which highlights the response of local officials and institutions to the outbreak. The authors discuss the need for additional information about the disease for effective disease control in the future and make a plea for improvement in the internal communication and culture of Hong Kong's public health institutions in order to achieve deeper and broader collaboration among the stakeholders involved in health management.

During the SARS outbreak, although medical professionals and virologists played a vital role in caring for the sick and identifying the coronavirus, experts in other disciplines could also have made an important contribution had they been more extensively involved in the fight against the disease. For example, aerosol scientists could have helped public health authorities to better understand the spread of infectious diseases. Statisticians could have helped to analyse trends in the outbreak. I was, therefore, particularly keen to have Alexis Lau and Stephen Ng contribute to this book. Dr. Lau is an aerosol scientist and a mathematician. His Chapter 6, **The Numbers Trail: What the Data Tells Us**, shows how non-medics could have helped to unravel some of the questions and controversy surrounding infection and death rates for the disease. Dr Ng, an epidemiologist, contributes a fascinating Chapter 7 titled, **The Mystery of Amoy Gardens**, Amoy Gardens was the housing estate where between 21 March and 1 April 2003, 187 residents and 142 households were affected by SARS. Dr. Ng helps us to understand various theories as to why this housing estate was so susceptible to SARS and why, despite studies by the Hong Kong Government and the WHO, this mystery has yet to be fully resolved.

In addition to the obvious impact of SARS on medicine, public health and science, the impact of SARS on Hong Kong politics also deserves serious consideration. Michael DeGolyer discusses the effect of SARS on local politics and the many challenges it posed for officials in Chapter 8, **How the Stunning Outbreak of Disease Led to a Stunning Outbreak of Dissent**. His chapter also looks at the relationship between SARS, Article 23 legislation and Government accountability from a political perspective, particularly in terms of the massive 1 July 2003 demonstrations. I have contributed a chapter focusing on the politics of Hong Kong and mainland China, including the role played by the

WHO. Chapter 9, **The Politics of SARS: The WHO, Hong Kong and Mainland China**, explores the relationships between Hong Kong and Guangdong, Guangdong and Beijing and Hong Kong and Beijing. Chinese efforts in terms of disease control and prevention were critical in the fight against SARS worldwide. China's initial denial of the severity of the disease contributed directly to the extent of the global outbreak. In Chapter 10, **SARS and China: Old vs New Politics**, YIP Yan Yan and I highlight what we believe are the inherent contradictions in the Chinese political system, which continues to favour secrecy over transparency even as national leaders seek modernity and global recognition of China as a responsible world power.

The next three chapters help to provide a more complete picture of Hong Kong's SARS experience. Economist Stephen Brown offers a useful discussion of Hong Kong's political economy in Chapter 11, **The Economic Impact of SARS**. He shows that SARS actually had little impact on the overall economic picture, although individual businesses, especially those in the travel and hospitality sectors, obviously suffered. Indeed, Hong Kong's amazingly successful external sector, which includes trade and global manufacturing, appears not to have been affected at all. William Chiu, Veronica Galbraith and I take a look at how Hong Kong was affected by international media reporting on SARS as well as the controversial role played by the Hong Kong media in Chapter 12, **The Media and SARS**. The local media felt conflicted by its role as objective bystander and its desire to use media channels to participate directly in fighting SARS.

Finally, Jennifer Welker and I examine the community response to the outbreak in Chapter 13, **SARS and the Community**. The disease had the effect of forcing individuals to reassess their personal priorities and companies to consider their social responsibility. The sense of community solidarity was one of the most enduring aspects of the SARS experience and may prove to be one of the most significant in terms of Hong Kong's future.

I provided the concluding Chapter 14 on **Lessons Learned**. This chapter summarises some of the key points noted by other authors as well as providing additional insights on the impact and legacy of SARS, particularly in light of the findings of the SARS Expert Committee Report, released on 2 October 2003, and the Hospital Authority Review Panel Report on the SARS Outbreak, released on 16 October 2003.

*　　*　　*

Like many organisations in Hong Kong, Civic Exchange sought to contribute to the fight against SARS in some way. How could we participate most usefully as a public policy think tank? In April 2003, we drew on our network of researchers to provide SARS data to the public as and when it became available. Later, we helped to found *Fearbusters*, a community campaign to develop short- and long-term projects related to disease prevention and improving public hygiene. We closely followed SARS-related events as they took place, both locally and globally. When Hong Kong University Press suggested that we consolidate this information and write about the lessons learned from SARS, we were delighted to do so. This book is the outcome of that suggestion.

Having the opportunity to help write and put this book together also represents the culmination of a very special personal experience. As the devastating impact of SARS on the community became evident, I found myself at a loss as to what I could do for Hong Kong. My feeling was that we needed to deal with our fear first and foremost so that we could assess the risk of catching the disease objectively and take effective preventative action, both on a personal and on a societal level. I believed strongly that providing the public with timely information at the outset would have helped to ease panic. Since I manage a research organisation, my focus is on informing people about issues and events from as broad a perspective as possible. This is how I thought I could contribute. I learned what I could about SARS and tried to provide information and analysis to others through Civic Exchange and the *Fearbusters* campaign. This became a personal journey through which I met many caring and energetic people who all wanted to help Hong Kong. Today, my most vivid and meaningful memories from the outbreak are of working together with people from all walks of life and being able to share my fears and hopes for the future with others. I am also aware of the pain and grief that SARS has left behind in the community. Each illness and death affected many lives. In recognising the positive aspects of SARS as a learning experience, we must not forget that there were irreparable losses.

Acknowledgements

We are grateful to all of the authors for their willingness to participate in this project and for writing so enthusiastically and speedily. Each played an important role, whether directly or indirectly, in fighting SARS. We also wish to thank Elizabeth Hutton, Veronica Galbraith and Joanne Bunker for their editorial advice and assistance, and Colin Day for his wise counsel and constant encouragement in helping us get this book out on time.

As a whole, we hope this book will tell the story of Hong Kong's SARS experience from a variety of perspectives. Civic Exchange believes that by considering this experience widely from the viewpoint of experts as well as generalists, the book provides an honest account of what life was like at the epicentre of the SARS outbreak. It looks at the question of how the people of Hong Kong perceived what was happening to them and whether this has altered their sense of identity and community. Hopefully, the experience of SARS and the lessons that can be learned from it will help Hong Kong and other cities to be more prepared for dealing with similar emergencies in the future.

Shortly before this book went to print, the government-appointed SARS Expert Committee released its report on the public sector's handling of SARS. That report was followed by the release of the Hospital Authority Review Panel report on the SARS outbreak two weeks later. Both reports point to a lack of leadership, absence of strategy and contingency planning and poor communication and crisis management skills as major weaknesses of Hong Kong's healthcare system. However, the finding by the Expert Committee that no one with the power to make decisions was responsible for error does little to address public demands for increased accountability and transparency on the part of the authorities. While the Review Panel report was highly critical of many aspects of Hong Kong's handling of SARS, it also avoided the issue of accountability. Had time permitted, I would have liked to include an additional chapter to this book that compared the findings of the two reports.

The Tung Chee-hwa administration needs to understand that its unpopularity, as demonstrated by the massive public protest on 1 July 2003, is due to its governance style and poor decision-making. Its abhorrence of fault finding is characteristic of its approach to running Hong Kong. In politics, those who hold power must to be able to move on from mistakes so that new opportunities for the renewal of public trust are created. Finding individuals to be at fault is never an easy task. Indeed, it is unpleasant and difficult. But to try and explain Government errors by saying that officials tried their best, that SARS was a new threat or that it is better for officials to stay in power because they have learned from past mistakes rings hollow to the public — particularly given the high human and economic cost of SARS for Hong Kong. Moreover, lingering doubts about the competency and transparency of officials will continue to fester and sap the credibility of the administration as a whole. It would be equally painful for the individuals concerned to remain in power and be forced to continue to defend their actions and decisions. A more effective approach would be to remove individuals responsible for error from office and signal a new beginning by introducing fresh faces.

Undoubtedly, there are important lessons to be learned from SARS. The question remains whether Hong Kong authorities are ready to learn them and change accordingly.

Christine Loh
Chief Executive Officer
Civic Exchange
October 2003

Calendar of Events

William Chiu and Veronica Galbraith

All events in Hong Kong unless otherwise indicated.

 Events in Mainland China

 International events (excluding Hong Kong and China)

To the greatest extent possible, all dates are in Hong Kong time.

2002

 16 November *First known case*
A chef specializing in exotic meats is treated in Foshan city. He is later identified as the first reported SARS patient.

2003

23 January *Confidential report issued about Guangdong outbreak*
A Guangzhou medical official delivers a confidential report to the Guangdong Department of Health describing an unknown respiratory disease outbreak.

31 January *SARS patient arrives in Guangzhou*
A man from Zhongshan is admitted to hospital, where he infects 30 people. He is transferred to another hospital, where he infects 26 others. He has also spread the disease to 19 family members.

8 February *Guangdong informs Beijing*
Guangdong informs the Central Authorities in Beijing about the outbreak and holds a press conference in Guangdong on 10 February about it. Officials state that everything is under control. For months, citizens of Guangdong have been using facemasks, antiseptic and traditional methods, such as vinegar and a herb called Isatidis Radix, to prevent infection.

11 February *WHO receives report*
The WHO receives a report from the Chinese Ministry of Health of an outbreak of acute respiratory syndrome in Guangdong listing 305 cases including 105 affected healthcare workers and 5 deaths. Calling the disease "a minor problem" officials emphasize that the disease is under control. On 12 February the WHO is informed that the outbreak in Guangdong affects 6 municipalities and that the disease is not a flu virus. On 14 February, Beijing tells the WHO that the outbreak in Guangdong is consistent with atypical pneumonia.

21 February *Super-spreader checks in at Metropole Hotel*
Dr. Liu Jianglun, who has treated SARS patients in Guangzhou, stays at the Metropole Hotel in Hong Kong. He spreads the virus to other guests in the hotel. They subsequently carry the disease to Vietnam, Canada, Germany, Singapore and Ireland, as well as locally to the Prince of Wales Hospital. Dr. Liu checks into Kwong Wah Hospital on 22 February, warning healthcare workers that he has a "very virulent disease." This warning allows them to take special precautions when treating him. Dr. Liu dies on 4 March.

23 February *WHO officials arrive in Beijing*
The team from the WHO requests permission to go to Guangdong to investigate the new disease.

26 February *Carlo Urbani reports first case of SARS in Vietnam to WHO*
Johnny Chen, an American businessman, is admitted to hospital under the care of Dr. Urbani after contracting the disease at Hong Kong's Metropole Hotel. The Vietnamese Government learns of the situation on 5 March. On 10 March, the affected hospital is shut down. Dr. Urbani is hospitalized on 11 March and dies on 29 March.

1 March *Woman admitted to hospital in Singapore*
A 26 year-old woman is admitted to hospital with respiratory problems. She stayed at the Metropole Hotel from 21 to 25 February while in Hong Kong.

5 March *Death in Toronto*
A woman dies in Toronto's Scarborough Grace Hospital after returning from Hong Kong on 23 February. She had stayed on the same floor as Dr. Liu at the Metropole Hotel. Five of her relatives have also been infected.

5 March *First case reported in Beijing*

6 March *Princess Margaret Hospital receives first patient*
Johnny Chen is transferred back from Hanoi to Hong Kong, where he had contracted the virus while staying across the hall from Dr. Liu on the ninth floor of the Metropole Hotel. Mr Chen dies on 13 March.

10 March *China asks for help from WHO*
Chinese officials request laboratory and technical support in investigating the cause of the Guangdong outbreak.

11 March *Outbreak Prince of Wales Hospital Ward 8A*
The Prince of Wales Hospital announces that more than 20 healthcare workers assigned to Ward 8A are showing symptoms of an unknown upper respiratory disease. The disease is suspected to be airborne and related to February's atypical pneumonia outbreak in Guangdong.

 12 March *WHO issues first global alert*
The WHO issues a global alert for an outbreak of a "severe form of pneumonia" in Vietnam, Hong Kong, and Guangdong province.

Hong Kong contacts WHO
Hong Kong government notifies WHO of the outbreak at the Prince of Wales Hospital.

13 March *Government announces measures to tackle the disease*
Saying that the public has no cause for worry, the Secretary for Health, Welfare and Food, Dr. EK Yeoh, announces that the government has identified Ward 8A of the Prince of Wales Hospital as the source of the outbreak and believes that the disease is spread by droplets. The government establishes a steering group to coordinate the fight against the disease and an expert group to investigate it further. The WHO is invited to provide support and advice. The government begins to give daily updates of the situation to the public.

14 March *No community spread*
Secretary Yeoh comments on the WHO's global alert on Hong Kong stating that there is no pneumonia outbreak in Hong Kong as all cases are limited to healthcare workers and their families. He warns that the press must report the situation accurately.

 15 March *WHO issues second global travel alert and names disease "SARS"*
With the disease spreading quickly via air travel, the WHO issues a second travel alert. It announces the case definitions for suspected and probable cases, providing guidelines for healthcare workers worldwide, and names the virus "Severe Acute Respiratory Syndrome" after its symptoms.

 Air China flight 112 starts string of infections
Hong Kong-Beijing Flight CA 112 is responsible for a string of SARS cases that spread throughout Asia. Twenty-two passengers and two flight attendants eventually fall ill.

17 March *HK Government accuses WHO of spreading panic*
Secretary Yeoh accuses the WHO of spreading panic over SARS while denying that the disease has spread in the community.

Professor Chung contradicts Yeoh

Professor Sydney Chung of the Chinese University informs the press that there are cases outside the medical community — a sign that the disease is in fact spreading in the community, directly contradicting Yeoh. The next day, Secretary Yeoh admits for the first time that there are cases of SARS outside the medical community.

China tells WHO: All under control

China issues a brief report stating that Guangdong's outbreak is under control.

SARS spreads to many countries

14 suspected cases of SARS are reported in the US, and first cases have been reported in Germany, Switzerland, Spain, Thailand, Malaysia and, on 18 March, the UK and Taiwan.

Laboratories worldwide collaborate to understand SARS

Under WHO's coordination, an international network of 11 laboratories involving 9 countries is established to determine the cause and treatment of SARS.

18 March   *Chinese University thought to have identified virus*

The Chinese University of Hong Kong announces that they have identified the SARS virus as paramyxoviridae, which later turned out to be wrong.

19 March   *Hong Kong's first SARS deaths confirmed*

The first five deaths are announced. Secretary Yeoh explains that it has taken the government several days to confirm that the deaths were indeed SARS related.

Prince of Wales ICU closed

The Hospital Authority (HA) decides that the Prince of Wales Hospital's intensive care unit (ICU) must close for 3 days. The ICU is eventually reopened on 29 March.

Different diseases

Zhang Wenkang, the Chinese Health Minister, states that the SARS outbreak in Hong Kong may have little to do with Guangdong's outbreak.

20 March   *Hong Kong learns of SARS spread in community*

The Hospital Authority receives confirmation that the virus is spreading in the community and subsequently informs the Department of Health the same day, according to an internal e-mail which is disclosed to the public on 29 March.

21 March   *University of Hong Kong devised first diagnostic test*

The University of Hong Kong announces that it has devised a diagnostic test that verifies the presence of the SARS virus in 1 hour. Also, the scientific team singles out a coronavirus as the likely candidate of SARS virus as it is found in 95% of the cases.

First case reported in Italy

23 March *Measures to protect possible spread of SARS in schools*
The government asks all students and school staff who have had contact with SARS patients to stay home for one week.

24 March *Measures to fight SARS in the community announced*
The government, declaring that it will be making a full effort to fight SARS, establishes an inter-departmental taskforce. It also announces that it will issue sector-specific guidelines to the public on how to combat the virus. Because the disease is spreading in the community, the government calls on "each and every citizen of Hong Kong" to help fight the disease.

 Singapore imposes home quarantine measures
Singapore requires all people having contact with SARS patients to spend 10 days at home in isolation.

 First case reported in France

25 March *Classes will go on*
Top government officials decide that classes will continue in all schools, despite the fact that 54 schools have decided to shut down for two days (26-27 March). Secretary for Education and Manpower Arthur Li says that the schools are safe, and closing schools might in fact increase the risk of contracting the disease.

 27 March *Further measures to combat SARS*
Invoking the powers under the Quarantine and Prevention and Disease Ordinance, Chief Executive Tung Chee-hwa announces that people who have been in contact with SARS patients are to stay home for 10 days and report for daily check-ups at designated clinics during that time. The media estimates that this measure will affect more than 1,000 people. In addition, the government will establish a liaison mechanism between Hong Kong and Mainland authorities to better coordinate measures to fight SARS. Also, all inbound passengers into Hong Kong are required to fill out a health declaration form at all immigration control points from 29 March. To help prevent the spread of SARS, classes in all schools other than tertiary institutions are closed until 6 April.

 SARS in Beijing, Shanxi
A Chinese spokesperson said that there had been 4 cases in Shanxi Province and 8 cases in Beijing, including 3 deaths. All cases in Beijing were imported cases, he said.

 27 March *First case reported in Romania*

28 March *Hong Kong Rugby Sevens continue as scheduled*
Although nearly all performers and artists scheduled to perform in Hong Kong have cancelled their tours due to concerns over SARS, the annual Rugby Sevens continues as scheduled. It is the last major public event to take place until SARS subsides.

31 March *Amoy Gardens Block E is isolated*
Block E of Amoy Gardens is put in isolation until midnight on 9 April. Of the 213 infected residents, 107 lived in the same wing of the same block.

HK$200m Funding
The Hong Kong Legislative Council approves HK$200 million (US$25.7 million) in funding for SARS education, prevention and treatment.

1 April *Amoy Gardens Block E residents relocated*
Believing that the virus has spread through the sewage system infecting residents, the government relocates all residents on Block E of Amoy Gardens to two holiday camps in Sai Kung and Chai Wan for isolation. The 250 residents return home on 10 April.

April Fool
A 14 year-old boy hacks on to a newspaper's website and posts a phony news story stating that the Hong Kong government will soon declare Hong Kong an "infected port" and thus be cut off from the world. This creates widespread panic, causing thousands of Hong Kong residents to line up in supermarkets for food supplies. Director of Health Margaret Chan calls an urgent press conference to deny the rumour. The boy was eventually charged for violating the Crime Ordinance.

 First case reported in Australia

2 April *WHO travel advisory imposed on Hong Kong and Guangdong*
For the first time in its history, the WHO issues a travel advisory recommending that global travelers postpone non-essential travel to Hong Kong and Guangdong.

HK exhibitors barred from Basel Fair
The Swiss government announces that exhibitors from SARS affected countries are not allowed to participate in one of the world's top watch and jewelry fairs, the Basel World Watch and Jewelry Show, scheduled for 3-10 April in Basel, Switzerland.

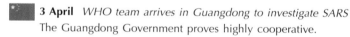 **3 April** *WHO team arrives in Guangdong to investigate SARS*
The Guangdong Government proves highly cooperative.

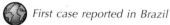 *Chinese Health Minister Zhang Wenkang states that China is "safe"*

 First case reported in Brazil

 5 April *First case reported in Malaysia*

8 April *Lower Ngau Tau Kok Estate*
The Department of Health instructs the Housing Authority to clean the Lower Ngau Tau Kok Estate, an aging public housing complex across the street from Amoy Gardens. Under pressure, the Housing Authority discloses that there are 30 cases of SARS affecting 27 families in the estate.

Statement by Jiang Yanyong is published in the international press
Dr. Jiang Yanyong, a retired Chinese surgeon, tells the foreign media that there are many SARS cases in Beijing's military hospitals, contradicting Health Minister Zhang Wenkang's 3 April statement that there were only 12 SARS cases in Beijing. International pressure on China to release accurate SARS figures increases after Dr. Jiang's statement is published.

9 April *Malaysia imposes travel ban on Hong Kong residents*
Malaysia freezes issuance of visas to Hong Kong residents and "Visa on Arrival". (Holders of the HKSAR passport have previously enjoyed a 30 day visa-free access to Malaysia.)

WHO releases report on Guangdong and Beijing
The WHO issues a report of the outbreak in Guangdong noting the strong medical system there is responding well to the outbreak, but such success is not expected should the virus spread to other parts of China. The same report is much more critical of the situation in Beijing, stating that few hospitals in Beijing have been reporting SARS cases daily, contact tracing is not monitored closely, and that rumours about SARS are not sufficiently pursued by authorities.

First case reported in South Africa

10 April *Escalating quarantine measures*
The Department of Health announces that all people in contact with SARS patients are to confine themselves at home for 10 days with no visitors.

Change of heart
Under intense public pressure, the government finally agrees to publish the partial addresses of SARS sufferers. Only the buildings' names are announced.

First case reported in Kuwait

11 April *Hong Kong and Guangdong pledge heightened cooperation*
Hong Kong and Guangdong officials announce an agreement to exchange disease information, cooperate on medical issues, create a disease notification system, and set up quarantine at the border.

12 April *High level meeting in Shenzhen*
Chinese President Hu Jintao meets Hong Kong's Chief Executive Tung Chee-Hwa in Shenzhen and states that China will provide "full support" to Hong Kong by delivering medical supplies and protective gear if necessary.

14 April *University classes resume*
Classes in all universities in Hong Kong resume.

First cases reported in the Philippines and Sweden

15 April *First case reported in Indonesia*

16 April *WHO confirm identity of SARS virus as coronavirus*
The WHO announces that a new form of coronavirus is the cause of SARS.

17 April *Hong Kong medical delegation visits Guangzhou*
Deputy Director of Health Leung Pak-yin leads a delegation of medical professionals to meet Mainland health authorities to discuss the treatment and prevention of SARS. Delegates discuss establishing a disease notification mechanism between Hong Kong and Guangdong province.

Amoy Garden Report released
The government releases the results of its investigation into the SARS outbreak at Amoy Gardens. The report indicates that dried U-shaped water traps in contaminated sewage systems are partly to blame for facilitating the spread of SARS virus within residential blocks. Not entirely satisfied with this report, the WHO sends a team to conduct an independent investigation.

China announces that all officials should give a candid account of SARS
Premier Wen Jiabao announces after a Politburo meeting that all officials must provide accurate and timely information about the SARS outbreak.

Temperature screening for outbound airport passengers begins

First cases reported in India and Mongolia

20 April *Chinese health minister and Beijing mayor sacked*
Health minister Zhang Wenkang and Beijing Mayor Meng Xuenong are fired. The Ministry of Health announces that there are 339 confirmed cases and 402 suspected cases of SARS in Beijing alone, nine times higher than the previously released figures. The nationwide death toll stands at 79 with 1,814 confirmed cases. Vice-Premier Wu Yi becomes the Minister of Health on 26 April.

No "Golden Week"
Chinese authorities announce that celebrations for the May First "Golden Week" vacation are cancelled. While admitting that this will have a major impact on tourism, health officials in Beijing say that their number one priority is the well-being of the population.

22 April *Malaysia lifts travel ban on Hong Kong residents*
After 13 days of negotiations between Malaysia and Hong Kong, Malaysia lifts the travel restriction imposed on residents of SARS-affected countries.

Classes resumed for students
Students and teachers are asked to wear masks during class, and parents are told to take their children's temperature on a daily basis. Classes in all secondary schools resume on 28 April; Primary Four to Six resume classes 12 May; and classes in all remaining primary and special schools resume 19 May.

23 April *Relief and economic revival measures*
The government announces a package of relief measures worth HK$11.8 billion (US$ 1.5 billion) in an attempt to help the community overcome economic difficulties resulting from SARS. The package includes waivers of rate payments and fees for various licenses targeting the travel, food, entertainment and retail industries, and rent concessions for most commercial tenants of the Housing Authority and government departments. The package also includes the reduction of water, sewage and trade effluent surcharges as well as a tax rebate.

 WHO extends travel advisory
WHO issues travel advisories to Beijing, China's Shanxi province, and Toronto, Canada.

24 April *Hong Kong's outlook downgraded*
Fitch Ratings change Hong Kong's sovereign outlook from stable to negative due to the impact of SARS.

WHO officials to study Amoy Gardens on site
A WHO expert arrives in Hong Kong to follow up the Hong Kong government's report on the Amoy Gardens outbreak.

25 April *Quarantine measures extended to suspected cases*
Families of suspected SARS patients must confine themselves at home for a period of 10 days.

Hong Kong-Guangdong meeting
Chief Executive Tung led a delegation of officials to meet Guangdong Governor Huang Huahua and other top Guangdong officials in Shenzhen to discuss SARS. They agree to improve communication between Hong Kong and Guangdong.

26 April *First medical worker dies of SARS*
A nurse at Tuen Mun Hospital who contracted SARS while treating SARS patient is the first medical worker to die of the virus.

Inbound visitors to have temperature taken
All people, including transit passengers, arriving at any of Hong Kong's checkpoints will have their temperature taken to further monitor the spread of SARS.

 27 April *Xiaotangshan SARS hospital is completed in Beijing*
7,000 workers complete a hospital dedicated to SARS patients in 8 days.

 28 April *Outbreak contained in Vietnam*
WHO officials remove Vietnam from the list of SARS-affected areas.

 29 April *Chinese Premier Wen Jiabao arrives in Bangkok*
The Premier takes part in a ASEAN-China Leaders' Meeting on SARS.

 First case reported in South Korea

30 April *WHO lifts Toronto travel advisory*
WHO states that local measures to stop the spread of SARS have been effective.

1 May *"We Love HK" campaign commences*
Amid the sharp decline of visitors in Hong Kong, the Tourism Coalition of Hong Kong looks to the people of Hong Kong to revive the local economy. The coalition, whose members include representatives from the hotel, tourism and airline industries, launches the "We Love HK" campaign which offers incentives for Hong Kong residents to spend at various businesses to get cash moving in the economy.

 2 May *First case reported in New Zealand*

3 May *WHO sends three officials to Taiwan with Beijing's consent*
Taiwan has been requesting help from the WHO from the beginning of their SARS outbreak.

5 May *Government announces "rebuild measures"*
The government announces new measures to fight SARS, which include possibly establishing a CDC-type organization specializing in fighting and preventing infectious diseases. The government also launches "Team Clean", a special taskforce headed by Chief Secretary Donald Tsang to provide long and short-term solutions to Hong Kong's hygiene problems.

 First case reported in Colombia

6 May *Serum treatment*
The Prince of Wales Hospital uses serum from recovered SARS sufferers to treat SARS patients who are not responding to Ribavirin and steroid treatment.

7 May *Number of new cases of infected medical staff drops to zero for the first time since the outbreak*

Hong Kong students not welcomed at US school
The University of California at Berkeley refuses to let students from SARS-affected countries attend their summer school programme. The decision is reversed on 17 May after a rebuke from the WHO. The university apologises to the affected students and their parents for making the decision.

More overseas exhibition trouble
Organisers of the JCK Las Vegas Show 2003, an international jewelry trade show, ask Hong Kong exhibitors to move their displays to a parking lot outside the exhibition hall. The Hong Kong government intervenes. The organizers reverse their decision on 13 May. Hong Kong exhibitors are still required to isolate themselves for 10 days upon arrival to the US.

 First case reported in Finland

8 May   *Mainland medical supplies arrive*
Chief Executive Tung asked for medical supplies from the Mainland and visits Shenzhen to receive medical supplies sponsored by the Central Government, including 110,000 protective suits. A second batch of supplies arrives in Hong Kong from the Mainland on 29 May.

Baptist Hospital admits cover-up
Baptist Hospital, a private hospital, admits that 5 patients suspected of SARS have been treated at the hospital without informing patients who share the same ward "to avoid panic." Upon receiving a full report from the hospital on 27 May, the Director of Health Chan publicly criticizes the hospital for not following instructions to report SARS cases on 2 June. On 4 June, the hospital replaces the head of hospital. On 6 June, the widow of a SARS victim infected in the ward sues the hospital of negligence.

 WHO extends travel advisory to Taipei, Tianjin and Inner Mongolia

10 May   *HK$1billion to re-launch Hong Kong*
Hong Kong to spend HK$1billion (US$129 million) to marketing Hong Kong internationally, including hiring a PR firm.

13 May   *SARS doctor dies*
Tuen Mun Hospital doctor Joanna Tse Yuen-man is the first doctor at a public hospital to die after contracting SARS on the job.

 14 May   *WHO removes Toronto from list of SARS affected areas*

 15 May   *Chinese Government passes new law*
The new law allows the death sentence and life imprisonment for those who break SARS quarantine and deliberately spread the disease.

16 May   *Hong Kong athletes banned from Special Olympics*
The Irish government decides to ban athletes from SARS-affected countries from participating in the 2003 Special Olympics World Summer Games. The games are to be held in Dublin, Ireland, beginning on 21 June. The Irish government reverses its decision on 7 June on the condition that athletes stay in a non-affected country for 10 days prior to their arrival in Ireland.

Temperature check for outbound land and sea travellers
All outbound travellers from the Hong Kong Macau Ferry Terminal and the China Ferry Terminal must have their temperature taken in an effort to monitor SARS. Starting 21 May, passengers departing from Hung Hom KCR terminus will also have their temperature checked.

WHO releases report on Amoy Gardens
The WHO's report mostly confirms the findings of the previous investigation conducted by the Hong Kong government, and adds that exhaust fans installed in bathrooms and the misuse of flush water might have played in part in spreading and breeding the virus.

17 May *WHO extends its travel warning to include Hebei Province, China*

 19 May *WHO's 56ᵗʰ General Assembly*
Secretary Yeoh speaks in Geneva, stating that Hong Kong's steps to control SARS have been and continue to be effective.

 21 May *First case reported in Macao*

 WHO extends travel advisory to all of Taiwan

23 May *WHO travel advisory lifted from Hong Kong and Guangdong*
52 days after issuing a travel advisory on Hong Kong and Guangdong province, the WHO announces that both regions have successfully controlled the SARS outbreak and lifts the travel advisory implemented on 2 April.

Civet cats believed to be possible source of SARS
The University of Hong Kong, together with Shenzhen Disease Control and Prevention Centre, discover that the genetic sequencing of the coronavirus found in civet cats is 99% the same as the SARS virus. On 24 May, the government announces that importing game meat from civet cats, a Chinese delicacy, is temporarily suspended as a precautionary measure.

24 May *Zero new infections*
No new cases are recorded in Hong Kong for the first time since the outbreak.

 26 May *WHO re-lists Toronto as affected area*
The WHO lists Toronto as an area where SARS has recently been transmitted locally after Canadian health officials report new clusters of 26 suspect and eight probable SARS cases linked to four Toronto hospitals.

28 May *Team Clean announces strategy to improve hygiene*
Chief Secretary Tsang announces measures to boost personal, home, and community hygiene. Short-term measures include a major cleanup of the city, including increasing fines.

Controversial SARS Experts Committee established
A SARS Experts Committee is established to review the government's handling of SARS but controversy arises as it is to be led by Secretary Yeoh. The legislature passes a motion on 30 May urging the government to establish an independent committee instead.

 31 May *Singapore removed from the WHO's list of "affected areas"*

 First case reported in Russia

5 June *Economic growth forecast halved*
Hong Kong revises its 2003 economic growth forecast from 3% to 1.5%.

13 June *WHO removes areas of China from list of affected areas*
Guangdong, Hebei, Hubei, Jilin, Jiangsu, Shaanxi, Inner Mongolia, Shanxi and Tianjin provinces are all removed from the WHO list.

 17 June *WHO SARS conference opens in Kuala Lumpur*
The conference assesses the SARS crisis and how different governments managed their outbreaks.

23 June *Hong Kong removed from WHO's list of SARS-affected areas*
100 days after Hong Kong was listed as a SARS-affected area, the WHO finally announces that Hong Kong is off the list. School staff and students are no longer required to wear facemasks in class. The government immediately announces a HK$400 million (US$51.5 million) promotion plan to attract Mainland and overseas tourists to Hong Kong.

 24 June *Beijing removed from WHO's list of SARS affected areas*

 2 July *Toronto removed from WHO's list of SARS affected areas*

 5 July *Taiwan removed from WHO's list of SARS affected areas*

WHO announces that SARS is under control worldwide

17 July *Secretary Yeoh removed as head of SARS Expert Committee*
Responding to public pressure, Secretary Yeoh is removed as head of the review committee "in order to further dispel public misunderstanding." The Committee will submit its report to the chief executive in October 2003.

 9 September **SARS resurfaces in Singapore**
The WHO confirms that a 27 year-old post-graduate medical student, who works in a virology lab, tested positive for SARS. The WHO stresses that this is a mild, isolated case that has not produced any secondary cases and "is not an international public health concern."

References

"Disease Detectives," Hong Kong University Convocation Newsletter, **www.hku.hk/ convocat/newsletter/0306/04-15_SARS.pdf**, 6 June 2003," pp. 4-15.

"Feature: A Doctor's Extraordinary April in 2003," *People's Daily*, **http:// english.peopledaily.com.cn/200306/13/eng20030613_118182.shtml**, 13 June 2003.

WHO SARS Update, **http://www.who.int/csr/don/2003_07_04/en/**, 4 July 2003.

HKSAR Government Press Releases, **http://www.info.gov.hk/isd/news/index.htm**

Media Reports

CHAPTER 1

Unmasking SARS:
Voices from the Epicentre

Alexandra A Seno and Alejandro Reyes

D ressed in a black sleeveless shirt and matching trousers, Virginia looked ready for a turn on a nightclub dance floor. But on the sweltering afternoon of 1 July 2003 — the sixth anniversary of the handover of Hong Kong from British to Chinese sovereignty — the restaurant manager was heading to Victoria Park to join a protest. Organisers billed the demonstration as a march against the national security bill that the Government of Chief Executive Tung Chee-hwa had proposed in accordance with Article 23 of the Basic Law, Hong Kong's constitution. Yet the controversial legislation was certainly not the only issue on the minds of the half a million people who turned up in spite of the 34-degree heat and strength-sapping humidity. "We have so many reasons to be dissatisfied," Virginia declared as protesters chanted for Tung to resign.

One popular poster printed by a local newspaper pressed home her point. It showed a caricature of a befuddled Tung surrounded by several signs, each representing one of the many problems bedevilling his administration: the sluggish economy, persistent deflation, the depressed property market, the mounting budget deficit, Article 23 — and, of course, severe acute respiratory syndrome, now better known as SARS. This mystery disease had arrived stealthily in Hong Kong more than four months earlier, smuggled across the border by a coughing, feverish passenger on a bus from Guangzhou. The virus would eventually infect thousands and kill hundreds in Asia, North America and Europe, triggering panic as it spread and battering East Asian economies.

While SARS appears to have originated in mainland China, it was only after the virus emerged in Hong Kong that the world began to take note. SARS spread quickly from Hong Kong's medical community into the general population and, via infected travellers, was exported to Canada, Singapore and Vietnam. Within the space of a few weeks, Hong Kong had become the epicentre of a global outbreak.

SARS struck Hong Kong at a moment when the confidence of Hong Kong citizens in the Government was already at a low. Since its transition from British colony to a special administrative region (SAR) of China in 1997, Hong Kong had endured the Asian financial crisis, the collapse of the property market and the effects of a global economic downturn, as well as the indirect effects of the 9–11 terrorist attacks and the wars in Afghanistan and Iraq. SAR residents were already worried about their future. SARS deepened those anxieties. The immediate concern, however, was the risk of infection. Many people wore surgical masks, even at home or in the car. Washing hands became compulsive as disinfectant spray dispensers appeared in shopping malls and office buildings. People avoided public places, leaving restaurants, cinemas, buses and sidewalks empty. School was cancelled, and meetings and conferences postponed. The sudden drop in activity in what is one of the world's most densely populated and frenetic cities was surreal.

At the same time, SARS also brought Hong Kong people closer together. The mask turned into a symbol of solidarity. "We shall overcome" became a rallying song. This community spirit seemed to persist, even after the World Health Organisation (WHO) lifted the travel advisory for Hong Kong and the number of new SARS cases dropped to zero. It was this sense of unity in the face of adversity that contributed to the massive protests on 1 July 2003. Watching the hundreds of thousands of protestors marching peacefully past the Government offices in Central, it was hard not to feel that the priorities and goals of Hong Kong people had shifted in the past four months.

*   *   *

There was a spring chill in the air on Friday, 7 March 2003, when Dr. Henry Chan Lik-yuen entered Ward 8A of the Prince of Wales Hospital (PWH) in Shatin. The 34-year-old associate professor at the Chinese University of Hong Kong (CUHK) was head of PWH's hepatitis treatment unit. With over a decade of experience under his belt, the sharp and affable physician was a rising star in the Faculty of Medicine.

That morning, Chan was serving as an examiner, observing and marking clinical students as they made their rounds in the wards. It seemed like a routine day. In reality, it was anything but that. In one of Ward 8A's 34 beds lay a 26-year-old airport worker with flu-like symptoms. In late February, he had gone to see a friend at the Metropole Hotel in Kowloon, where Dr. Liu Jianlun, a visiting doctor from Guangzhou, was staying in Room 911. On Saturday, 22 February Liu checked himself into Kwong Wah Hospital, telling doctors that he had "a very virulent disease," and demanded that special precautions be taken when treating him. Liu died 10 days later.

The Ward 8A patient, who had somehow come into contact with Liu at the Metropole, was having difficulty breathing. He was being treated with a nebuliser, a device that changes liquid into a mist so that patients with respiratory problems can inhale medicine into their lungs more easily. What healthcare workers did not realise was that the apparatus also sprayed droplets into the air around the patient, spreading his disease to nearby patients, nurses and doctors.

Unaware that he had been infected, Dr. Chan worked out at his gym for two hours the next day, then played an hour of badminton and an hour of basketball with friends. On Sunday, his muscles were aching. Too much exercise, he thought. On Monday, 10 March, he was still hurting down to his bones and running a fever. He called in sick. The following day, Chan could not get out of bed. He felt "cold from the inside." When he phoned PWH to say he was still unwell, he was told to go to the hospital immediately so that he could be monitored. A number of doctors, nurses and medical students had reported similar symptoms, he was told.

Chan was admitted to PWH with a fever above 39 degrees Celsius. The next day, when his temperature dropped to 37.8 without paracetamol treatment, he was discharged. He returned to his flat where his wife, also a physician, took care of him, believing he had the flu. But later that day, after his fever shot up again, Chan took a taxi back to the hospital. He would remain there for the next three weeks.

*   *   *

Professor Clive Cockram also remembers Monday, 10 March. At midday, the 54-year-old endocrinology lecturer was in a routine meeting with colleagues in an office at PWH. They were discussing incoming postgraduate students when they were interrupted. "We were called into a conference by the chief of service — and then we heard the news," Cockram recalls. A large number of hospital staff and students were ill with flu-like symptoms, with more and more falling sick. "From the get-go," says Cockram, "we knew we were dealing with something serious."

Cockram and other healthcare workers at PWH who were still healthy dropped everything to tend to the growing number of infected patients, forming the front line of defence at what would become ground zero of the SARS outbreak in Hong Kong. "It's been non-stop," Cockram said one week later. "It's been scary. It's been psychologically tough and harrowing." Initially, visitors were allowed to come in and out of the wards and medical workers were allowed to go home to their families at the end of their shifts. Via these contacts, the virus spread to the community, despite Government claims that the outbreak had been contained in the hospital.

Meanwhile, the growing number of patients with similar symptoms in Hanoi, Singapore and Toronto was raising concern. On 12 March, the WHO issued a global alert warning of the emergence of a "severe form of pneumonia" in Vietnam, Hong Kong and China's Guangdong Province. The WHO released a second advisory three days later, dubbing the virus "severe acute respiratory syndrome," or SARS — a name that many in Hong Kong saw as a cruel pun on the fact that the virus had come to international attention in the SAR.

The first response from Hong Kong Government officials was to minimise local and international concerns about the new disease. On 17 March, Hong Kong Secretary of Health, Welfare and Food Dr. Yeoh Eng-kiong accused the WHO of spreading panic, denying that the disease had broken out into the community.

But health professionals like Professor Cockram knew that the situation was serious. The affected patients demonstrated a variety of symptoms, including sharp muscle pain, headaches and high fever. Some required a respirator in order to breathe. In the absence of any real information about what they were dealing with, doctors were forced to experiment with different treatments to keep patients alive.

The task was made even more difficult because the wards were filled with familiar faces, colleagues whom Cockram and other staff knew well. Seeing so many students fall ill was particularly distressing. At one point, Cockram broke down and cried. "They are like our children," he later explained. "We're teaching them to be doctors. It was heartbreaking. This is a new disease and so we didn't know what to do. We felt so helpless."

During those difficult days, tears were not uncommon among PWH staff. "I have seen real selfless heroism," Cockram recalled later. "We are so proud of our frontline staff. They did everything they could do. Young doctors went to the wards without thinking of themselves, even if they were all scared."

*   *   *

One young doctor fighting for his life was Henry Chan, now in one of the beds in Ward 8D. He says he hardly remembers his first few days in hospital. Shivering with chills and running a high fever, he was always exhausted. "I would close my eyes and the next thing I knew, I had fallen asleep for four hours," he says. He was under the care of Dr. Joseph Sung Jao-yiu, Chairman of CUHK's Department of Medicine and Therapeutics, whose office one floor up was across from Chan's. Sung, who later authored one of the first scientific journal reports on SARS, visited his colleague-turned-patient at least twice a day.

After he did not respond to antibiotics, Chan was prescribed oral Ribavirin, a powerful antiviral agent. When he found out how high the dosage was he was shocked. "They were giving me three times the amount I give to my Hepatitis C patients. This regimen was going to be toxic but I had had fever for many days and we had to try." Chan, of course, was well aware of the side effects of the drug: a decline in red blood cells and a further drop in energy levels. His situation would deteriorate quickly and easily.

As the days passed, breathing became more difficult for Chan. Just taking a shower required considerable effort. He could not turn on his side by himself. One colleague who rang him on his mobile phone to see how he was doing cried as she listened to him gasping for air. She thought he was going to die.

Chan's chest X-rays raised serious concern on his tenth day in hospital. After the doctor-patient saw the film, for the first time he was scared. The lower and middle parts of his lungs were almost completely white, an indication of the extent of the build-up of mucus. "This is the bad thing about being a doctor," he says. "I knew it was very serious." He called his wife, who was looking after their 16-month-old daughter, to let her know.

Chan was administered an even larger dose of Ribavirin intravenously. He now laughs when he recalls how "very busy" his IV drip was as it fed him a potent cocktail of Ribavirin, steroids and antibiotics to combat a disease about which there was still very little information. The treatment worked. On Day 12, his fever broke. Four days later, an X-ray showed his lungs had almost cleared. Looking back weeks later, Chan says: "I'm a very aggressive person. This is why I conquered it." But at the time, even as his breathing became less laboured, the doctor, known among his colleagues for his energy and enthusiasm, lay exhausted in his hospital bed, barely able to react to the good news.

Chan was kept under observation for another week and put through a regimen of physical rehabilitation. Because the Ribavirin had lowered his red blood cell count, he was suffering from anaemia. The steroids caused his muscles to atrophy. During convalescence, he and some of the other recovering SARS patients — many of them colleagues — would play cards but were generally too tired to play more than a few hands. Chan spent hours reading newspapers and watching television. "I never knew Hong Kong TV programmes were so bad," he joked.

*   *   *

As the SARS outbreak unfolded, the medical community around the world nervously watched the developments in Hong Kong and China. Many wondered whether the mystery disease would prove to be the twenty-first century equivalent of the global influenza epidemic of 1918, which led to the deaths of tens of millions of people. Public health experts, including WHO specialists, have long feared the outbreak of a major flu pandemic. Airplane travel means that a contagious, airborne flu could spread across continents in a period of hours.

In 1982, the British medical journal *The Lancet* published the seminal article, "An Influenza Epicentre?" by Dr. Kennedy Shortridge, a microbiologist then working as a professor at the University of Hong Kong (HKU), and C.H. Stuart-Harris, a colleague. The article discussed the links between all recorded influenza epidemics and southern China, a region that has long been a crucible for viruses. Shortridge, who began his research career in Australia in the 1970s, moved to Hong Kong in 1975 to study influenza viruses, particularly their presence in poultry and other animals. In 1992, he collected blood samples from farmers in Taiwan, Hong Kong and China's Jiangsu and Guangdong provinces. His analysis showed that mainland farmers had antibodies for every known flu virus, suggesting that farms in these areas were a locus for multiple pathogens — the agents of disease.

Weather is, of course, a factor in the proliferation of viruses and bacteria. "The very humid and warm weather in southern China makes it easy for pathogens to grow," says Chen Kow-tong, an epidemiologist with Taiwan's Centre for Disease Control (CDC). Temperatures rarely sink below 2 degrees Celsius and the humid, rainy autumn and spring seasons provide perfect breeding conditions.

But there are other factors that make this part of China a natural petri dish for pathogens. Flu viruses can mutate, allowing them to hop from human to animal and vice versa. This tendency, called zoonosis, has accelerated over the last two decades in the Pearl River Delta region due to the proliferation of poultry and pig farms, often in cramped conditions — a result of growing prosperity in the area. Says Shortridge: "The flu virus is a promiscuous virus that can swap around genes with so many others." The H5N1 avian flu virus that in 1997 caused six deaths in Hong Kong was a combination of chicken, duck and quail influenza strains to which people did not have immunity. A flu virus that is harmless in animals can become dangerous to people when it joins with human genetic material or another animal gene.

Did SARS emerge from a farm in mainland China? If so, says David Bell, a member of the WHO's public health team in Manila, "it would not be a surprise. But we do not know where SARS originated and may never know." The first known SARS case appears to have been a chef specialising in exotic meats. He was treated for flu in Foshan, a city in Guangdong Province, in November 2002. Bell notes that "contact tracing [for this case] would be difficult — like finding a needle in a haystack."

*   *   *

On 23 February 2003, a team of WHO officials arrived in Beijing to investigate reports of an outbreak of an unknown respiratory disease, or atypical pneumonia, in Guangdong Province. The Chinese Ministry of Health had informed the Geneva-based UN agency of the outbreak on 11 February, but insisted the situation was under control.

The WHO team sent to China included Dr. Hiroshi Oshitani, a communicable diseases specialist from the organisation's Western Pacific regional headquarters in Manila. While in Beijing, Oshitani received a call from Dr. Carlo Urbani, a colleague at the Hanoi French Hospital in

Vietnam. Urbani wanted to discuss the growing number of strange pneumonia cases he was seeing, wondering if perhaps this might be an outbreak of avian flu as one of his patients — Chinese-American businessman Johnny Chen — had visited China and Hong Kong. Urbani wanted to send some specimens to Oshitani for analysis. The soft-spoken Japanese doctor was worried but not alarmed by Urbani's news.

But in quick succession, far more troubling developments took place. On 1 March, 26-year-old Esther Mok, a former flight attendant who had been on a shopping spree in Hong Kong in late February, was admitted to Tan Tock Seng Hospital in Singapore with respiratory problems. Four days later, 78-year-old Kwan Sui-chu died in Toronto's Scarborough Grace Hospital. She too had been in Hong Kong during the past two weeks and, along with Mok and Johnny Chen, had stayed at the Metropole Hotel on the same floor as Liu Jianlun, the doctor from Guangzhou. Chen was airlifted to Hong Kong from Hanoi and brought to Princess Margaret Hospital on 6 March. He died a week later. On 11 March, as healthcare workers at PWH, including Henry Chan, were beginning to become sick, Urbani fell ill and was hospitalised in Bangkok. The 46-year-old Italian epidemiologist, one of the first doctors to identify the SARS virus as a new disease, died less than three weeks later. On 13 March, Kwan's son Tse Chi-kwai, 44, died in the same Toronto hospital as his mother.

By this time, alarm bells were ringing. On 12 March, the WHO issued the first global alert warning of an outbreak of "a severe form of pneumonia" in Hong Kong, Vietnam and China's Guangdong Province. The same day, the Hong Kong Government informed Geneva of the mounting number of cases at PWH. By 17 March, two days after Geneva released its second global advisory, the detective work to track down what was now known as the SARS virus began as the WHO mobilised a network of 11 research laboratories located in nine different countries. (The number of laboratories cooperating in the investigation later increased to 13 in 11 countries.)

Concerns were only heightened by the fact that little if anything was known about the disease. "Influenza is more serious and kills more people [than SARS] yet we are not so scared of it because it has been out there for a long time and it is known," says Dr. Barbara Ebert, scientific coordinator of the Bernhard Nocht Institute for Tropical Medicine in Hamburg, one of the WHO labs.

Members of the public in Hong Kong were especially fearful. The

Hong Kong Government had initially chosen to play down the outbreak, claiming that the WHO alerts were exaggerating the situation and causing unnecessary panic. The Government assured the public that the outbreak was limited to healthcare workers and their families. But on 17 March, Professor Sydney Chung, dean of the CUHK medical school, stated in a press conference that this information was incorrect and that the disease had now spread to the general public. On 18 March, Secretary of Health, Welfare and Food Dr. Yeoh admitted for the first time that there were SARS cases outside of the medical community.

*   *   *

As the situation at PWH worsened, the Department of Health asked for an immediate investigation into the cause of the outbreak. Director of Health Dr. Margaret Chan Fung Fu-chun suspected avian flu. She was familiar with the disease due to her work during the 1997 outbreak. At that time, the Government implemented drastic measures, including the slaughter of millions of chickens, to stop the disease from spreading beyond Hong Kong.

But within days of the PWH outbreak, avian flu was ruled out. Investigators now focused on identifying the causative agent for the disease. They had to move fast. "We had this sense of urgency," Chan recalled later. "With international travel, a disease can spread all over the world in 48 hours. We had to work as a team."

Chan knew that Hong Kong had to tap the best public health and infectious disease experts in the world. She contacted the WHO, which was already beginning to investigate similar cases at the Hanoi French Hospital. Chan also called the US Centres for Disease Control (CDC) in Atlanta. "Tell me what it takes [to deal with this]," she told them. Tissue samples taken from Johnny Chen, the Chinese-American businessman who was hospitalised in Hanoi and later died in Hong Kong, were sent to the CDC for testing.

Along with her superior, Secretary of Health, Welfare and Food, Dr. Yeoh, Dr. Chan soon became a familiar face to Hong Kong people. Both were present at the numerous press conferences and briefings on SARS. A slight, bespectacled figure, Chan possesses a steely determination barely concealed by her elegance and quiet dignity. During the crisis, she never seemed to lose her composure, though she shed tears during several interviews with the media. Behind the scenes, Chan was impatient for results and spoke constantly with her counterparts in Hanoi, Geneva,

Singapore, Beijing and Manila. She spoke with Dr. David Heymann, then the WHO's executive director for communicable diseases, at least once a day.

Chan, Yeoh and other Hong Kong officials conferred daily to pore over the latest SARS data. The "war council" usually met at the Department of Health offices in Wanchai over boxed lunches or at Chief Executive Tung's offices in Central. "Every day, we asked, 'what are we dealing with? What do we know?'" Chan recalled later. With a population of only seven million people and access to a highly organised modern medical system, gathering information on Hong Kong's SARS cases was not too difficult. The Government tracked the outbreak by residence using a computer programme on loan from the Hong Kong Police Force that alerted authorities when more than two cases appeared in one building. This tool was particularly useful after the outbreak at Amoy Gardens, a Kowloon housing estate, in April as the authorities sought to prevent similar SARS "hotspots" from developing elsewhere.

Indeed, while SARS may have caught Hong Kong health authorities off guard, the SAR had the capacity to mount an effective defence against the virus — at least once the Government got organised. For that, Chan was thankful. "We are pretty well resourced," she said in the middle of the outbreak. "We are open. And we have the infrastructure and a first-world medical system. Many places cannot dream to have what we have. By comparison, others will have a tough job."

*   *   *

Within the community, anxiety continued to mount. By 1 April, as the number of SARS cases continued to climb, masked faces had become common on Hong Kong streets. Rumours swirled endlessly, passed on at lunchtime gossip sessions and through e-mail and mobile phone text messages.

After large numbers of residents at Amoy Gardens were infected with SARS, the Government quarantined Block E of the complex as a SARS hotspot. Of the 213 infected residents, 107 lived in the same wing of the building. All residents were relocated to two holiday camps and kept in isolation. The reasons for the Amoy Gardens outbreak were unclear, with baffled investigators blaming everything from the sewage system to rats. Initial studies by the Hong Kong Government and the WHO concluded that the problem probably lay in the plumbing system and the inflow of droplets of infected sewage into apartments when bathroom fans were running. However, the exact cause of the outbreak is still unknown (see Chapter 7).

The situation at Amoy Gardens added to the confusion and tension. On the face of it, Hong Kong seemed calm and quiet, with many people choosing to avoid public places and staying at home. Yet beneath the surface, the community was at a breaking point.

The high level of public anxiety in Hong Kong became obvious following a cruel April Fool's Day prank by a 14-year-old boy. Hacking onto the website of the Ming Pao newspaper, he posted a fake report that Hong Kong would be closed down to contain the spread of SARS, meaning that no one would be allowed to enter or leave. By noon, the news had spread throughout the community. More masks appeared on the streets, and panic-stricken residents rushed to supermarkets to stock up on basic necessities. By the afternoon of 1 April, Dr. Margaret Chan was forced to call an impromptu press conference to deny the story.

In a tragedy unconnected to SARS, at about 4.30 p.m. on the same day, Leslie Cheung, 46, a famous Hong Kong pop star and idol, walked into the Mandarin Oriental Hotel in Central and rode up the lift to the 24th floor. Just after 6.30 p.m., he leapt off the building. He was found on the pavement at the front driveway of the hotel. In his pockets were a mobile phone, a wallet, a lighter, a car park ticket and a green surgical mask. Already depressed, Hong Kong plunged into deep mourning.

*   *   *

Meanwhile, local and international efforts to contain the spread of the virus continued. The war on SARS was a unique global campaign waged on many fronts. It was, says Dr. Ebert of the Nocht Institute, "the first time the WHO has coordinated such a large number of laboratories with scientists talking by phone, e-mail or videoconference at least every second day to share information. We are using all this brain power." Involved in the detection work were research facilities in North America, Britain, Europe, Japan and Hong Kong. HKU and CUHK were both included in the international consortium.

Initially, the strategy was little more than trial and error. Researchers tested a variety of theories using specimens — blood, tissue or nasal swabs — from confirmed SARS patients. Samples usually arrived at the labs locked in multi-layered plastic cases, labelled with biohazard warning stickers and packed in ice. Specimens had to be opened in sealed chambers constructed to allow the use and testing of "Biosafety Level 3 or Level 4" material. This means that the facilities, equipment, safety precautions and work procedures in place are designed for the handling of life-threatening agents, including those that are transmissible through the respiratory system or are airborne. Lab workers must wear protective airtight suits. When they emerge from the inner chamber, they go through an acid and water shower to clean the suits before going into the dressing chamber where they change to regular clothes. After use, the rooms are steam cleaned with chemicals.

The first mission of the lab teams around the world was to identify the virus causing SARS. Some researchers analysed antibodies taken from patients, while others grew the virus on kidney tissue from monkeys or put samples through a polymerase chain reaction (PCR) test to track the genetic material of the causative agent. The work of the Hong Kong teams proved central in unravelling the mystery. Local researchers benefited from Hong Kong's recent experience with the avian flu, as well as the pioneering work of scientists such as Kennedy Shortridge.

HKU scientists led by microbiologist Professor Malik Peiris determined that the SARS virus was unique. Working non-stop, the team took blood samples from patients and found antibodies that reacted with the infectious agent they had isolated. On examining the virus under an electron microscope, they detected spikes on the cell surface that indicated what they were looking at was a coronavirus, the same type of virus that causes the common cold. This conclusion was bolstered when, on the 39th foray of his genetic "fishing expedition," Peiris's colleague Dr. Leo Poon, a molecular virologist, sequenced genetic material from infected cells and compared the partial genome with those of known coronaviruses. They were strikingly similar.

This discovery, announced by HKU on 21 March, generated considerable excitement within the international scientific community and did much to showcase Hong Kong's research capacity. While labs in Canada and the US completed the genetic sequencing of the SARS virus first, Hong Kong's microbiologists were not far behind, their efforts validating other results. The SARS outbreak also highlighted the excellence of Hong Kong's healthcare system. Two teams of doctors from the SAR were the first to publish scientific reports describing SARS symptoms and indicators as well as treatments. Health professionals elsewhere closely watched how Hong Kong's healthcare workers were treating SARS patients in order to learn how to deal with their own cases.

Hong Kong also benefited, of course, from cooperation with

international organisations like the WHO and public health authorities in several countries. By any measure, the global network mobilised by the WHO to combat SARS was incredibly successful — and efficient. By comparison, in the 1980s, it took labs in France and the US three years to identify the AIDS virus.

*   *   *

As scientists around the world gathered information about the virus, the fight to save lives continued. By mid-April, at least the mood among healthcare workers at PWH had much improved, although their lives had changed drastically. To make their rounds, doctors now had to put on protective gear — a gown, a heavy-duty N95 surgical mask that filters out most germs, covers for their head and shoes and gloves. Staff had to be careful not to tear any of the gear when moving around. They washed and scrubbed their hands constantly.

Out of concern that they might spread the virus to their families, many doctors slept at the hospital. Some, like Dr. John Tam, CUHK's star virologist, checked into hotels. While Professor Cockram continued to return home when he could, he and his wife slept in separate rooms and used different bathrooms. For as long as he was treating SARS cases, he wore a surgical mask around his apartment. He managed to stay in good health but was exhausted. "This is a very dangerous and vicious virus," he said. "But now it seems containable, though there is a long way to go."

*   *   *

Dr. Henry Chan was finally discharged in early April, three weeks after entering hospital. Upon returning home, he discovered that his daughter Jasmine, who had no idea what her father had been through, had learned several new words. Says Chan: "She grew so much while I was away."

Required to stay at home for two weeks, he put himself on a rigorous exercise regimen. When Chan was finally able to go back to work at PWH, he found a Lunar New Year decoration — two Winnie the Pooh figures framing the Chinese character for "good fortune" — still stuck on his office door. Chan was certainly lucky. The fact that he had received treatment early increased his chances of recovery. One of his patients, a middle-aged woman, came to his clinic that day. "It's good to see you again," she said as she greeted him. It was good to be a physician again, good to be alive, Chan thought.

*   *   *

On 1 July, the anniversary of the handover, the Hong Kong Government presented honours to 315 people. Six public-sector medical workers who lost their lives in the battle against SARS were posthumously awarded medals for bravery. Some had left behind young children and spouses.

Among those recognised was 35-year-old Dr. Joanna Tse Yuen-man, who had volunteered to treat SARS patients in the ICU of Tuen Mun Hospital. A Christian, Tse wanted to make a difference. She was still mourning her husband, Albert Chan, also a doctor, who had died of leukaemia in 2002. The couple had no children.

Tse was probably infected while performing a messy procedure: the insertion of a ventilator tube into the throat of a patient to assist with breathing. She fell ill on 3 April. Twelve days later, she was moved to the ICU, where she died early in the morning of 13 May.

About 2,000 people, including top Government officials, attended her funeral. Tse's medical school graduation portrait was on display at the front of the room. Draped in white fabric, the room was filled with flowers, mostly bouquets from family members, friends and colleagues. Friends and fellow church members launched a website at www.joannatse.com to pay tribute to her. "Little Sister Cousin," as hospital colleagues fondly called Tse, had been the girl-next-door who was too young to be a widow; she died a Hong Kong hero.

*   *   *

Throughout the SARS crisis, Hong Kong people seemed to be seeking heroes — role models who embodied the spirit and energy that the community seemed somehow to have lost since the handover. Some now describe SARS as Hong Kong's "9–11." Certainly, citizens were desperate for a confident, charismatic, Giuliani-style leadership that they could trust. Neither Secretary of Health, Welfare and Food Dr. Yeoh nor Director of Health Dr. Chan proved sufficiently reassuring. Chief Executive Tung rationed his public appearances, preferring to manage from his inner sanctum as usual. His wife Betty did tour the area around Lower Ngau Tau Kok Estate, a second SARS "hotspot," but lost points for wearing heavy protective gear as hospital workers claimed that authorities were failing to provide them with adequate supplies. Tung's poll numbers, already low, dipped even further.

Questions continue to be raised about what the Hong Kong Government did or did not do, should or should not have done, in response to the outbreak. Did the lack of action at the start make the situation worse? By choosing to downplay the extent of the crisis, had the Government lost the chance to contain the virus at an early stage? Could the outbreak within the community have been better contained? Were medical workers provided with adequate protective gear when they went into SARS wards? Would a stronger, more visible and more decisive leader have made a difference during the most difficult days of the crisis?

What does seem clear is that the experience of SARS has brought about important changes in the way that Hong Kong people see themselves. If SARS gave them a new and unwelcome sense of vulnerability, it also reminded them of Hong Kong's strengths and abilities, which extend far beyond its capacity as an international financial centre. This reminder has, in turn, affected attitudes towards the community, the Government and the future of Hong Kong. The tremendous turnout of citizens from all walks of life at the 1 July protests were an indication that Hong Kong people were seeking to play a more active role in determining how Hong Kong would develop and who its leaders would be.

CHAPTER 2

At the Frontline:
The Medical Challenge

Moira Chan-Yeung

The first new disease of the twenty-first century posed the threat of a major global epidemic. Within a week of reaching Hong Kong in February 2003, SARS spread to 11 countries in Asia, Europe and North America. Its relatively long incubation period — up to 10 days — meant that infected air travellers, many of whom did not show any symptoms of illness prior to boarding their flights, unknowingly carried the virus around the world.

Scientists quickly identified the coronavirus as the culprit and broke its genetic code just five weeks after the onset of the SARS epidemic in Hong Kong (see Chapter 4). Still, much remains unknown about how the virus behaves and spreads, and how the disease develops in the body.

SARS presented a major medical challenge in the most severely affected areas — Canada, mainland China, Taiwan, Singapore, Vietnam and, of course, Hong Kong — for several reasons. First, there was — and is still — no treatment to cure the disease or a vaccine to prevent it. Isolation and quarantine remain the best ways to control the disease. Second, SARS can be virulent. During the outbreak, between 10 to 25 percent of patients required intensive care treatment, while 5 to 15 percent died.[1] Third, hospital staff — the vital human resource for treatment and control of the disease — were at high risk, with many becoming infected. Finally, the phenomenon of the "super-spreader," someone who infects 10 or more people, was and remains a worrisome puzzle.

Countering the attack

Each of the first five SARS patients in Hong Kong was treated in a different hospital. Four had been to the Metropole Hotel in Kowloon, three as guests. They included Liu Jianlun, the doctor who brought the virus across the border from Guangzhou. The fifth case was a man who had travelled to southern China.

Here is a summary of how each hospital handled its SARS cases:[2]

Kwong Wah Hospital

When 64-year-old Liu Jianlun arrived at the Accident & Emergency Department (A&E) of Kwong Wah Hospital on 22 February, he was already extremely unwell. He mentioned to hospital staff that he had been infected with pneumonia on the mainland but had recovered. Liu told them that he had a highly infectious disease and should be isolated. He was immediately admitted to the intensive care unit (ICU). Liu died on 4 March.

Liu infected one healthcare assistant who was in the A&E when he arrived. On that day, the hospital reported the case to both the Hospital Authority (HA), which oversees all of Hong Kong's public hospitals, and the Department of Health.[3] Later, Liu's brother-in-law would end up in Kwong Wah's ICU with the same symptoms. He infected a nurse who spent six hours looking after him.

By 3 March, the hospital began to admit clinically confirmed and suspected SARS patients directly to isolation beds, of which the hospital had 28. By 12 April, Kwong Wah had 57 confirmed SARS patients. Five more hospital staff had become infected.

Pamela Youde Nethersole Eastern Hospital

On 2 March, Pamela Youde Nethersole Eastern Hospital admitted into a general ward a patient with fever, an abnormal chest X-ray and diarrhoea. He had recently been to southern China. The patient's condition deteriorated rapidly. Unable to breathe on his own, he was put on a ventilator in the ICU, where he eventually died.

While in the ward, he infected seven hospital staff. The hospital quickly implemented a new infection control policy, with confirmed and suspected SARS patients isolated immediately on admission. From 2

March to 12 April, Pamela Youde admitted 46 SARS patients. Four additional hospital workers became ill. Three had been exposed to the first infected staff member, while the fourth had been cleaning a room used to develop X-ray films of SARS patients.

Prince of Wales Hospital

On 4 March, a 26-year-old airport worker was admitted into Ward 8A of the Prince of Wales Hospital (PWH) in Shatin with a high temperature, muscle pain and cough. He had visited the Metropole Hotel to see a friend. His chest X-ray showed a small shadow in the right upper lung. The illness progressed rapidly to the point that both lungs were affected. Tests for micro-organisms, including the common respiratory viruses, were negative.

He was treated with antibiotics for typical pneumonia and also received a bronchodilator, a drug to open up narrowed airways, through a jet nebuliser, a machine that generates an aerosol to deliver medicine to a patient through inhalation.[4] Two days after his admission, doctors, nurses and medical students who had examined or cared for him began falling ill. By 10 March, 11 healthcare workers were complaining of fever, coughing and difficulty in breathing. Ward 8A was immediately closed to new patients and visitors. The HA reported the outbreak to the Department of Health on that day.

By the following day, 11 March, the number of sick hospital staff had increased to 50. Admission to Ward 8A was stopped, although the no-visiting policy was modified to restricted visiting, with visitors required to wear surgical masks, disposable gowns and gloves. On 12 March, the eighth floor of the hospital was made a restricted area. Specific medial wards were designated as isolation wards for probable and suspected SARS cases. On 13 March, further measures were introduced to contain the outbreak. These included suspension of non-emergency surgical operations, day services and cardiac specialist outpatient clinics. Droplet infection control measures and guidelines were upgraded. Training in infection control was provided for staff. Despite these efforts, by 17 March, 166 staff had come down with the disease, some requiring intensive care.[5]

Hospital operations were paralysed due to the lack of healthy staff. Repeated requests by Professor Sydney Chung, Dean of Medicine at the Chinese University of Hong Kong (CUHK), for which PWH serves as a teaching hospital, and the Chief Executive of the New Territories East Cluster of HA hospitals, to close isolation wards to visitors and the hospital to new admissions were denied by the HA and the Department of Health.

In a press conference on the evening of 17 March, Chung revealed that the mysterious pneumonia was no longer confined to hospitals but had spread into the community.[6] He suspended all non-urgent surgery, speciality clinics and teaching activities at PWH. His announcement finally forced the authorities to close the emergency room. However, despite the closure of the hospital and the introduction of an infection control policy, more staff members were infected after 25 March. It remains unclear how many of Hong Kong's SARS cases were linked to the PWH index patient, both directly and indirectly.

The total number of SARS cases at PWH alone arising as a result of contact with the index case was 238.[7] Lack of knowledge about the disease, the use of a jet nebuliser (which spreads aerosols in the air) to treat the index case, the high viral load in the environment due to the large number of SARS patients, lack of experience with infection control procedures plus the fear and stress of healthcare workers were some of the reasons why so many hospital staff became infected in the first two weeks of the PWH outbreak. Moreover, because Ward 8A and other isolation wards were kept open to visitors and patient admissions were not halted, SARS spread rapidly from the hospital to the community.

On 13 March, a patient with chronic kidney disease went to PWH for treatment and spent the night in Ward 8A while waiting for the results of a blood test. After being discharged the next day, he visited his brother at Block E of Amoy Gardens, a private residential estate in Kowloon, and did so again on 19 March. As he had diarrhoea, he used his brother's bathroom several times. On 22 March, he was readmitted to the hospital with fever and pneumonia. His visits to Amoy Gardens resulted in 321 cases of SARS within the housing development. The Amoy Gardens outbreak prompted the World Health Organisation (WHO) to issue an advisory regarding travel to Hong Kong on 2 April.

Princess Margaret Hospital

On 6 March, Princess Margaret Hospital (PMH) admitted a patient who had been transferred from the Hanoi French Hospital. The Chinese-American businessman had spent a night at the Metropole Hotel and then travelled to the Vietnamese capital, where he became sick. When he arrived at Princess Margaret, the patient was already gravely ill. He was admitted directly into the ICU, but died shortly after.

No hospital worker at PMH was infected, probably because staff members were well trained in handling infectious diseases. The hospital had Hong Kong's largest infectious diseases unit, with 86 isolation beds. Between 17 and 30 March, daily SARS admissions varied from three to 10 a day. Many were family members and visitors of patients at PWH who were infected at that hospital. The Amoy Gardens outbreak contributed to an increase in admissions, with a peak of 58 admissions on 31 March. PMH became the first Hong Kong hospital designated for SARS patients.

Although PMH staff withstood the stress of the SARS outbreak and managed particularly well, some inevitably succumbed. On 7 April, some workers began to report symptoms. In total, 62 staff members became infected — a very low number considering that the hospital handled 593 SARS cases, 34 percent of all cases in Hong Kong.[8] However, even though they performed remarkably, PMH staff members were under extreme stress and after 12 April, subsequent new cases were sent to the United Christian Hospital.

Queen Mary Hospital

Affiliated with the University of Hong Kong's medical school, Queen Mary Hospital (QMH) is a major public healthcare facility on Hong Kong Island. On 7 March, it admitted a Chinese-Canadian executive who had been a guest at the Metropole Hotel. His stay overlapped by a day with that of Liu Jianlun, although there was apparently no direct contact between them. Previously, for six days the businessman had been treated for pneumonia in a general ward at St. Paul's Hospital. After his transfer to QMH, his condition deteriorated and he was put in the ICU.

Fortunately, none of the staff that attended on this patient were infected, but a nephew who visited him at the Metropole and at the ICU contracted the disease. While at St. Paul's, he infected three nurses who had spent five eight-hour shifts with him. They had not worn facemasks or gowns when they cleaned him after faecal incontinence. The nurses were eventually admitted to the Pamela Youde Nethersole Eastern Hospital.

Isolation wards were established at QMH within one week of the admission of its first SARS patient. All clinically confirmed SARS patients were admitted directly from the emergency room to the SARS isolation ward. Suspected SARS patients went first to a pneumonia-patient ward for observation and isolation. Those subsequently confirmed to have SARS were transferred to the SARS isolation ward. Those not likely to be suffering from SARS were sent to a "step-down" isolation ward and quarantined for three days after their fever had subsided and chest X-rays proved clear.

All suspected SARS patients had daily chest X-rays and complete blood and liver function tests. A SARS team was formed and a senior doctor reviewed the condition of each suspected patient in the pneumonia ward every day. The wards were closed to visitors. Although it admitted 24 clinically confirmed SARS patients between 4 March and 12 April, none of the staff were infected during this period. But in the middle of May, two nurses contracted SARS. A thorough investigation traced the cause to the administration of high-flow oxygen to SARS patients in a room with inadequate ventilation.

How SARS spread

SARS spread through the Hong Kong community in several ways. First, the virus was brought in from southern China, as in the cases of Liu Jianlun and the first case at the Pamela Youde Hospital. Second, the virus spread among hospital workers through contact with SARS patients. Third, it spread within hospitals to patients being treated for other illnesses. Fourth, SARS infected the families and friends of healthcare workers, as well as hospital visitors.

In the case of the kidney patient at PWH, no one could have predicted that he would become infected while undergoing routine testing and then infect hundreds of people just from visiting his brother's home. "Super-spreaders" like this may carry a high viral count in their secretions, which would account for their capacity to infect many other people.

The causative organism was a previously unknown coronavirus. In humans, this virus attacks the lungs and gut. It is believed that transmission occurs through direct contact or via droplets generated by coughing and sneezing. Contact with surfaces contaminated by droplets can also be a source of infection. The virus can survive in stool and urine at room temperature for at least two days and for up to four days in the stool of patients with 'loose' bowels. Fortunately, it loses its ability to infect after exposure to several commonly used disinfectants such as bleach, 75 percent ethanol (rubbing alcohol) and fixatives such as formaldehyde and paraformaldehyde.[9]

The fact that a large number of residents at Amoy Gardens developed the disease within a short period of time raised suspicions that other modes of transmission such as the air or the oral-faecal route were possible (see Chapter 7). An investigation by the Department of Health concluded that droplets containing the virus were carried into bathrooms as a result of contamination of waste drainage pipes and the drying up of the U-shaped pipe in toilets, which should be water-filled. The Government's report ruled out airborne transmission, but did not provide conclusive evidence for doing so.[10]

Clinical features and diagnosis

Incubation and symptoms

The incubation period — the time between exposure to an infected individual and the development of symptoms — is from two to 10 days. Most patients were admitted to hospital about five days after the onset of symptoms. Because they were much more aware of the disease, healthcare workers were usually hospitalised sooner.[11]

Practically all patients except a few elderly cases develop a high fever, usually higher than 38 degrees Celsius. Other common symptoms include chills, a dry cough, shortness of breath, muscle pain, headaches, dizziness and a general feeling of being unwell. Diarrhoea occurred in only about 20 percent of all patients in Hong Kong, but in 60 to 70 percent of those who lived in Amoy Gardens. A sore throat and runny nose were present in less than a quarter of cases.

Some people with SARS, particularly older patients, do not develop a fever or respiratory symptoms. Instead, they lose their appetite and feel generally unwell. Such patients pose a threat to healthcare workers and residents in old age homes or staff and other patients in hospitals as diagnosis is difficult and isolation not usually practised.

X-rays

Chest X-rays show pneumonia in the lungs of a majority of SARS patients. In a small number of cases, an abnormality shows up only when more sensitive high-resolution computed tomography (HRCT) — another form of chest X-ray — is used. In general, the disease attacks the lobes of the lungs, progressing rapidly. Lung condition may worsen for another five days after a course of treatment has started before there is any improvement.[12]

Laboratory findings

Unlike typical pneumonias, a high white blood cell (lymphocyte) count is rare in SARS patients despite the high fever. Most patients have a low lymphocyte count, which is consistent with viral infection. Abnormal liver function and disturbances in electrolytes may also be present. All standard microbiological tests for bacteria, fungi, respiratory viruses and other less common micro-organisms are negative.[13]

The diagnosis of SARS remains a clinical judgment based on the features of the patient and the ruling out of other community-acquired pneumonias and lung diseases. A rapid diagnostic test to demonstrate the presence of the coronavirus is not yet available.

Defining SARS

For an accurate count of cases, the diagnosis of SARS should be carried out according to a consistent definition. The HA defines SARS as having these characteristics:

1. The presence of new chest X-ray shadows compatible with pneumonia,
2. A fever higher than 38 degrees Celsius at any time in the past two days, and
3. At least two of the following: chills sometime in the last two days, new or increased coughing or breathing difficulty, muscle pains and a general feeling of being unwell, or a history of exposure to a SARS patient.[14]

The World Health Organisation (WHO) defines a suspected case as:

A person presenting after 1 November 2002 with a history of high fever (greater than 38 degrees Celsius) and cough or breathing difficulty and one or more of the following exposures during the 10 days prior to onset of symptoms: close contact with a person who is a suspect or probable case of SARS, history of travel to an affected area, or residing in an affected area.[15]

Laboratory test results are not included in the case definition.

Antibodies

The demonstration of the presence of antibodies to the causative coronavirus, a marker of the body's immune response, or of the coronavirus itself in body secretions of the patient confirms the clinical diagnosis.[16]

Two methods have been developed to detect antibodies against the virus: the enzymatic assay (ELISA) and the indirect immunofluorescence antibody (IFA) tests. Blood specimens have to be collected during acute illness and convalescence, at least 21 days after the onset of symptoms. It takes time for the body to mount an immune response, thus the conversion of the antibody test from negative to positive or a four-fold rise in the antiviral antibody confirms the diagnosis. The test is specific, as none of the sera from 200 blood donors had antibodies to the new coronavirus, but it was not useful for doctors in making a rapid diagnosis during acute illness.[17]

The virus can be isolated in body secretions but this is difficult to do. One way is to demonstrate the presence of the ribonucleic acid (RNA) of the coronavirus using a molecular biology technique known as reverse transcriptase-polymerase chain reaction (RT-PCR). Viral RNA can be detected in various body secretions, including those obtained from the back of the nose and throat, saliva, urine and stool. The test was found to be positive in 32 percent of secretions from the back of the nose and throat three days after the onset of symptoms, and 68 percent by day 14. With stool, 97 percent of samples collected on day 14 were positive. The test is very specific for SARS, as it is negative in individuals without the disease. However, the test is not sensitive enough to detect all patients with the virus. Several specimens of various body secretions from one patient should be sent for checking to improve the diagnostic yield.[18]

Disease management

SARS is a completely new infectious disease. There is, at present, no specific treatment. All current regimens are based on clinical experience and have not undergone any randomised controlled clinical trials. In these kinds of trials, patients are randomly assigned to one of two groups. The first group takes the drug to be tested while the second group takes another drug or a placebo without any active ingredient for comparison. Many questions regarding management of SARS remain to be answered, including the choice of anti-viral drugs such as Ribavirin used in Hong Kong; the role, dose and timing of corticosteroid treatment or other modes of treatment such as the use of convalescent serum (from the blood of patients who have recovered from SARS as they have antibodies against the virus); and the use of Traditional Chinese Medicine (TCM).

Isolation and barrier nursing

With a highly infectious disease such as SARS, strict hospital isolation is necessary. Isolation facilities should be created not only for confirmed SARS patients but also for suspected patients. There should be no visitors to any isolation ward.

Strict barrier nursing should be carried out. This means all staff should wear a facemask, gown, eye-shields, goggles and gloves. They should be taught how to wash their hands meticulously before putting their protective devices on and how to take them off and to wash their hands afterwards. There should be clear demarcation of "dirty" and "clean" areas for staff to get into and out of protective gear. They should follow instructions on how to gown and de-gown. Staff should be trained properly in these procedures before being assigned to isolation wards.[19]

Antibiotics

A combination of antibiotics for the treatment of community-acquired pneumonia should be given to patients. Patients with symptoms of this kind of pneumonia usually respond clinically and their chest X-rays improve within two to three days. For those who fail to respond, or deteriorate, treatment as for SARS should be initiated. Anti-viral therapy should be implemented in the early viral replication phase.[20]

Ribavirin

Ribavirin has been used in Hong Kong to treat SARS. A high dose is given intravenously for at least three days or until the clinical condition becomes stable, followed by oral administration of the drug twice daily for a total of 10 to 14 days. There is considerable controversy surrounding the use of Ribavirin, which is a broad-spectrum antiviral drug used to treat a number of RNA and DNA viruses. In the laboratory, it has no demonstrable effect on the coronavirus[21] but it has been shown to act as an immunomodulator (a drug that can alter the body's immunological response) in mice. The prevalence of side effects at the recommended dose, especially destruction of red cells, is high. It can also cause congenital abnormality if given during early pregnancy. The outcome of those who received Ribavirin was not different from those who did not receive the drug, but the latter group is rather small. Some physicians in Hong Kong have now abandoned the use of Ribavirin because of its lack of efficacy and the high prevalence of side effects. Unfortunately, there are no anti-viral drugs with activity against the SARS coronavirus.

Corticosteroids

Most SARS patients show a clinical and chest X-ray response to corticosteroids with resolution of fever within 24 to 48 hours. Physicians differ in the way they prescribe corticosteroids. Some start using corticosteroids only when there is no response to antibiotics while others give high doses of corticosteroids together with Ribavirin early in the clinical course. The majority of SARS patients improved on the above regimen. The remaining patients, about 20 to 25 percent of patients requiring admission to the ICU, appeared to have a more severe form of the disease.

These patients usually deteriorate towards the beginning of the second week of illness or develop a recurrence of pneumonic changes. A second course of high-dose corticosteriod therapy often leads to improvement in these patients clinically as well as in their chest X-rays, although some cases continue to deteriorate. A few such patients have responded to other immunomodulating therapies, such as intravenous administration of immunoglobulins, which aid in fighting illness, or convalescent serum from recovered patients. Secondary chest infection is a complication at this stage, and may lead to death. In some patients whose chest X-rays have cleared after corticosteroid treatment, the reduction of the dose resulted in a recurrence of pneumonia, supporting the notion that corticosteroid treatment is beneficial. Most physicians in Hong Kong agree that despite the side effects, early treatment with an appropriate dose of corticosteroid prevents irreversible lung damage.[22] However, as a randomised placebo-controlled clinical trial, which is the "gold standard" for determining the usefulness of a new drug or new form of treatment, has not been carried out, the role of corticosteroids in the treatment of SARS is still not clear.

Course of disease

The severity of the disease varies for different individuals. Some patients rapidly progress to acute respiratory distress syndrome over the course of two to three days while others worsen more slowly over the course of their second week of hospitalisation. This phase occurs at a time when the viral load is actually decreasing.[23] Those who progressed rapidly to respiratory failure were transferred to the ICU for treatment and about half of these patients required assisted ventilation. At the end of May 2003, Hong Kong's overall fatality rate (the percentage of SARS patients who died) was around 16 percent. It was highest among those over the age of 65 years (55.8 percent), but older patients accounted for only 14 percent of all cases. Children under the age of 10 years old tended to have milder infections.[24] Men were more at risk of dying than women.[25]

In Hong Kong, patients were usually discharged after their chest X-rays had improved and fever had subsided for one week. They were asked to monitor their temperature at home. Of the 800 SARS patients discharged from hospitals up to 30 April, 12 had recurrence of fever and chest symptoms. Chest X-rays showed some abnormalities within two weeks of being discharged. Most of these patients, however, had other problems such as chest infections caused by micro-organisms other than the coronavirus. None of them died.

The long-term functional and psychological effects of SARS are not yet known. Chest X-rays of some patients requiring admission to the ICU and taken before discharge from the hospital showed scarring in the lungs, indicating the severity of the disease.

Ongoing research

In May 2003, the HA set up the Chinese Medicine Expert Panel on SARS Exploratory Treatment, comprising local and mainland experts. Two specialists from the Chinese Medicine Hospital of Guangdong Province came to Hong Kong to provide advice on the use of TCM in the treatment of SARS and the application of an integrated Western-Chinese Medicine approach. The specialists collaborated with TCM experts at three Hong Kong universities to develop clinical and research protocols for the treatment and prevention of SARS.[26] There is also an ongoing international effort to discover more effective antiviral drugs and to develop an effective vaccine for SARS.

Infection of healthcare workers

In Hong Kong, healthcare workers accounted for 22 percent of all SARS cases by the end of May.[27] In Canada and Singapore, the proportion of infected healthcare workers was much higher as these countries had far fewer SARS cases in the community. As an outbreak in hospitals may lead to the spread of a virus within the general public and because healthcare workers are in the frontline in fighting disease, it is critical to understand why so many were infected.

Three factors explain the high number of affected health staff:

Process

This includes the degree of awareness among healthcare workers, how they handled patient admission and transfers and how high-risk procedures were applied. When SARS first struck, health workers did not know what they were dealing with. This was evident in the treatment of the first index patients to be hospitalised.

Moreover, Hong Kong had let down its guard in the prevention and management of infectious diseases. After all, diseases such as smallpox and cholera, rampant during the first half of the twentieth century, had practically disappeared in Hong Kong. As such, there was a general lack of familiarity and training regarding infection control measures.

A study by the HA showed that most hospital workers were infected during the first fortnight when they worked in SARS isolation wards.

Video cameras in the wards also captured the times when staff did not comply with infection control measures. Some workers reused protective gowns and masks as the supply of protective gear was inadequate during the early part of the epidemic. While healthcare workers at PMH were experts in handling infectious diseases, the rapid influx of SARS patients after the Amoy Gardens outbreak meant staff had to cope with an excessive workload. The high levels of stress led some of them to become infected.

When PMH could no longer admit any more patients, those suffering from SARS were sent to the United Christian Hospital, where health workers lacked training in handling infectious diseases. This resulted in the spread of the virus among healthcare workers at the United Christian Hospital. Furthermore, it was not always easy to execute hospital admission and transfer procedures in a way that minimised the risk of transmission.

The outbreak at the Alice Ho Mui Ling Nethersole Hospital showed how hard it could be for healthcare workers to determine what to do in specific cases. One patient was transferred to the hospital from PWH and was not suspected of having SARS. He had a history of abdominal pain and loose bowels and was admitted to a general ward. Three days later he developed a fever. An X-ray showed a worrying shadow on his lungs, at which point he was transferred to a medical ward. He did have SARS and went on to infect 16 hospital staff and eight patients. Another patient with rectal bleeding was identified as a SARS case only after all patients in the same ward were screened for the disease using chest X-rays and blood counts.[28]

In terms of treatment, certain types of procedures have been shown to be high risk because they lead to extensive spreading of droplets from the patient — for example, the use of the jet nebuliser, intubation and assisted ventilation outside the ICU. The release of high-flow oxygen in a room without adequate ventilation was found to be responsible for the infection of two nurses at QMH.

Environmental

When a patient with SARS was sent to a general ward, where beds are only about three feet apart, it was easy for the disease to spread. Inadequate air ventilation may also have been a contributing factor. Air exchange may not have been sufficient to clear a high viral load.

Furthermore, many public hospitals do not have sufficient facilities to enable staff to wash their hands frequently, let alone provide a place for them to shower after removing used protective gear. It could be said that when Hong Kong's hospitals were designed, little thought went into coping with infectious diseases.

Human nature

Finally, the behaviour of the patients themselves proved to be a critical factor in the infection of healthcare workers. It is never easy to care for the elderly and those who require extensive care. Patients can be uncooperative and may refuse to wear a facemask or maintain good personal hygiene. As has already been pointed out, some patients did not show typical SARS symptoms and so remained in general wards for a period of time before being isolated. While there, they spread the disease to others.

Lessons for the future

The south China region, including Hong Kong, has been the birthplace for several viral illnesses in the past — the Hong Kong flu, Asian flu and avian flu, to name just a few. SARS is likely to be followed by others. Hong Kong needs to learn from the 2003 SARS outbreak to prevent the occurrence of something similar — or worse.

To prevent the spread of SARS in hospital settings:
- Physicians must stay alert for the emergence of SARS or other new infectious diseases.
- SARS patients should be kept in isolated units with barrier nursing practices in place. Probable and suspected SARS cases should be admitted directly to isolation wards to minimise staff exposure.
- High-risk procedures should be avoided unless absolutely necessary.
- Hospital staff should be trained in infection control, the handling of masks and frequent and thorough hand washing, with a daily reminder to comply with such procedures.
- Hospital and health authorities and the medical profession should respond swiftly to establish clear guidelines for isolation, infection control and admission policy. Staff should be trained to deal with the enormous demands involved in caring for SARS patients in order to prevent hospital infection.

- There should be improved co-ordination between hospitals within regional clusters and between clusters. No general hospitals should be allowed to take in large numbers of infectious patients within a short period of time.
- Rapid sharing of experience between hospitals and updating of hospital staff on new developments in treatment and infection control measures are of vital importance in dealing with epidemics in hospital settings.

For the general prevention and control of infectious diseases:
- The reporting of an outbreak of infectious disease as early as possible to the WHO is absolutely essential for containment and control. The WHO disseminates information, alerts health authorities in other countries and enlists international experts to assist in investigating an epidemic and identifying the causative agent.
- There should be a much greater communication between the health authorities of neighbouring regions when an outbreak of infectious disease is suspected. The medical profession should be alerted to a potential problem without delay.
- Early quarantine of those who have had close contact with patients is necessary for controlling an epidemic.
- The teaching and training of the medical profession in infectious diseases and the capacity of the public health sector to deal with these diseases must be strengthened locally. The establishment of a centre for disease control similar to that in mainland China or the US is one way to address this need.
- The environmental conditions that led to the spread of disease must be dealt with. The public must be educated and reminded about maintaining personal and public hygiene. Only when every citizen realises the importance of a clean environment can better living conditions be sustained and the chances of diseases like SARS spreading reduced or eliminated.

Acknowledgements

The author wishes to thank Dr. WH Seto, Professor Joseph Sung, Dr. Sek-to Lai, Dr. Wilson Yee, Dr. Loretta Yam, Dr. Kenneth Wah-tak Tsang and Dr. Alice Sheng-sheng Ho for providing information on their respective hospitals.

CHAPTER 3

Healing Myself:
Diary of a SARS Patient and Doctor

Gregory Cheng

D
r. Gregory Cheng is a Consultant Haematologist at the Prince of Wales Hospital (PWH). In early March 2003, he was one of a number of health workers at PWH to be diagnosed with SARS. The following is an account of his experiences and reflections during the outbreak.

Symptoms and diagnosis

9 March 2003, Sunday

Have developed severe chills, rigour and muscle ache. Diagnosed myself as having the flu. Still went out for dinner, but had an early night.

10 March, Monday

Many of the nursing staff and physicians [at Prince of Wales Hospital (PWH)] had similar flu-like symptoms. Joked around with them, saying, "You guys are not much better than me." Had blood and nasal swabs taken for investigation.

11 March, Tuesday

Some colleagues developed more severe symptoms and shortness of breath. This was not an ordinary infection. The hospital set up an emergency clinic that evening. Many of the staff had hypoxia [deficiency in oxygen to the body] and an abnormal chest X-ray, requiring admission to hospital. I did not have any shortness of breath. Did not have a chest X-ray taken. Went home and started myself on [the anti-flu virus drug] Tamiflu and [the antibiotic] Levofloxacin.

12–18 March

No more fever and chills, but still had severe muscle ache. Finally had an X-ray, which showed haziness in right lung. Little was known about the causative agent of the disease. Some of my colleagues were treated with Ribavirin and a high dose of steroids at PWH. Decided to treat myself with Ribavirin and [the high-dose steroid],Dexamethasone at home, hoping that I would recover without having to be admitted to hospital.

19 March, Wednesday

Rested at home in the evening. Hospital issued an "arrest warrant" for me to be admitted immediately. Very reluctant. Claimed that I was already getting better through self-treatment. I could continue medication at home since it had already been a week after the onset of symptoms and none of my close family members had developed any signs of illness. My most contagious period had already passed and self-quarantine at home was sufficient, I argued.

Eventually agreed to be admitted after much persuasion by my department head and colleagues, as well as lecturing and coercion by the Dean. Was finally convinced by the coaxing of my beautiful medical officers. They promised to visit me and buy me four newspapers each day.

*   *   *

Looking back, it was very fortunate that I did not spread the disease to my family or any of my patients. It is still an enigma as to why some patients, such as the "index case" patient who was at the Metropole Hotel and our index patient in Ward 8A, became "super-spreaders" who infected hundreds of people, while others like me, and many of my colleagues, had low infectivity and did not pass the virus on to any close friends or family. Why did some patients have a more severe form of the disease? Is it the viral load? Is it possible that in the severely affected patients, there is co-infection with a second virus that is very difficult to isolate?

Unravelling these puzzles will help a great deal to control infectious diseases in the future. Patients with a mild case and low infectivity may not need to be admitted to hospital. Being quarantined at special camps or even at home may be sufficient. However, the Department of Health did not contact my family members until I was admitted to hospital — more than one week after the outbreak! If another outbreak occurs, the policy of tracing contacts should be implemented much faster in order to ensure that potential patients are treated quickly.

*   *   *

Treatment and cure

My daily hospital routine: Get out of bed at 6.30 a.m. Wait for my medical officers to deliver the newspapers. What a pity that their beautiful faces were hidden behind masks. Have breakfast and read until noon. Lunch. Wander around the ward. Dinner at 6–6.30 p.m. Watch TV for news about SARS and the Iraq War — then some boring television soap operas. Go to bed early.

I really missed home — and sports on cable TV!

19–23 March

For the first three days, family members were still allowed to visit. While I longed to see my family, especially my wife, I was strongly against hospital visits. If the main reason for my hospitalisation was to be quarantined in order to protect my family, allowing them to come defeated that purpose. They would have been exposed to me, the other patients and contaminated objects in the ward. Finally, on 22 March, the hospital banned visitors.

I was saddened to hear that more people were getting infected. Was very concerned that members of the PWH "Dirty Team" [a team of medical workers fighting SARS,] would get infected too [a number of team members, including Professor Joseph Sung, nurse Hidy Chan, surgical ward manager Chui See-to, Dr. Tam Lai Shan and Dr. Gavin Joynt, did subsequently get infected].

Some of my co-workers and fellow patients were getting worse, requiring oxygen supplements. They were short of breath just walking to the washroom. I worried about them. My close colleague, Raymond, did not even have the energy to speak to me.

I was very fortunate — my symptoms were mild and I never required oxygen. I insisted on treating myself with my own steroid regimen instead of a more prolonged sequence of a less powerful steroid. Requested chest X-rays and blood tests be done every two or three days, instead of daily. A very naughty and uncooperative patient!

The hospital outfits really made you feel like a sick patient. The trousers were too short and the shirts too small. You were never in the mood for anything. Couldn't stand the toilets so I avoided having a bowel movement for as long as possible.

Received get-well cards from many of my patients, friends and the public. Very touching and encouraging. Plenty of food and fruit baskets. The medical officers brought us roasted pigeon, ice cream, snacks and a mah-jong set. But the hospital environment deprived me of any appetite and I was in no mood to play.

Each morning, I hoped that Professor Sung [head of the Department of Medicine and Therapeutics] would discharge me early because I felt I was recovering well. Very disappointed when I was told I had to stay until 29 March, 21 days from the onset of symptoms. But I had to accept my fate.

24–28 March

My colleagues were recovering, and the ward became more lively. Thanks to my medical officers, I was able to manage some of my patients by phone. Raymond came over to my bed and chatted with me for the first time since my admission. We played cards, but neither of us really enjoyed it. We wanted to go home as soon as possible.

On the 26th, I couldn't bear it any longer. Had to rush to the toilet for a bowel movement. As it turned out, it was my only BM during my entire hospitalisation. Up to 20 percent of SARS patients developed severe diarrhoea. I couldn't have survived if I had.

Started a countdown to the 29th, discharge day. Each day seemed so long; each temperature measurement so stressful. I feared that I would develop a fever again and my leaving hospital would be delayed.

*   *   *

What is the most appropriate time to start steroid therapy in SARS patients? Would a short course (four to five days) of high-dose steroids be as effective as a prolonged course (three to four weeks) of less potent steroids? Should steroids be given only to patients whose illness has progressed rather than to those at an early stage of treatment? I took Dexamethasone, a high-dose steroid, for four days, starting on Day Seven of my illness and recovered well.

There were concerns about the clinical effectiveness and side effects of Ribavirin and steroid treatment, but unfortunately during the SARS epidemic in Hong Kong, it was not possible to perform a random control study. At World Health Organisation meetings on SARS in Hong Kong and Kuala Lumpur, there was no consensus on steroid therapy.

How long should patients stay in hospital? In Hong Kong, hospitalisation had to be for at least 21 days from the onset of symptoms, with the patient showing clinical improvement. Elsewhere such as Canada, the period was much shorter.

We did not know how long a recovered patient remained potentially infectious. Coronavirus was still detectable in the stool and urine of some asymptomatic patients and recovered patients for several weeks, yet their infectivity seemed quite low. In Hong Kong, there was no documented case of a clinically recovered patient spreading the disease to other people after discharge from hospital. Moreover, lengthy hospitalisation can have a detrimental effect on a patient's physical and psychological recovery.

The banning of hospital visits is essential to prevent the spread of the disease in the community during an epidemic. This policy should be implemented early. Of course, a lengthy separation from family and loved ones is difficult to bear. One could argue that visits could be permitted under special circumstances, such as to see dying relatives. While this may be humane, it is not good for effective infectious disease control. First, visitors may not know how to put on protective gear properly. Any mistake could significantly increase the risk of infection. Second, visitors may not know how to take off the gear correctly. This is even more of a problem. One error could lead to the virus being brought back into the community through contaminated clothing and other belongings. Objects brought into the ward from outside — thermos flasks containing soup, for example — must be sterilised before being taken out.

*   *   *

Recovery

29 March, Saturday

Finally discharged! Home! To resume a normal life, I hoped.

30–31 March

Photos of me made the front pages of all the major newspapers. I also made numerous television appearances. Suddenly I became a spokesman for SARS. Felt uncomfortable with my sudden "celebrity" status; luckily, my face was hidden behind a mask.

I realised that things would never be the same. People would still avoid close contact, fearing that I might be infectious.

Depressing news about the uncontrolled outbreak at Amoy Gardens.

1 April, Tuesday

Wanted to resume duties, but again the hospital was uncertain about infectivity and did not allow me to go back to work. Very frustrated.

2 April, Wednesday

Played tennis for the first time since being discharged. Poor coordination, unable to serve, slow to react. Could not even hit a running forehand — my favourite shot. I feared that I would never again play as well as I used to.

The first week of discharge was full of disappointments, heart-breaking news and frustrations, but I told myself that I must stay optimistic.

Second week after discharge

Marked improvement physically. Able to play tennis at 80 to 90 percent of my previous level.

Allowed back to my hospital office, but not permitted to see patients yet. Managed my patients through a "middleman" and appointments outside the hospital setting. What an undisciplined doctor!

11–18 April

Chest X-ray completely clear. Resumed duties and began to look after patients again. I finally considered myself fully recovered — a real doctor once more.

Resumed ward duty. Had to gown up and gown down every time I entered and left a medical ward. To prevent the spreading of infection, the air-conditioning was turned off. Wearing the protective gowns, facemasks and eye shields, you felt like you were inside a furnace. I fully understood the discomforts that the frontline staff had to put up with.

Two months after discharge

Fully recovered — I am very lucky. Some of my colleagues have still not resumed full duties because they have abnormalities in their chest X-ray and are taking steroids. Out of frustration, many of them have turned to traditional Chinese medicine for additional treatment.

Looking back

There are so many questions we need to answer before the next outbreak: When should patients who have recovered return to work? Are such patients with anti-coronavirus antibodies immune to future coronavirus infection? If so, for how long would the immunity last? If another outbreak occurs, should I go and work on the frontline since I have immunity? Or is there a possibility that a second coronavirus infection may lead to an exaggerated attack of the disease and a harder hit? If that is the case, then should healthcare staff who have recovered from SARS be allowed to go to the frontline in the event of another outbreak?

What kind of personal protective equipment (PPE) should medical staff wear? During the outbreak, frontline staff often complained that the PPE was not up to standard or in short supply. The Hospital Authority (HA) said that PPE had been delivered to the hospital. The staff said that the hospital administrators withheld such equipment. There seemed to be a breakdown in communication between the frontline staff and the HA. Staff had to vent their frustrations through the media.

Should the Government have closed down PWH in early March? Should there have been a complete "blockade," with all patients and medical staff prevented from leaving and no outsiders allowed in? Should all doctors and nurses, whether infected or not, be barred from going home and made to stay in quarters close to the hospital? The HA and the Department of Health must have a clear policy on this for the next outbreak.

During the crisis, emotion prevailed over rationality. We could not practise evidence-based medicine, as we lacked information. At a time of panic, should we play into the emotions of the public and frontline staff, rather than be strictly rational? Perhaps the HA should have supplied staff with what they wanted in the first place, rather than arguing over whether the equipment was necessary. Healthcare workers should not have been given the impression that they could use only a limited number of protective suits each day. The issue of the effectiveness of the gear could have been debated later. The HA must show that it cares more about promoting staff well-being and morale than saving costs.

Each hospital treated SARS patients differently. Mistakes at one facility were repeated at another. The HA had no clear-cut guidelines on treatment and infection control. Staff teams and hospital chief executives set their own policies. The intensive care units at some hospitals were full, while others had empty beds. Those with space had to be begged to take SARS patients from other hospitals.

The Government must set up a crisis team comprised of infectious disease experts. Whenever an outbreak occurs at any hospital, this group would go to that facility immediately, assess the situation, talk to frontline staff and provide clear instructions on protective gear, infection control and treatment. The team would have the authority to close down a hospital and manage the recruitment and deployment of staff.

Ideally, there should be uniform policies for all hospitals. The Government and HA must take to heart the bitter lessons learned from this outbreak. Issues to cover include the use of protective equipment, ward and hospital closure, the shutting down of schools, quarters for medical staff, hospital visits, quarantine camps, the deployment of pregnant healthcare workers, disease definition and reporting and experimental treatments. In setting policies, the Government and HA should hold extensive consultations with medical professionals and the public to reach a consensus before final implementation.

Should SARS return, we know what to expect and we need to be prepared. Perception is key. Medical equipment must not only be available in sufficient supply, but must be perceived by the public and hospital staff to be readily available. Policies must be effective and perceived to be so.

SARS vaccines will take at least two years to develop and may not be available if the virus strikes again. Although there were over 8,000 cases of SARS worldwide, with a mortality rate of more than 10 percent, there is no consensus on treatment. When the next outbreak occurs, we will be back to square one as far as treatment is concerned. Good personal hygiene, isolation and quarantine remain the most important ways to control SARS.

Final thoughts

Having been one myself, I now understand better how a patient feels. I fully appreciate why some want to go home as soon as possible. I couldn't have endured one extra day of hospitalisation. A word of care and encouragement can mean a lot to patients.

Through this ordeal, some of my friendships have become stronger and healthier while other relationships have faded. After being discharged, I became an instant celebrity, but fortunately people could recognise me only with a mask on! Still, I really want to contribute to SARS research. I have already donated my blood and plasma several times to help in the development of diagnostic kits, monoclonal antibodies and vaccines.

Above all, I should learn to be a more disciplined doctor and a more obedient patient — but that is easier said than done.

CHAPTER 4

The New Coronavirus:
In Search of the Culprit

Moira Chan-Yeung and Christine Loh

Virologist Klaus Stohr first had an inkling that trouble was brewing in November 2002. On a business trip to Beijing, the influenza programme manager for the World Health Organisation (WHO) was attending a routine meeting on China's flu vaccination policy. Stohr heard a report from a Guangdong health care worker that several people in the southern province had contracted a severe flu with unusual characteristics. The WHO requested a sample of the virus from the Chinese, but testing of the specimen received by the UN agency did not show anything out of the ordinary.[1]

By January 2003, Hong Kong virologists began to receive news of peculiar cases of pneumonia in neighbouring Guangdong. When health authorities in Guangdong announced on 10 February that a form of atypical pneumonia had infected 305 people since November 2002, five of whom had died, Hong Kong experts knew the situation across the border had to be watched closely.

Scientists initially suspected that the mysterious disease was somehow linked to a flu that mainly affects birds, particularly fowl. Several geese in a Hong Kong park had recently died from the H5N1 virus. A team of scientists at the University of Hong Kong (HKU), led by Professor Malik Peiris and Dr. Guan Yi, had been studying this strain of influenza since the 1997 outbreak in Hong Kong. The outbreak began with the sudden death of thousands of farm chickens. When the virus crossed over to

43

infect humans, 18 people fell seriously ill with what was termed as the avian or bird flu. Six of the patients died.[2] Hong Kong slaughtered over a million chickens and other poultry to stop the disease from spreading.

Up until this point, scientists had believed that the bird influenza virus could not infect humans. The 1997 outbreak proved that the crossover from animal to human hosts was possible. The good news was that transmission from person to person was not efficient. Had it been more efficient, the avian flu would have affected many more people. The virus re-emerged in Hong Kong in 1999 but in a less severe form.

On 11 February 2003, China's Ministry of Health informed the WHO of the atypical pneumonia outbreak in Guangdong. After the announcement, Hong Kong's Department of Health and the Hospital Authority (HA) set up a Working Group on Severe Community-acquired Pneumonia and launched an intensive surveillance operation to locate any unusual cases of severe pneumonia. Peiris' laboratory was one of the facilities involved in the investigation. The next day, China reported that the outbreak in Guangdong had affected six municipalities. But laboratory analysis of blood and saliva samples from patients did not indicate the presence of any influenza viruses.

China informed the WHO on 14 February that similar cases in Guangdong had been reported as far back as 16 November 2002.[3] Dr. Guan Yi and Dr. Zhen Bojian, colleagues in HKU's Department of Microbiology, travelled to Guangzhou to learn more about the outbreak and obtain samples for testing back in Hong Kong. A few days later, Hong Kong officials told the WHO that two people, a father and son, who had visited Fujian Province and travelled through Guangdong back to Hong Kong had contracted the H5N1 flu.[4] The daughter of the family had developed the disease and died while in Fujian, where she was buried.[5]

Because of these cases, there was uncertainty as to whether the illness reported in Guangdong in February 2003 was a new disease or simply a return of the avian flu. Peiris and his team suspected the latter. They were therefore screening samples from flu patients for evidence of H5N1 infection.

On 21 February, a Guangdong doctor, Liu Jianlun, arrived in Hong Kong. He was admitted to Kwong Wah Hospital the following day. Liu's brother-in-law, a Hong Kong resident, who had accompanied Liu shopping and sightseeing also became infected and was admitted to hospital. Kwong Wah sought the help of Professor Yuen Kwok-yung of

HKU as Liu had told staff that he had been in contact with suspected atypical pneumonia patients in Guangdong. Both Liu and his brother-in-law eventually died from the infection.

There was insufficient evidence that these cases were different from other pneumonia cases. By the end of February, however, scientists became more certain that they were dealing with a new virus. "We stopped wondering and started worrying," Stohr said.[6] On 5 March, Hong Kong's Department of Health announced it was investigating reports that healthcare workers were falling ill with atypical pneumonia at the Prince of Wales Hospital (PWH). At about the same time, reports of similar cases emerged in Hanoi, Singapore and Toronto. (Chapter 2 provides a detailed account of what happened at each of the hospitals in Hong Kong and in other cities.)

In a 15 March global advisory, the WHO for the first time referred to the new disease as "Severe Acute Respiratory Syndrome." By this time, over 150 people in countries around the world had become infected with SARS. The WHO believed that what it was dealing with was the first readily transmissible disease to emerge in the twenty-first century.

The hunt for the virus

By mid-March, the race had begun to find out everything possible about SARS. The WHO devised a two-pronged plan of attack. On the ground, it sent teams of experts and specialised protective equipment for infection control in affected hospitals to areas requesting assistance. In the "air," it used its electronically linked global influenza network as a model to quickly establish a similar "virtual" connection among 11 leading laboratories around the world through a shared secure website and daily teleconference calls. The number of labs involved in the investigation was eventually increased to 13. Their mission: to work around the clock to identify the SARS causative agent and develop a robust diagnostic test.[7]

Stohr was the mastermind behind the network. He invited the world's top research laboratories to do something unprecedented — to collaborate in a virtual global laboratory. Scientists at the three Hong Kong institutions involved in the consortium — HKU, the Chinese University of Hong Kong (CUHK) and the Department of Health — were among the first to agree to cooperate. Stohr carefully selected which laboratories to tap, taking into account the expertise of each research team. His decision to include the laboratory at Erasmus University in the Dutch port city of Rotterdam due to its experience in working with non-human primates would prove crucial.

The priority for the virus hunters was speed. With the virus spreading quickly, Stohr needed answers fast. If he had been forced to wait for each research team to come up with its own results, it would have taken considerably longer than if the teams worked together. "We needed people to share data and set aside Nobel Prize interests or their desire to publish articles," Stohr said.[8]

From his operations centre in Geneva, Stohr chaired daily teleconferences during which researchers from around the world shared their findings. "Good morning, good day and good evening!" was his standard greeting.[9] Genetic sequences, photographs and other data were posted on the secure website. Chemicals required for experiments and cultures were shipped around the world within hours of a collaborator's request.

On 18 March, laboratories in Germany reported the presence of the paramyxovirus in a tissue sample of a patient from Singapore.[10] This virus can cause respiratory disease and belongs to the same family of microbes that causes measles and mumps. In 1999, an outbreak of paramyxoviruses in Malaysia and Singapore killed more than a hundred people and devastated Malaysia's pig industry. The causal agent, the Nipah virus, named after the place in Malaysia where it was first detected, was now a suspect in the SARS investigation.

At the same time, CUHK found the human metapneumovirus, or hMPV, also a pathogen that causes respiratory disease, in samples from patients in Hong Kong. The virus causes respiratory tract infections, including croup in children. Samples from Hanoi, Singapore and Frankfurt patients were negative for hMPV, but two patients from Canada tested positive. The initial conclusion: the new virus was from the hMPV family. These findings were immediately shared with the other labs.

Discovery of the SARS-coronavirus

Working day and night, the HKU team had been trying a range of tests for new viruses, using clinical specimens from two patients with SARS, one of whom was Dr. Liu's brother-in-law. Since pneumonia is a common disease, one problem they faced was determining which pneumonia patients had the disease reported in Guangdong. On 10 March, Dr. Peiris and a colleague from Queen Mary Hospital, Dr. Chan Kwok-hung, spotted something growing in cells inoculated with the two specimens. They found that serum from other patients with probable SARS also reacted with these viruses. This convinced them that they had found the virus causing the disease.

The team then used two approaches to identify the culprit. HKU pathologist John Nicholls and Dr. Wilina Lim, head of the Virus Unit in the Department of Health, used a powerful electron microscope to observe the virus. What they saw looked like a coronavirus, so named because of the unmistakable crown-like spikes on the surface.[11]

At the same time, HKU team members Dr. Leo Poon Lit-man and Dr. Guan Yi set off on what they called a "fishing expedition" to discover the genetic make-up of the virus. Poon, a molecular virologist, started random genetic screening of infected cells in order to find some piece of information that might provide clues to the nature of the disease. Guan, also a virologist, exposed cells normally not used for virus testing to blood and tissue samples from sick patients. "Just like fishing," Poon explains, "you catch something but you really do not know what fish it is until you pull the whole thing out."[12] Over a period of four 15-hour days, the two scientists pieced together a partial genetic fingerprint of the virus. Their results also indicated that it was a coronavirus.

On 21 March, Peiris sent an e-mail to the international network to report his team's discovery. Their findings were quickly reproduced in other laboratories. Two days later, Dr. Julie Gerberding, director of the US Centres for Disease Control and Prevention in Atlanta, announced the same result, as did the Bernhard Nocht Institute for Tropical Medicine in Hamburg, Germany, headed by Dr. Christian Drosten.[13]

The outcome of the hunt came as a surprise to the medical community because coronaviruses generally cause only mild cases of the common cold in humans, as well as illnesses in cattle, pigs and poultry. To double check their results, the Atlanta team sent genetic material from the virus to Dr. Joseph DeRisi, a biochemistry and biophysics professor at the University of California at San Francisco, for further examination.[14] Using a virus-detection tool he had developed, DeRisi determined the presence of a coronavirus that had not been seen before.

Further confirmation came from work done at Erasmus University. Koch's Postulates are a series of conditions formulated in 1882 by German physician Robert Koch, considered one of the fathers of modern bacteriology, to prove that a microbe is the cause of a disease. To show that the new coronavirus was responsible for SARS, scientists had to see whether injecting it into animals led to symptoms similar to those in humans with the disease.[15]

Researchers at Erasmus infected monkeys with a SARS-associated virus from cell cultures and found that the animals developed a lower respiratory tract disease similar to SARS. By contrast, monkeys infected with hMPV developed only mild nasal problems, but not lower respiratory disease. And those infected with both the coronavirus and hMPV did not develop a more severe lower respiratory tract disease than those infected with the coronavirus alone. Therefore, the new coronavirus met Koch's criteria.[16] This boosted the confidence of the researchers at the various labs in the WHO network that they had indeed found the virus that causes SARS.

From animal to human

A virus is made up of a strand of nucleic acid — either deoxyribonucleic acid (DNA) or ribonucleic acid (RNA) — that contains its genetic blueprint. In the case of the coronavirus, this information is coded as RNA. The nucleic acid is enveloped in a protein coat. When a virus infects a living cell, it releases its genetic material and, using the cell's resources, replicates itself. Some viruses kill the cells they infect, possibly producing more infectious viruses in the process. The common flu is a good example. Other viruses disrupt normal cell division, making the cell cancerous. Still other viruses, such as those associated with herpes and shingles, incorporate their DNA with the host's nucleic acid and then remain dormant until conditions are ripe for the virus to re-emerge.

Most viruses have a preferred host. Some are commonly transmitted from person to person, while others, such as rabies, infect mainly animals. In rare instances, as with the avian flu, a virus can cross over from fowl or other animals to humans.

The first coronavirus was isolated in 1937. The virus caused bronchitis in chickens, leading to the death of thousands of birds.[17] It has subsequently been found in cattle, pigs and other animals. Since 1960, coronaviruses have been responsible for about half of all common colds in humans, with two strains — OC43 and 229E — accounting for up to 30 percent of all cases. Until the 2003 outbreak of SARS, no links to pneumonia, a severe form of respiratory disease, had been found.

So where did the SARS-coronavirus come from? Scientists are still unsure, although the current thinking is that it jumped from birds or some other animal to humans.[18] Researchers believe that the virus probably emerged in one of two ways. First, the new virus may be a hybrid that resulted from the recombination of two forms of coronaviruses in animals. But it is unclear how such a virus could have jumped from animals to humans if neither of the parent viruses infects humans. The other explanation is that after spreading among one animal species for a long time without causing disease, the virus accidentally jumped to humans, where it found a favourable environment to replicate and cause trouble.

The most recent research by an international team of scientists, led by Dr. Guan Yi, indicates that civet cats in Guangdong animal markets could have provided "a venue for the [virus] to amplify and transmit to new hosts, including humans."[19] The HKU team also found that eight of 20 wild-animal traders, three of 15 animal slaughterers and one of 20 vegetable sellers in Guangdong tested positive for antibodies to the SARS virus, showing that they had been exposed to SARS. However, none of these individuals reported feeling unwell, indicating that humans may be able to carry and spread the disease, even if they do not show SARS symptoms.[20]

Most coronaviruses cause respiratory disease, intestinal disorder or both.[21] Mutation can change a virus that originally causes intestinal disorders in piglets to one that causes respiratory problems in humans. Furthermore, those taking immunosuppressive drugs may shed virus for prolonged periods, as their bodies' natural defences are less effective at fighting it off. The virus could also multiply in the body and possibly produce a mutant strain. Co-infection with other viruses, parasites or bacteria exacerbates some animal coronavirus diseases.

In animals, infection by a coronavirus is associated with a range of problems, including a lack of protective immunity, persistent infection and immune enhancement, in which antiviral antibodies fail to halt the progression of disease. The latter may explain in part the relatively high mortality rate associated with coronavirus infection. The features of the SARS outbreak indicate that these characteristics have to a certain extent been replicated in humans.

Breaking the code

Uncovering the identity of the SARS pathogen only raised more puzzling questions. To get answers, investigators knew that they had to crack the genetic code. This would provide essential insight into how the virus replicates and its role in the pathogenesis of disease. Sequencing the genome for the virus could also lead to the development of tests to detect the SARS-coronavirus, drugs to combat the disease, such as inhibitors that block enzyme activity and limit viral replication, and perhaps a vaccine.

The coronavirus has a relatively large genome made up of more than 30,000 nucleotides, the building blocks of nucleic acids. Coronaviruses can be grouped into three categories based on genetic data and the reactivity of the antibodies they produce. The two previously known human coronaviruses, OC43 and 229E, fall into different groups.[22] Other animal coronaviruses represent a third group. The partial genome deciphered by HKU researcher Poon suggested that the SARS coronavirus did not fit into any of the three existing categories but rather belonged to a fourth group.

On 2 April, the Atlanta team began to fish segments of genetic code out of the virus, posting the information they gathered on the network website so that others could use it. Meanwhile, the Michael Smith Genome Sciences Centre in Vancouver, Canada, a research facility under the British Columbia Cancer Agency, decided to try and sequence the full genome. Under Dr. Robert Holt, a group of its scientists had already been studying fast-growing diseases for a year. While their work had originally started as a response to the global bio-terrorism threat, they viewed the SARS investigation as an opportunity to apply what they had learned.

The Canadian team received its first sample on 5 April. It was taken from the lung tissue of the first SARS patient infected in Toronto, a man who became sick in March, several days after his mother fell ill on her return from a trip to Hong Kong. Both died. The son was a "super-spreader" who had infected many people. Once his specimen arrived, nearly half of the 90 staff at the Vancouver laboratory worked on sequencing the virus.

In the early hours of 12 April, Holt's team finished the sequencing, posting the genome map on the website later that day. On 14 April, the researchers in Atlanta completed their genome map. The two genetic blueprints were practically identical.[23] Just days later, an HKU team led by Department of Zoology professor Frederick Leung and a CUHK group headed by chemical pathologist Dennis Lo Yuk-ming completed the sequencing of two SARS virus strains obtained locally.

On 17 April, exactly a month after Stohr set up the virtual research network, the collaborators announced conclusive identification of the SARS causative agent: a new coronavirus. Scientists now had a complete genetic map for the virus. Dr. David Heymann, then the WHO executive director for communicable diseases, described the pace of the research as "astounding."[24]

Analysis of the sequence revealed that the genome of the SARS-coronavirus is different from all previously known coronaviruses. Researchers concluded that it probably evolved separately from a coronavirus ancestor. It had likely infected some animal host for some time before infecting humans.[25] Before SARS surfaced, there were 11 known animal coronaviruses. According to epidemiologist Arnold Monto, a coronavirus expert at the University of Michigan School of Public Health, the new virus does not behave like the others. One possible explanation for this difference is that it underwent a major genetic change when it jumped from animals to humans.[26]

In order to validate this hypothesis, it would be necessary to carry out serological tests of wild and domestic animals, including birds, in the south China region where the outbreak first occurred. Serological tests are used to detect the presence of antibodies or antigens, substances that are recognised by the body as a threat, in a sample. Comparison with the genetic sequence of the virus in animal samples with those from SARS patients could then be used to determine how the virus spread to humans. If there were no reservoir of the virus in animals, the chances of eliminating it in human hosts would be better.

The HKU team began screening exotic animals for coronaviruses. In preliminary tests, they found six masked palm civets, or civet cats, that were carriers of a coronavirus almost identical to that found in SARS patients, except that its genomic map had 29 extra nucleotides.[27] Mainland Chinese experts have also found the SARS-coronavirus in monkeys, snakes and bats.[28] Much more research is needed to reach any firm conclusion.

The genome of the SARS-coronavirus from Toronto differs from genetic material obtained from SARS patients in Vietnam by only eight nucleotides. This suggests that the genetic material remained stable during human-to-human transmission. Minor nucleotide changes found in viruses from different clinical samples may prove useful markers for epidemiological studies. But their significance cannot be fully understood until more is known about the functions and antigens of the viral proteins. Most of the mutations in the genome of the SARS virus probably resulted from adaptation to cells used for cultures before sequencing.

Infection, incubation, illness

Scientists knew that the SARS virus is transmitted from person to person by inhalation of droplets. This typically occurs when a sick person sneezes or coughs. The microbe is carried in saliva spayed in the air. Another person nearby who breathes in the saliva may become infected. Droplets can easily travel a meter or more. They may also land on a surface such as a table, doorknob or elevator button. When somebody touches these surfaces with his hand, he may become infected if he then puts his hand to his eyes, mouth or nose. Some studies showed that the SARS virus could survive for at least 24 hours on a plastic surface at room temperature.[29]

Other tests indicated that the virus was also present in human excrement. A kidney patient who had been treated at the PWH and was infected with the SARS virus suffered from diarrhoea. He discharged the virus when he used the toilet in his brother's flat at Amoy Gardens, a private housing development that later became a SARS "hot zone" when many of its residents were infected (see Chapter 7). The virus was found to be able to survive in loose human stool for up to four days, whereas it could survive for up to only six hours in normal stool.[30] Heat of 56 degrees Celsius or higher kills the virus quickly. And it is no longer infectious when exposed to disinfectants such as bleach and 75 percent ethanol or rubbing alcohol, and chemical fixatives such as formaldehyde and paraformaldehyde.

The SARS virus has a long incubation period that varies from two to 10 days before symptoms begin to show. The average incubation time is about five days. The quarantine period for people suspected of having SARS is 10 days, although during the outbreak the WHO recommended two weeks. The infectivity of individuals during the incubation period is unclear. Within three days of the onset of symptoms, the virus is present in the nose and throat secretions of about one-third of patients. By the tenth day, it is evident in stool samples from almost all patients. Traces may be found as late as one month after the patient becomes ill. Viral secretion is usually highest near the end of the second week.

However, despite fears about transmission of SARS, the SARS-coronavirus has a relatively low infectivity. It does not transmit from person to person efficiently and a fairly large dose of virus appears to be needed for transmission to occur. SARS is much less infectious than the typical flu. The concern is the virulence of the SARS-coronavirus, which can cause rapid and serious damage to human organs. A high number of patients require intensive care. At the height of the outbreak in Hong Kong, 14 percent of SARS patients were in intensive care units (ICUs). This put considerable pressure on the healthcare system.

Will SARS return?

In the middle of June 2003, the number of new cases of SARS dwindled to a handful and by the beginning of July, the chains of local transmission were broken in all affected areas. The dramatic drop in the number of cases was the result of monumental efforts by the Government and healthcare staff with the cooperation of the public.

But SARS is likely to re-emerge. Other pathogens that have crossed over from animals to infect humans, such as the Ebola virus, periodically resurface and then fade away again. SARS may return when conditions are ripe for it to spread to humans from some animal or environmental source. Indeed, on 9 September 2003, the Singapore Government announced that a medical researcher was confirmed as a SARS case after going through two rounds of tests. The 27-year-old researcher worked in a microbiology laboratory and was doing work on the West Nile virus. He had not recently travelled outside Singapore. While this was regarded as a "single isolated case" it provided a timely reminder that SARS is still lurking.[31] As soon as the case was confirmed, the Department of Health in Hong Kong alerted laboratories at the HA, HKU and CUHK to tighten safety procedures.[32]

The world's public health systems have gained considerable experience from this outbreak, demonstrating their capacity to respond quickly and cooperatively. They now know how to control an infectious disease using isolation and quarantine measures. What is needed is better preparation and even faster action at the first sign of danger. While intensive research on SARS is under way, more time is required to develop a rapid diagnostic test, possibly an effective vaccine and a cure. Should the disease that caused so much panic around the world appear again, the global impact will be milder. SARS is no longer such a mystery. Still, this is no time for health authorities, healthcare workers and the public at large to let down their guard.[33] SARS is surely not the only hidden virus lurking out there. The next pathogen to launch a surprise attack may be more virulent and possibly more deadly. The lesson for all of us: Be prepared.

Acknowledgements

The authors wish to thank Professor Malik Peiris and Dr. Leo Poon Litman for their assistance in the preparation of this chapter.

CHAPTER 5

The Public Health Viewpoint

Gabriel M Leung, Anthony J Hedley, Edith MC Lau and Tai-Hing Lam

The SARS epidemic is already regarded as a defining moment in the evolution of communicable disease and will undoubtedly be seen as a milestone in the history of global public health. In 1969 the then US Surgeon-General confidently announced that "the book of infectious disease was now closed" and "that antimicrobial war had been won." We have since been forced to acknowledge many times over just how flawed that optimistic vision was. The history of newly emergent communicable disease during the past three decades should be a caution to any health professional or government official who is tempted to declare that we are free of the health risks presented by micro-organisms.

It appears that the SARS epidemic originated in Foshan, Guangdong Province in November 2002. The epidemic then spread to the cities of Heyuan and Zhongshan before causing a large outbreak in the provincial capital of Guangzhou in January 2003 (Figure 1). It is believed that a single highly infectious index patient, also known as a "super-spreader," from Guangzhou who visited Hong Kong in mid-February and stayed at the Metropole Hotel transmitted the SARS coronavirus to a number of Hong Kong people and to 16 other tourists from Vietnam,[1] Canada[2] and Singapore, who in turn triggered outbreaks in their home countries. The subsequent admission and treatment of this initial cohort of infected Hong Kong people at two of Hong Kong's busiest public hospitals initiated an infectious cascade that ultimately led to 1,705 cases locally.[3,4]

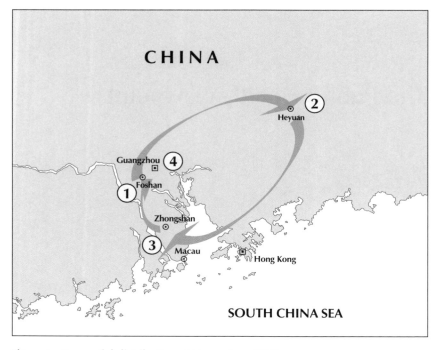

Figure 1   Geospatial distribution of Guangdong SARS cases

In an ideal situation, how should and could public health authorities have responded to the beginnings of this outbreak? For example, in Hong Kong, an initially small and apparently unrelated cluster of cases at Kwong Wah Hospital and Prince of Wales Hospital (PWH) provided the first indication that something unusual was happening by the third week of February. However, the World Health Organisation (WHO) did not officially declare the situation to be an outbreak until three weeks later, by which time the disease had already spread into the community and been exported to 11 other countries. What kinds of disease surveillance and communication systems were needed to alert public health practitioners to the emerging infection within days, as opposed to weeks, of its arrival into Hong Kong? Once the epidemic was acknowledged, what sorts of information were essential in guiding the formulation of public health policies? How best might such information be captured and studied? How could direct evidence of the growth potential and trajectory of the infection in the community be obtained? How long should the quarantine period be? Who should be isolated and where? How might health authorities determine whether the various personal and public hygiene measures, such as wearing of facemasks, school closures and frequent hand washing, were sufficient or could have been more effective in halting the spread of the virus, both before and after they were implemented? How might different scenarios in combating SARS on the community level, as the epidemic evolved, be modelled to better prepare for future outbreaks?

While these and related questions may not have the same popular appeal as the microbiological detective stories of the discovery of the SARS coronavirus, or the apparent immediacy of developing a vaccine, they are nonetheless crucial in the control of any epidemic. SARS has been no exception. The world has contained the present outbreak not because of genetic breakthroughs or high-technology solutions, but through painstaking implementation of classic and simple public health principles. These measures were instrumental in bringing the global epidemic under control.

This chapter examines some of the core principles of public health as they apply to the SARS epidemic in Hong Kong. First, we look at the possible origins of SARS, tracing its roots from rural farms to city markets and beyond. Then we dissect the early actions, or lack thereof, of public health authorities in affected areas worldwide and discuss how and why they handled the outbreak differently. The third section deals with the generation of scientific evidence and how it can be and has been usefully employed to control the epidemic. We conclude with a discussion of more generic systems issues, problems and potential solutions for Hong Kong to consider in better preparing itself for the next infectious disease outbreak.

The origins of SARS — markets, farms and migration

Human beings were mainly nomadic until after the last ice age, about twelve thousand years ago. Once human settlement began, animals were domesticated. Animal husbandry contributed to the process by which animal pathogens jump from species to species and become a cause of disease in humans. Due to this evolutionary process, humans share a large number of diseases with those animals that are either common companions or of major economic importance. It is notable that relatively recent changes in the management of certain animal populations, such as cattle, have been associated with new diseases such as bovine spongiform encephalopathy and its human variant Creutzfeld-Jakob Disease ("Mad Cow Disease").

Southern China has high-density human and animal populations that exist in close proximity to each other. In particular, the demand for chickens and ducks as food is almost insatiable, leading to intensive rearing and marketing practices. Avian species have long been recognised as an important source of new viruses, particularly those that cause influenza. Over 20 years ago Shortridge and Stuart-Harris[5] discussed the findings of a meeting between scientists from mainland China and Hong Kong on this issue. They described how "the closeness between man and animals could provide an ecosystem for the interaction of their viruses." Shortridge and Stuart-Harris noted that poultry were raised in the suburbs of Guangzhou as well as in villages, "and the rate of isolation of influenza virus from ducks there is the same as that for birds on the farms…" They suggested that an exchange of viruses between animals and humans might occur even in densely populated urban areas. This was a critically important observation for the south China region. In the 1970s, renowned virologist Robert Webster and his colleagues demonstrated that animal reservoirs of viruses could facilitate the reassortment of genetic material between animal and human influenza viruses. The phenomenon of avian flu viruses mutating to become the cause of serious disease in humans is common knowledge in Hong Kong.

Hong Kong researchers were therefore well acquainted with the idea that viruses could jump from one species to another before SARS appeared, but as the then Director of Health Dr. Margaret Chan stated on 6 June, they were looking for influenza rather than a lethal coronavirus from a civet cat. The animal reservoir remains to be confirmed but the filthy wild animal markets of Guangdong would meet the criteria as vectors for the cross-species evolution of a new disease. Moreover, the regular, massive migration back and forth between rural areas and the various thriving coastal cities in Guangdong would facilitate the rapid spread of any potential new viruses that have jumped from domesticated animals in the villages to humans. It is this unique mix of rural-urban migration, intensive animal husbandry (especially involving avian and other wild species, such as civet cats), slaughtering practices on village farms as well as in urban markets and the lack of proper hygiene standards that has made Guangdong and southern China a likely epicentre of new emerging viruses.

We need to acknowledge however the myriad remaining uncertainties associated with the origins and spread of SARS. The most perplexing alternative epidemiological proposition has been put forward by astrophysicists in the new field of astrobiology. Professor Chandra Wickramasinghe, a protégé of the legendary Cambridge astronomer Professor Sir Fred Hoyle, and his colleagues have published evidence that supports the theory that earthly epidemics have inter-stellar origins. They argue that the emergence of SARS in south China is consistent with precipitation of stratospheric viral particles in the thinnest part of the upper atmosphere as seen in previous epidemics. As further proof of this theory, they point out that although during the 1917–18 influenza pandemic person-to-person spread did occur on a large scale, the disease appeared on the same day in different parts of the world, but took days to weeks to spread short distances.[6]

Early actions (or lack of them) — who did what and when

While hindsight may be perfect and *post hoc* armchair criticism easy, it is essential to review key public health measures adopted in controlling the SARS outbreak by authorities in different locations worldwide if lessons are to be learned for the next epidemic.

Figure 2 shows the daily number of new SARS cases in Hong Kong and highlights key events in the control of the local epidemic. Following formal recognition of the outbreak at PWH, the first and most extensive nosocomial (within-hospital transmission) cluster in Hong Kong, on 11 March, health authorities implemented several measures to combat the spread of SARS including:

- Public-service announcements about personal protection (17 March);
- Addition of SARS to the list of notifiable diseases and requests for close contacts of cases to attend designated medical centres for screening (27 March) until the later introduction of mandatory home quarantine;
- A two-week suspension of schools (announced 27 March and implemented 29 March) and universities (29 March);
- Introduction of health declarations for all incoming residents and visitors (29 March);
- Isolation of residents of Block E of the Amoy Gardens estate due to

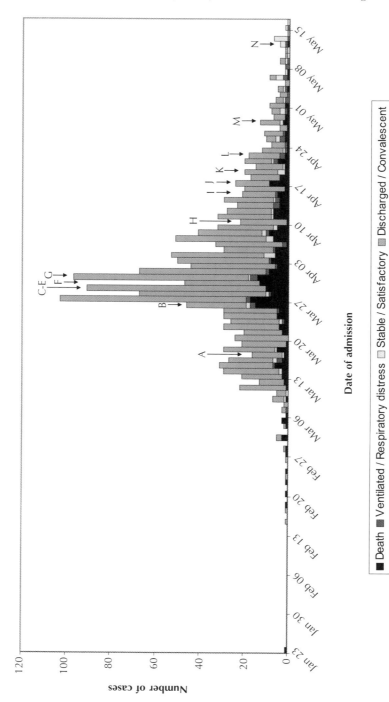

Source: Government statistics and newspaper reports

Figure 2 Temporal pattern of SARS epidemic in Hong Kong, as of 26 May 2003

Figure 2   Temporal pattern of SARS epidemic in Hong Kong, as of 26 May 2003

A: Public-service announcements about personal protection (17 March)

B: Addition of SARS to the list of notifiable diseases and requests for close contacts of cases to report to designated medical centres for screening (27 March), continued until the later introduction of mandatory home quarantine

C: Two-week suspension of schools (announced 27 March, implemented 29 March)

D: Two-week suspension of universities (29 March)

E: Introduction of health declarations for all incoming residents and visitors (29 March)

F: Isolation of residents of Block E of the Amoy Gardens estate, at the centre of a cluster of about 300 cases (31 March)

G: Subsequent relocation of residents of Amoy Gardens to rural isolation camps for 10 days (1 April)

H: Home quarantining of close contacts of cases and restrictions on their travel out of Hong Kong (10 April)

I: New public announcements urging those with symptoms to seek medical attention (15 April)

J: Body-temperature checks for all air passengers (17 April)

K: Two-day city-wide cleanup campaign (19–20 April)

L: Form 3 to 7 resumed classes after three-week break beginning 29 March (22 April)

M: Form 1 and 2 students resumed classes (28 April)

N: Primary 4 to 6 students resumed classes (12 May)

O: Lower primary and kindergarten students resumed class (19 May)

P: WHO lifted its travel advisory against Hong Kong (23 May)

Q: Government's 'Team Clean' launched to keep city hygienic (28 May)

R: US Centres for Disease Control (CDC) lifted its travel advisory against Hong Kong (5 June)

S: US State Department lifts travel note against Hong Kong (10 June)

a community cluster of about 330 cases (31 March) and the subsequent relocation of residents to isolation camps for ten days (1 April);

- Home quarantining of close contacts of cases and restrictions on their travel out of Hong Kong (10 April);
- New public announcements urging those with symptoms to seek medical attention (15 April);
- Body-temperature checks for all air passengers (17 April); and
- A territory-wide clean-up campaign over the long Easter weekend (19–20 April), followed by the subsequent formation of a high-level Government committee ("Team Clean") to develop and implement a sustainable hygiene and environmental health policy (28 May).

While this series of public health measures is comprehensive, there are concerns that authorities could have acted more quickly and more decisively, especially during the first two weeks following formal recognition of the outbreak, to curb the explosive growth of the epidemic. However, as we explain later, it is uncertain if such earlier action on the public level would have made a major difference to the eventual spread of the SARS virus in Hong Kong. Nevertheless, infection control measures at certain hospitals could have been better organised thereby minimising the chances of exporting infectious individuals to the community setting. As the Hospital Authority's own internal review report points out, "there appears to have been a lapse as the Amoy Gardens index case was discharged home from a ward housing confirmed and highly suspected SARS patients with neither a period in step-down ward, nor any follow up."[7]

In the city-state of Singapore, officials acted swiftly early on in the epidemic to impose controls. In many cases their actions preceded implementation of corresponding measures in Hong Kong, such as: listing SARS as a notifiable infectious disease (17 March in Singapore vs 27 March in Hong Kong); implementing home quarantine for contacts of cases (24 March vs 31 March for Amoy residents and 10 April for other Hong Kong residents); and announcing the closure of all schools (27 March vs 27 and 29 March). On 30 May, Dr. David Heymann, then executive director for communicable diseases at the WHO, said, "from the start Singapore's handling of its SARS outbreak was exemplary. This is an inspiring victory that should make all of us optimistic that SARS can be contained everywhere." However, although some have credited Singapore's quick response measures as being responsible for limiting the extent of the outbreak there, it is unclear whether a direct causal inference can be made. In any comparison of the control of the epidemic in Singapore and in Hong Kong, a number of additional factors must be considered, especially given the differences in the way the population responded to the epidemic, in the density of housing and the overall environmental situation and not least in the very unusual circumstances surrounding the large Amoy Gardens outbreak in Hong Kong. Moreover, Singapore's decision to impose controls was at least partly based on insights gained by observing developments in Hong Kong, where the epidemic started earlier (Figure 3).

Vietnam has been similarly complemented for its quick, transparent and decisive response to the SARS outbreak, which has been traced to a single imported index case: a Chinese-American businessman who arrived from Hong Kong. However, given the random nature of the transmission pattern of the disease, chance almost certainly played a role as well, as most of the cases were confined to two hospitals (Hanoi French and Bach Mai Hospitals) and there was little community spread.

To further illustrate the often unpredictable nature of disease transmission, Toronto's outbreak appeared to be under control by early May but towards the end of the month further hospital clusters totalling more than 60 cases signalled a resurgence, despite rigorous adherence to preventative and control measures in healthcare facilities.

Lastly, China is widely acknowledged to have been slow and opaque in dealing with the SARS outbreak early on, first at the provincial level in Guangdong and later at both municipal and national levels in Beijing. The lack of transparency and Government action probably contributed significantly to the subsequent global spread of the disease, until mounting international pressure and criticisms led to the removal of Health Minister Zhang Wenkang, who was later replaced by Vice Premier Wu Yi. After this point, the Chinese Government made substantial and effective improvements in transparency, implemented infection control measures at the hospital and community levels, built a 1,000-bed hospital in less than ten days and improved cooperation with international health agencies and national governments. This series of concrete actions led to the rapid containment of the outbreak within the next few weeks.

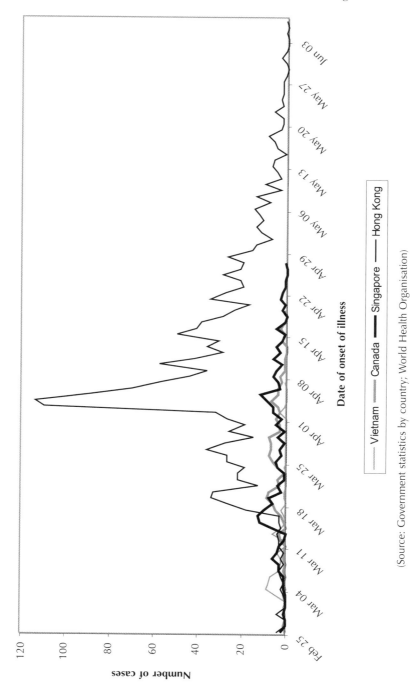

(Source: Government statistics by country; World Health Organisation)

Figure 3   Epidemic curves for Hong Kong, Singapore, Vietnam and Canada

Measuring the epidemic

Epidemiological parameters: What they mean and why we need to measure them

Incubation period: Consider this scenario. Kathy Chau, an intensive care nurse working in a SARS ward, has just been confirmed as a SARS case. In accordance with the Government's home quarantine orders, her husband, James Chau, will need to be quarantined and observed to prevent potential spread to the community. But how long should he be kept in isolation? This depends on the duration between infection and the first appearance of clinical symptoms, or the average "incubation period" of SARS.

The incubation period (estimated as the time between the last exposure and the onset of symptoms) is a key piece of information for the management of communicable disease outbreaks. With SARS, it proved to be difficult to estimate with high precision. Although Hong Kong's estimates were based on the largest number of cases, even towards the end of the epidemic (8 June) information on only 90 out of 1755 cases met the necessary criteria for making this calculation. The evidence indicates that a small proportion of SARS cases had a much longer incubation period than the rest. Knowledge of the distribution of incubation periods and possible changes during the epidemic should guide quarantine arrangements (Figure 4).

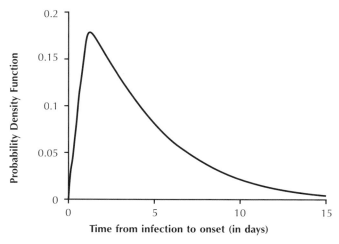

Figure 4 Incubation period, estimated at different intervals during the epidemic

There are real difficulties in acquiring high quality information for epidemiological work from sick people given the turmoil of hospital admission and treatment. New protocols, documents, procedures and training should be developed and tested to ensure good data collection.

The onset-to-admission interval: Unfortunately Mr. Chau has been infected through household contact with his wife and falls ill with SARS. Moreover, he has not complied with the home quarantine guidelines and has gone back to work for fear of losing his temporary job, an understandable concern given the difficult economic climate. From the time of the onset of his symptoms, he has been infectious and could have transmitted the SARS virus to those around him. The sooner he is admitted to hospital and removed from the general community after first showing symptoms, the lower is the likelihood that he will spread the virus. This critical time period, important in determining the rate of spread of the infection, is termed the "onset-to-admission interval."

Reducing the period during which infected individuals can transmit the disease is an important target for health authorities engaged in outbreak control. The interval for each patient can be measured by carefully recording the date of onset of the first symptoms and the date of admission to hospital. The problem again is getting access to patients and deploying skilled interviewers using standardised procedures to ensure that the measurement of onset times is reliable. Rapid analysis of this data is then needed so that policies such as encouraging people to report symptoms and seek medical care at the earliest opportunity can be evaluated and if necessary modified to achieve greater efficacy.

In fact, by April there was an overall reduction in the onset-to-admission interval from 5.4 days in late February/early March to 3.5 days by 9–15 April (Figure 5).[8] By the third week of May, at the tail end of the epidemic, this number dropped further to 2.2 days. In any future outbreak, continuous statistical analysis of the interval measurements should be a high priority.

Still for even these two apparently straightforward characteristics of the disease and its management, there are major personnel and resource challenges involved in obtaining good information during an epidemic. With many hundreds of both probable and suspected cases, a well organised, sustained and continuously audited approach is needed. Significant advances were made in developing systems for the rapid capture of information during the outbreak, particularly by the

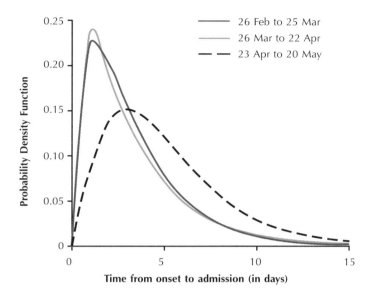

Figure 5 Onset-to-admission intervals during the epidemic

Department of Health (DH) and the Hospital Authority (HA), but a careful audit will show what more needs to be done. In addition to the investment of new resources in data systems, Hong Kong undoubtedly needs regular operational reviews and rehearsals based on simulated epidemics, followed by detailed evaluation. There is scope for much greater intersectoral sharing of this responsibility and collaborative work rather than defensive positioning.

The reproduction rate of the epidemic: Through contact tracing, the regional community physician of the DH has determined that Mr. Chau has infected three co-workers during the five days between the appearance of first symptoms and eventual hospital admission and isolation. If this pattern proves typical of the spread in the community generally, then we can expect the epidemic to grow exponentially where each infected individual "reproduces" three additional cases. Thus it is important to measure, on the population level, the reproduction rate of the epidemic at various points in time as it evolves. Once this is achieved, it is also possible to model and project the impact of different control measures on the reproduction rate or growth trajectory of the epidemic.

The rate of spread of an epidemic, and whether such spread is self-sustaining, depends on the magnitude of a key parameter called the basic reproduction number or R_0. It is defined as the average number of secondary cases generated by one primary case, or in simple terms, how many people a typical diseased individual infects *in a completely susceptible population in the absence of any control measures.*[9] This statistic is mainly determined by the nature of the micro-organism itself. In the case of SARS, R_0 has been estimated to be between 2.7 and 3, with upper bounds of 3.6 to 3.7.[10,11] This shows that SARS is a moderately transmissible disease. By contrast measles and influenza have basic reproduction numbers of about 13 and 5, respectively.[12,13]

A related quantity, the effective reproduction number (R_t), represents the number of infections caused by each new case occurring at any particular point in time, i.e. how many people a typical diseased person infects at different time points during an epidemic *with various control measures in place.* This is usually smaller than R_0 due to the effects of public health interventions. It is influenced by disease-specific parameters including the infectiousness of the agent and the length of time for which a diseased individual remains infectious to others. Other social factors are also important, such as contact rates in the population or effective mixing between infected and susceptible groups, and environmental attributes such as population density and geographic heterogeneity of people who are susceptible (or immune) to the virus.

The effective reproduction number or R_t needs to be reduced to below 1.0, the self-sustaining threshold, in order for the epidemic to be controlled.[14] A value above this critical level indicates that the epidemic is on a growth path and will expand — the larger the value, the faster the growth rate. Conversely, a value less than 1.0 means that eventually the epidemic will taper off — the lower the value, the quicker the rate of decline. In the Hong Kong SARS epidemic, the combined effects of reductions in the time interval between symptom onset and isolation by hospitalisation, in population contact rates and in hospital transmission are estimated to have caused R_t to drop to 1.0 by 26 March. Slippage at this stage in the management of the disease, such as poor hygiene or delays in reporting symptoms and providing treatment, could have "pushed" the reproduction number back up above 1.0. However by 10 April R_t had fallen further to 0.14,[15] meaning that the epidemic was already under control at a point weeks before the WHO lifted its travel advisory (Figure 6).

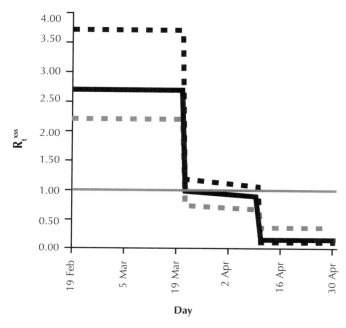

R_t^{xss}

Day

(Source: Riley *et al*, Science, 2003)

Figure 6   Changes in the estimated effective reproduction number in the absence of super-spreading events

Criticisms of and uncertainty regarding the efficacy of the Government's actions during the epidemic may be put into perspective by estimating what would have happened in the absence of the actions taken.[16] Figure 7 shows:

(A) The effect of no control measures or change in population behaviour; it is predicted that this would result in a catastrophic epidemic with over 100 cases a day and increasing.

(B) No change in behaviour but a reduction in the time elapsed from the onset of symptoms to admission to hospital; this would temporarily increase the numbers admitted but would reduce transmission of the disease by up to 19 percent.

(C) As for (B) but with complete cessation of movement between Hong Kong's 19 districts on day 45 (approximately 5 April); this would reduce transmission by 76 percent and control the epidemic even without change in population behaviour.

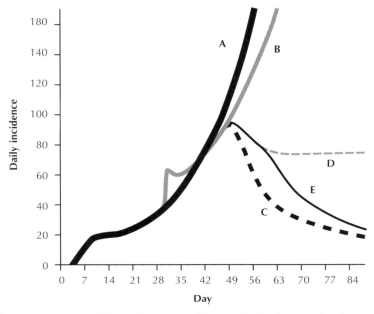

Figure 7   What would have happened without effective interventions?

(D) Again as for (B) but with a 50 percent drop in contact rates and hospital infections from day 45; this would be just sufficient to prevent growth of the epidemic.

(E) As for (D) but with a 70 percent reduction in hospital transmission from day 55 (approximately 15 April); the effect would be rapid control of the epidemic.

At least one international newspaper has trumpeted that earlier school closures and quarantine arrangements would have contained the outbreak. Although the epidemic was clearly sensitive to the level of population mobility, given the very marked self-imposed restrictions on movement in the community by the general public, it is possible but unlikely that school and university closures *per se* made a major contribution to the reduction in transmission. While open, the educational institutions were subject to rigorous cleaning of all surfaces and promotion of hygiene measures including hand washing, wearing of masks and checking of body temperature. Arguably, the risks of transmission to young people would be increased when out of school and out of a supervised environment.

Quarantine is unquestionably a necessary intervention in the event of an epidemic, but we need more analyses of the transmission of the disease between actual cases and their contacts before we can assess and quantify its benefits. The self-imposed restrictions on movement and the WHO travel advisory were not welcomed by the travel, retail and hospitality industries, but we believe these restrictions made a major contribution to removing key modes of transmission for the disease and to shortening the epidemic. Such measures should be implemented early and urgently in any future outbreak.

New evidence needed from this epidemic

Tools for diagnosis

The early diagnosis of SARS is very dependent on bedside observations and clinical judgement based on history taking and physical examination, chest X-rays and standard laboratory tests of blood and other specimens. An accurate diagnosis can be obtained by testing two blood samples taken 28 days apart for the presence of specific antibodies to the SARS-associated coronavirus. However, there is as yet no tailored diagnostic test developed for the rapid and accurate diagnosis of SARS when a patient first presents symptoms. As a consequence, the correct early diagnosis of SARS is fraught with difficulties because of the relatively subjective way in which a SARS case is defined. For instance, on 29 May, acting at the request of the WHO, the Toronto health authorities made a slight change in the X-ray criteria used in the clinical definition of a SARS case. Consequently, half of all suspected cases in Toronto were immediately reclassified as probable SARS patients.[17]

Even if and when an accurate and valid test becomes available and obviates the need for individual clinicians to diagnose SARS based on bedside information alone, it is unlikely to be available, affordable and practical in developing regions of the world. This would at present include mainland China, which was hardest hit by the SARS epidemic (especially rural areas and villages), and other regions where resources are scarce and the healthcare infrastructure does not support the application of such technology. Therefore, it is important that a highly sensitive clinical prediction rule be developed and validated using the detailed SARS case data accumulated in Hong Kong, in order to identify patients as likely SARS cases quickly and effectively and implement necessary quarantine and treatment. This is likely to lead to improved illness and mortality outcomes at the individual patient level and would also contribute to the effective control of the spread of the disease in the community.

Tools for prognosis

Estimates of the number of cases who die from the disease vary from 4 to 6 percent in mainland China and up to 15 to 20 percent in Hong Kong, Singapore and Canada.[18] These estimates have generated controversy in the media and among the public. Clearly, it is important to study the underlying factors that may be responsible for the widely divergent mortality outcomes in different communities. We can point to several potential contributory factors:

1. Differences in the characteristics of infected individuals in different places. For example, the relative distribution by age, sex and the presence of other serious health conditions (such as diabetes, chest and heart disease) among SARS cases;

2. Infective viral loads (i.e. dose of the virus) and the mode of transmission (e.g. heavy droplets through person-to-person contact or faecal-oral contamination through environmental point source infection) at the time the patient was exposed;

3. Differences in treatment protocols such as the use of the antiviral drug Ribavirin in over 90 percent of patients in Hong Kong compared with much less frequent use in Toronto patients, or the timing (initiation and duration) and use of high-dose "pulsed" steroids;[19, 20, 21] and

4. Possible natural evolution of the SARS virus and resultant changes in its virulence.

The aim of a comprehensive study of possible prognostic factors will be to identify and quantify predictors of survival or of adverse outcomes including admission to an intensive care unit (ICU), need for intubation (i.e. assisted respiration with a breathing tube) and ventilation (i.e. mechanical respiratory assistance) and extended hospital stays. There is also a strong case for a well-designed follow-up programme to study the longer-term physical, emotional and psychological effects of SARS on survivors.

In order for these initiatives to succeed, it is crucial that all 14 public hospitals and clinicians taking care of SARS patients, the two local medical schools, the HA, the DH and the Health, Welfare and Food Bureau contribute clinical, radiological, laboratory and contact tracing data to a central, integrated SARS database. Only then will sample size and statistical power be sufficient for rigorous examination, detection and elaboration of the finer nuances of clinical associations underlying the diagnostic and prognostic indices or measures. Hong Kong, which so far has the largest reliable set of SARS case data in the world, should seize this unique opportunity to demonstrate that different sectors of the community can collaborate and that it has the expertise to produce valuable data to guide research on both the prevention and treatment of SARS worldwide.

The public health tool box

Information and information systems

The aphorism "no decisions without information" is nowhere truer than in the management of communicable disease outbreaks. The SARS epidemic has sent a clear signal that Hong Kong needs a much greater and sustained investment in health informatics: public health information systems, the skills to use them and networks to share them.

In response to calls for this kind of investment, there are likely to be assertions that these measures are indeed in place, or at least in hand, but we do not agree. An in-depth review and analysis of the management of information during the course of this epidemic is needed. It is well recognised that health information systems in most countries are inadequate for the kind of management and decision-making that is needed at different levels of the healthcare system, from the bedside level through to systems planning at the macro-level. Hong Kong is not immune from this gap despite much investment in technology and hardware.

For several reasons Hong Kong failed to develop a fully integrated operational database on SARS patients and contacts. It came very close, but failed at the final hurdle because of generic problems that plague the establishment of all information systems. These include the lack of standardisation for data capture documents, and for procedures and protocols for information management, delays in transferring and updating information and a lack of rapid analysis and audit of databases.

In addition, while recognising the importance of maintaining the privacy and confidentiality of affected individuals and the potential for confusion when multiple parties are involved, good information needs to be shared freely and completely between all relevant parties. In Hong Kong, this includes the DH, which is responsible for public health; the HA, which provides over 90 percent of total inpatient bed-days; and the academic departments of public health, microbiology and relevant clinical specialties, which have the expertise and capacity to perform real time analyses to inform policy decisions and management options. Mainland and overseas health agencies such as the Chinese Ministry of Health and its provincial counterparts, the WHO and the Chinese and US Centers for Disease Control and Prevention (CDC) should also be involved. Findings should be efficiently fed back to frontline clinicians and those who are responsible for collecting information to improve data quality, reliability, relevance, validity and timeliness. In parallel, important results must be subjected to rigorous, international scientific peer review, be it via the WHO or medical periodicals, and then disseminated widely. More generally, there should be greater transparency in the data collection, collation, analysis and dissemination processes.

The development of efficient information systems will only be achieved if shortcomings are acknowledged and not denied or glossed over. The call for an appraisal of the need for tools to support control of communicable disease outbreaks in Hong Kong should not be seen as a criticism of local capacity or resources, but rather as necessary recognition of a generic issue in the development and maintenance of modern health databases and active information systems. SARS has brought this into sharp relief — but it could equally have been influenza or dengue fever.

Intelligence and risk communication

Additional issues concern how case data on SARS can be best used, and who should be involved in the analysis, in order to extract the best possible intelligence from available information. Coming from the academic sector we will be seen to have a clear bias. In fact, we believe analysis can and should be carried out jointly by teams from the service and academic sectors. However, the SARS epidemic demonstrated the real problems involved in establishing effective working relationships between many different parties and not only between the academic and service sectors. Different groups are seen to be motivated by different agendas rather than a common purpose. There is no doubt that they do in part have different needs and goals, but this should not negate the sharing of knowledge and skills for maximum benefit. There is no question that this cooperative approach is needed, but it was not always accepted or applied during the outbreak. No one party had overall supervision of information acquisition, management and analysis. As a result, at the time of writing some tasks still remain incomplete, such as a full and proper analysis of the transmissibility of disease between cases and their contacts.

In times of crisis, health information often becomes politically sensitive. The internal politics of public health emergencies such as the SARS epidemic remain an outstanding problem for the Government. Official objectives should include the efficient and carefully calibrated communication of risks to the public, information sharing and maximum utilisation of all skills and resources available for problem solving.

For example, during the SARS outbreak, the use of certain epidemiological terms and predictions about the course of the epidemic was sometimes inappropriate, causing confusion among the media and members of the public. Those from different sectors should form multidisciplinary teams to prepare and provide carefully worded daily profiles on epidemiological, social and political issues during the course of the epidemic. Such an approach would require a degree of openness (even in confidence) between the different groups involved that would go well beyond past and current norms of behaviour in Government departments.

Public support and involvement is crucial in the control and prevention of epidemics. During the SARS epidemic, both the mass media and the community made important contributions in mitigating the impact of the disease. In the early stage, the media and the public took a proactive stance in opposition to governmental prevarication and pressured the authorities to adopt more stringent public health measures. Community action eventually reached a climax during the middle stage of the epidemic as many groups such as non-governmental organisations, organised public information and support campaigns. These initiatives resulted in the wearing of surgical masks by most people and improvement of hygiene measures in households, workplaces, restaurants and commercial and residential buildings. There was also a marked increase in the feeling of solidarity in the community and a groundswell of opinion that everyone should unite and work together to fight SARS. Towards the end of the epidemic, several fundraising campaigns successfully raised many millions of dollars to support the victims, research and other causes (see Chapters 12 and 13).

Public health measures implemented during an outbreak must include good communication of sound information so that the public has a correct perception of the risks of contracting the disease and of the value of preventive measures. Misinformation and rumours can trigger widespread community panic, while public complacency results in non-action and non-acceptance of stringent measures such as quarantine. Recognising that there was a lack of knowledge about public perceptions and behaviour during the outbreak, several tertiary institutions carried out population surveys, the results of which were widely disseminated to the mass media. As these surveys were conducted as part of individual institutional initiatives, using limited resources, there was no coordination. Such efforts are unlikely to be sustainable. However, the surveys demonstrated that a moderate level of public anxiety is needed for the widest adoption of preventive measures. With improved understanding, changes in behaviour, including mask wearing and hand washing, did occur. Public health messages relayed to the community must strike a delicate balance between being overly reassuring and unnecessarily alarmist. Understanding the public's perceptions, emotional state, knowledge, attitudes and behaviour is essential so that public health messages, policies and actions meet the needs and expectations of the public, generate the greatest support from the community and will be effective public health instruments.

Deficiencies in communicating health information rather than shortfalls in diagnostic or therapeutic skills were undoubtedly among the reasons why the mainland health minister and the mayor of Beijing were dismissed. Although concealment of available information by those working under these officials may also have been a major factor, it is unlikely that anyone had access to all of the relevant data needed for effective epidemiological management. The deficit in public health intelligence on the mainland continued even after the decision by authorities to cooperate fully with international agencies and on 4 June the WHO stated that it was still "concerned" by how SARS cases were being counted and accounted for on the mainland — and that the credibility of mainland data remained an issue in interpreting the course of the epidemic.

It is now widely accepted that Hong Kong needs to renew its public health surveillance system for both infectious and chronic diseases. An essential part of such a system should be the monitoring of public behaviour, including risk factors and preventive measures. In addition, the public's perception of different risks and its understanding of diseases and control policies and measures should be regularly measured. There is an urgent need to review all of the surveys conducted during the SARS epidemic. In the short-term, resources are needed so that these surveys can be continued to monitor trends. For long-term planning, the experiences and knowledge gained should form the foundation for a public perception and risk factor surveillance system that can be used to monitor trends periodically between outbreaks, and activated to collect new and urgent information when there is a new outbreak.

Organisation and integration — problems and solutions

Was Hong Kong adequately prepared for this outbreak? The answer is clearly in the negative. The more pertinent question should be — "why not?" While it is always possible, in fact easy, to hide behind political grandstanding, finger-pointing and making a scapegoat of individuals, the real problems for Hong Kong lie in the macro-organisation of the system, and how our public health and healthcare infrastructure is financed.

As with any initiative, the prevention of disease and promotion of health requires the allocation of resources. Close examination of Hong Kong's latest available Domestic Health Accounts for 1996–97 reveals that only 2.3 percent of the total health expenditure was targeted at disease prevention and health promotional activities.[22] This minimalist approach to disease prevention, whether the disease is a communicable disease such as SARS or one of the many silent chronic conditions such as obesity or diabetes, remained unchanged for years before 1996–97 and has not changed appreciably since then. More generally, the extent to which the entire reimbursement structure in the healthcare sector is tied to diagnosis and treating disease, rather than to preventive health, deserves special attention and reconsideration. The HK$1 billion SARS fund earmarked for the establishment of a Hong Kong Centre for Disease Control and Prevention (CDC) or Centre for Health Protection (CHP), possibly based on the US CDC or UK Health Protection Agency models, and for research on the scientific and health implications of SARS is a much welcomed development. However, despite the immediate benefits this lump sum may provide, single injections of resources, however large, are usually insufficient unless sustained by a recurrent operating budget. The litmus test of Hong Kong's disease prevention capability will be whether we can prevent the *next* epidemic of infectious disease. To achieve better environmental health for more people in Hong Kong on a broader level, a major realignment of priorities is needed, including fair and equitable remuneration for health professionals in preventive disciplines to provide health education, disease prevention counselling, risk assessment monitoring and evaluation. Provided that we can measure impact and outcomes, the Government should encourage all third party payers, public and private, to reimburse it for disease prevention and health promotional activities. Such activities should no longer be an afterthought.

Hong Kong's two departments of public health medicine can play an important role in training, service and research if they are allowed to do so, but they are particularly vulnerable to the current higher education cuts. Both departments are small and ageing. Unless better opportunities and incentives to attract young specialists to public health are made available, this academic specialty will be dead within about ten years.

Arguably, the legacy of the Scott Report,[23] released in 1985, which ultimately led to the establishment of the HA, is at least partially responsible for the suboptimal response to the SARS outbreak. While it is widely acknowledged that medical care and amenities have been drastically improved due to management reforms by the HA, these changes were generously financed during a time of abundance in the 1990s, at the expense of a commensurate and necessary expansion and strengthening of the public health function. To this day, the DH, which is responsible for all public health functions in Hong Kong, is only allocated about 10 percent of the total public health care budget while the remaining lion's share is channelled to the HA. Of the approximately HK$3 billion the DH receives annually, a large proportion goes towards direct patient care services, such as the Maternal and Child Health Service and the Elderly Health Service. This resource allocation structure and the consequent chronic under-funding of crucial public health functions may explain, in part, Hong Kong's response to the SARS outbreak.

Moreover, there are inconsistencies in the public health regulatory powers delegated to the DH. For instance, the apparent concealment of the cluster of SARS cases at the Baptist Hospital prompted a strong and appropriate reprimand from the Director of Health, who oversees quality control and licensing of all 12 private hospitals in the territory. However, the 44 HA-run hospitals fall outside the DH's purview under legislative ordinance. In essence, this creates a triple role for the HA, with purchaser, provider and regulator all under one roof. This situation is untenable. By comparison, the US has a Joint Commission on Accreditation of Healthcare Organizations (JCAHO) that operates independently of any hospital board, while the UK has the Commission for Healthcare Audit and Inspection (CHAI), which is separate from the National Health Service (NHS). The same organisational independence and structural integrity is needed for healthcare regulation in Hong Kong.

To be truly effective in detecting and controlling the next infectious disease outbreak, whether it is SARS, dengue fever or avian flu (H5N1), cross-border collaboration is essential. As previous sections have shown, the Pearl River Delta is a crucible for the emergence of new viruses. Hong Kong should push for structural integration with the relevant public health and disease control and prevention agencies in Guangdong, at both the municipal and provincial levels. More important, however, is genuine operational collaboration, including the unconditional and routine sharing of micro-level surveillance datasets and information (not just aggregate numbers), harmonisation of data standards and collaborative training and posting of personnel. All these changes will be possible only with regular dialogue, mutual understanding and trust and greater political openness. At a lower level, the same willingness to cooperate and work together is needed within separate jurisdictions of the country. At least one major international newspaper has attributed the research and outbreak control failings in China's handling of the SARS epidemic to entrenched bureaucratic inflexibility, intramural bickering and government-directed agendas in Beijing.[24] Similar anecdotes abound in other quarters. The tasks and approach needed to avoid this situation have now been clearly set out for our politicians and public servants.

Hong Kong urgently requires the resources needed to develop new programmes in order to rebuild and maintain an efficient public health function. These resources should be directed at training public health professionals, funding additional posts in both the service and academic sectors, strengthening existing organisations and establishing new ones such as a Centre for Disease Control and Prevention and facilitating the further integration of public health with clinical medicine on the one hand and society-at-large on the other.[25, 26]

Finally, it is important to remember that the *post-mortem* on the handling of the SARS outbreak should not focus on individuals. Rather, contemporary systems theory informs us that human beings and organisations, in all lines of work, behave according to the macro system's inherent incentives and disincentives.[27] 1While doctors, allied professionals and healthcare organisations should have the highest level of integrity and concern for their patients, they should not be expected to function at a superhuman level. Instead, the system should be structured and resourced so that it is easy for people to do the right thing and hard to do the wrong thing. Cars are designed so drivers cannot start them while in reverse because this prevents accidents. Work schedules for pilots are designed so they do not fly too many consecutive hours without rest because the level of alertness wanes and performance is compromised by over-work. It is high time to re-examine Hong Kong's macro health system infrastructure, its organisation and how it should be funded so that we can be well prepared for the next epidemic.

CHAPTER 6

The Numbers Trail:
What the Data Tells Us

Alexis Lau

S ARS affected the daily routine of almost every person in Hong Kong — from schoolchildren kept at home for weeks to cleaners forced to work longer hours. The virus infected 1,755 people, with 299 dying of the disease.

Many important lessons must be learned from this experience. Infectious disease experts predict that SARS will most likely recur. Even if it does not, many more unknown viruses will surely emerge.[1] To help the community fight any similar public health threat, information and data should be as accurate as possible and released in a timely fashion. The more data there is, the more accurate the conclusions and predictions. And statistical studies should be done even as an outbreak is playing out — not just after it has ended.

This chapter explores what can be learned from the very little publicly available information on the SARS outbreak in Hong Kong and elsewhere. Analysing this data should help in understanding how SARS spread — and how another outbreak might develop.

Access to information

Citizens typically trust the government to tell them the truth and to refrain from generating panic. But often, authorities choose to be economical with the facts, often claiming that secrecy is necessary to ensure stability. They frequently assume — incorrectly — that the public is unable to handle certain situations reasonably and peacefully.

In withholding facts, leaders belittle the ability of citizens to act rationally, undermining public trust in the government. It is therefore important for a government to take the time and make the effort to educate people and provide them with clear explanations of important data and information. Once officials have hidden facts even once, they may never again enjoy the full confidence of citizens.

During the SARS outbreak, data was withheld not only from the public but in some cases also from the doctors who were expected to treat patients, from certain branches of the Government, from other health authorities dealing with the virus and from the media, which often could only report rumours or describe how people were reacting. In China's Guangdong Province, where SARS is believed to have originated, the earliest case can be traced back to 16 November 2002.[2] By January 2003, there were many cases of atypical pneumonia. While hospitals were warned to watch out for symptoms and treat patients with extra care,[3] no official announcement of the outbreak was made until 10 February.

In Guangdong, rumours began to spread. Shops quickly raised the price of vinegar, which many people boiled in the belief that this would ward off germs. The Guangdong authorities informed the Central Government in Beijing of the situation on 8 February and finally gave a press conference on the outbreak two days later. China's Ministry of Health then advised the World Health Organisation (WHO) on 11 February that there had been five deaths and 305 infections in the province but that the situation was under control.

Because of the tradition of secrecy in China as well as the long delay in acknowledging the SARS outbreak in Guangdong, people did not believe the first official reports and claims. This scepticism proved detrimental not only to Guangdong but also to Hong Kong in the months that followed. In both places, members of the public worried about whether SARS could be contained, as they had insufficient information. In Hong Kong, fear and panic began to grow.

Even worse, the control measures implemented in Guangdong were not taken seriously by the health authorities in Hong Kong during the early stages of the outbreak there. Had information been made available earlier and on a regular basis, trust would have grown among all parties — government, media, the public and the international community. The level of fear and panic would have been greatly reduced, both locally and abroad.

In Hong Kong, the lack of information about the outbreak in Guangdong meant that hospitals did not go on high alert. When the "index" patients checked in, no precautions were taken, except in the case of Liu Jianlun, the Guangzhou doctor who asked staff at Hong Kong's Kwong Wah Hospital to take special precautions when treating him. At the Prince of Wales Hospital (PWH), SARS spread rapidly through the wards, infecting many people.

Once news of SARS broke in Hong Kong, some people chose to leave. Now that the truth was out, the Government mobilised its resources to check the spread of the disease through improved control measures, such as effective contact tracing, isolation and quarantine measures, the closing of schools and community clean-up campaigns. The public also took action, with many taking special precautions and adopting better hygiene.

Tragically, it was not possible to prevent infections or deaths. But in such a densely populated city where public transport is crowded and widely used, SARS could easily have done more damage.

Even after the danger receded and Hong Kong returned to normal, the release of data to the public remained an issue. Some important information has still not been released. As of August 2003, for example, the public had not been told how many people had contracted SARS through community contacts and how many from hospital visits. It is also not clear whether the high death rate in Hong Kong was due to the large number of elderly patients, the stress on the healthcare system or the treatment that patients received. Many questions need to be answered.

The death rate

During the outbreak in Hong Kong, many were asking one question: "If I get SARS, what are my chances of dying?" This was not easy to answer. Age, health, when the disease is diagnosed and other factors affect whether a patient survives. In many ways, the SARS death rate is different for every person.

The medical community often uses two death-rate measures:

- Case Fatality Rate (CFR) = total deaths/total cases
- Outcome Rate (OR) = total deaths/(total deaths + total recovered cases)

Once the outbreak of any infectious disease is over, all the cases can be sorted into two categories — those that have recovered and those that have died. Both the CFR and OR should be the same. But during an outbreak, the CFR can be deceivingly low as hospitals are filled with patients struggling to stay alive, while the OR can be misleadingly high if patients take a long time to recover.

Estimating the death rate for SARS early in the outbreak was difficult since there were only a few cases identified and little was known about how the disease was transmitted. Hong Kong authorities adopted the CFR to calculate the death rate, an approach that was also used by the WHO. Initially, the death rate was thought to be between 4 and 5 percent.[4] As time passed, the number of cases mounted and deaths increased. The death rate crept up to 10 percent and then 15 percent, presenting a much gloomier picture.[5]

The rise led many in the public to believe that the Government had deliberately sought to downplay the seriousness of SARS.[6] The decision to use the CFR to report the death rate gave the impression that the truth had been hidden early on in the outbreak and that the authorities were not as transparent as they claimed. Some suggested that the OR should be used instead. To alleviate the growing mistrust of official reports, the Government issued a press release to explain the difference between the two death rates.[7] The Government emphasised that the CFR was a better measure since it was also used by the WHO. It also noted that the OR would be meaningful only *after* the outbreak was over.

Figure 1 plots the two death rates in Hong Kong over the course of the SARS outbreak using the data released by the Government. The OR, though initially high, stabilised at 16 to 17 percent within the first two weeks, presenting a realistic picture within a short time. In contrast, the CFR reached 10 percent at the beginning of May, converging with the OR only in June.

Which death rate is more meaningful? The OR is always higher because it includes only patients with a known outcome. Those under treatment in hospital are not included. While the CFR seems more credible because it is used by the WHO, the OR stabilises much more quickly. As Figure 1 shows, the OR more efficiently predicted the eventual death rate in Hong Kong. In fact, by using the CFR, the Government inadvertently misled the public about the actual SARS death rate throughout much of the outbreak.

Several factors affect the outcome of SARS cases, including a patient's

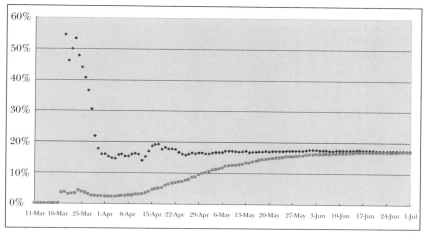

Figure 1 Case fatality rate (grey dotted line) and outcome rate (black dotted line) of SARS in Hong Kong from Government data

age, history of chronic illness and treatment received. Only with complete information on these measures can anybody make an accurate risk assessment.

Table 1 is taken from a Hong Kong Government press release indicating the number of SARS cases and deaths as of mid-April 2003 according to age. The release noted that 68 percent of patients had other illnesses.[8] It was clear early on that the elderly and chronically ill were at high risk and needed to take special precautions to avoid infection. By the end of May, nearly 80 percent of the patients who had died were over 65 years old or suffering from chronic disease.

How the healthcare system coped

During the outbreak, another important issue in which the public was interested was whether Hong Kong's healthcare system could cope as the number of SARS cases rose. From the initial growth rates of the disease, it appeared that, had transmission been more effective, hospitals would have come under much greater stress and may well not have been able to manage.

Early on, it was not clear how the disease would progress. One German newspaper went so far as to predict that everyone in Hong Kong

Table 1 SARS cases and deaths in Hong Kong as of 15 April 2003

Press Release Following is a list of Clinical SARS Cases and Details as at 15 April 2003:			
Age (years)	Number of cases	Numbers of deaths	Age-specific death rate
0–14	72	0	0.0 percent
15–34	467	2	0.4 percent
35–54	476	17	3.6 percent
55–64	92	6	6.5 percent
65–74	90	17	18.9 percent
Over 75	56	16	28.6 percent
Overall	1253	58	4.6 percent

Overall 68 percent of all deaths have co-existing illneses.

End/Saturday, 19 April 2003

would be infected![9] In fact, SARS spread relatively slowly. Dire predictions based on initial data were inaccurate because nobody knew how effective transmission of the virus would be. There were also other factors that affected the spread of the disease, including the community's response and the build-up of immunity among the population.

Apparently, Hong Kong authorities did not bother to analyse the trends of the outbreak in Guangdong. This would have been useful since Hong Kong closely followed the pattern exhibited by the spread of SARS in Guangzhou. Had the Government spent time to understand how the disease waxed and waned across the border, it would have had a better idea of which control and prevention measures would be most effective. Unfortunately, few people took the reports from across the border seriously, because of a lack of trust either in China's capacity in disease control and prevention or in the accuracy of data.

To be better prepared for an infectious disease outbreak, Hong Kong must assess the stress SARS put on its healthcare system. Figure 2a shows the daily change in the number of SARS cases (grey line) and the number of patients in hospital (black line). As indicators of stress on the medical system, the numbers of patients in hospital and in intensive care are the most significant.

At the height of the outbreak, about 1,000 patients were in the hospital. The vertical line on the left marks the date, 29 March, when

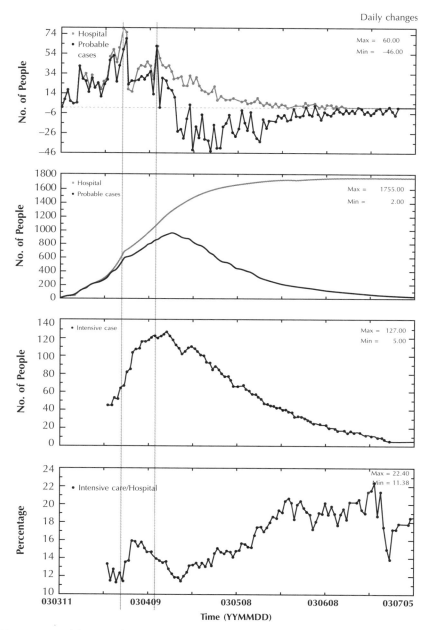

Daily changes

Note: Vertical lines mark the introduction of the first set of isolation measures on 29 March 2003 and the implementation of compulsory home confinement on 11 April 2003.

Figure 2   (a) Daily change in number of SARS cases and number of patients in hospital, (b) Number of SARS cases and number of patients in hospital, (c) Number of SARS patients in ICU, (d) Percentage of SARS patients in ICU

the first set of partial isolation measures were put in place. The vertical line on the right indicates the implementation on 11 April of the second, more stringent set of measures. Compulsory home confinement was ordered for anyone in close contact with SARS patients.

In Figure 2b, we can see that, from 11 March to 17 April, the number of people in hospital rose. From 17 April, six days after the tougher measures were implemented, there was a steady drop. Obviously, the additional isolation measures were critical to bringing down the infection rate. The first effort was less successful, probably because people were still asked to go to local clinics for daily health checks. Total home confinement, together with health monitoring and police visits, underscored the seriousness of the situation and did much more to slow the spread of the virus.

The true stress on the health system during the height of the SARS outbreak may be observed in Figures 2c and 2d, which show the number and percentage of SARS patients in intensive care. At first glance, the curve in Figure 2c looks similar to the one in Figure 2b that plots the number of people in hospital. In fact, the intensive care unit (ICU) patient curve peaks earlier and is also flatter near its peak. The ICU patient data became available in late March, when about 12 percent of SARS patients were in intensive care (Figure 2d). This proportion rose to about 14 percent on 2 April.

This figure would have remained stable if the virus had not weakened. But from 2 April to 20 April, the percentage of patients in intensive care dropped. This is statistically significant.[10] Assuming that the virus had not weakened — no change in virulence was indicated by the death rates — the conclusion must be that doctors were reluctant to place patients in intensive care during this period. This suggests that intensive care resources were stretched to full capacity, or at least close enough to the maximum, to cause grave concern.

If the rising tide of SARS infections had not been controlled by the mandatory isolation measures, Hong Kong's ICU system might have broken down. The resulting inability to house all the patients requiring intensive care or the inability to care properly for those already admitted could have caused a collapse in public confidence. The results could have been disastrous. There could have been a mass exodus of residents trying to leave the city. Apartment buildings or housing estates might have stopped strangers from entering, fearing they might be carrying the disease. Just how close did Hong Kong come to that situation?

The effectiveness of control measures

Despite the limited information released so far, much can still be learned about the virus and the effectiveness of the control measures by fitting the data against epidemiological models with varying degrees of complexity.[11,12] Figure 3a shows the number of new confirmed SARS cases as a function of time. Figure 3b plots the same data, but with the y-axis on a logarithmic scale. The changes in slope (noted by the straight lines) highlight the three phases of the Hong Kong outbreak: the initial stage from early March until 29 March, during which the number of cases rose sharply; the intermediate stage from 29 March to 11 April, during which health authorities battled to control the virus; and finally the control and decay stage from 11 April onwards.

During the first phase, the initial infections caught Hong Kong by surprise. Everyone involved, even experts in contagious disease, needed time to identify and learn how to deal with the new menace. The virus spread relatively freely, resulting in a rapid rise in cases. The rate of increase depended on the infection rate, the population density in affected areas and other factors.

During the intermediate stage, heightened public awareness, improved hygiene practices and the implementation of control measures started to slow the spread. Due to a lack of knowledge, not all control measures were effective. Nevertheless, the rate of increase of new cases reduced, an indication that initial efforts to counter the virus had some success.

Finally, effective control measures including home confinement for people who had been in contact with SARS patients were implemented, resulting in the control and decay of the outbreak. Figure 3a and 3b show that the number of new cases in Hong Kong decreased exponentially after 11 April (in Figure 3b the straight line on the right sloping down, equations in Figure 3a). A characteristic decay time scale can be fit from the slope of this line in Figure 3b. This decay time scale is a measure of the overall effectiveness of the control measures: the more effective the control measures, the faster the drop of new SARS cases, the steeper the line, and the shorter the decay time scale. For Hong Kong, the decay time scale was about 13 days. This measure will prove useful when we compare the effectiveness of the control measures of other countries fighting SARS.

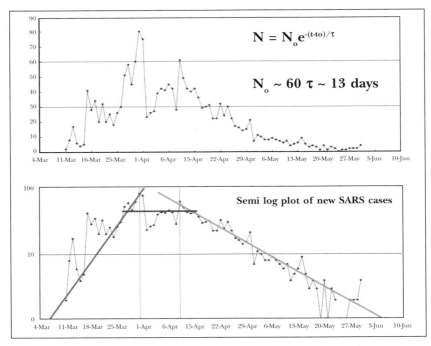

Figure 3   (a) Number of new SARS cases in Hong Kong over time, (b) New SARS cases on a logarithmic scale

Reading between the numbers

We can also learn from the data released by the health authorities in other places affected by SARS. Table 2 lists the total number of cases, deaths and recoveries reported to the WHO (as of 11 July 2003) by all countries and territories that had more than 50 infections.[13] The OR and CFR for each place are included. As expected, the two rates are practically the same, given that the outbreaks had waned in most areas by the time of data collection. The exceptions are Taiwan and Canada, both of which still had a considerable number of patients in hospital. Yet even in these two places, the OR and CFR were within 2 percent.

The lowest fatality rate — 7 percent — was in mainland China, with Vietnam close behind at 8 percent, substantially lower than in Canada, Hong Kong, Singapore and Taiwan. The reason for this notable difference is unclear. While some may believe that different reporting criteria in China could be partly responsible for the low death rate there,

Table 2   SARS cases and deaths, recoveries, case fatality and outcome rates for areas reporting more than 50 cases to the WHO as of 11 July 2003

Country	Cases	Deaths	Recovered	Case Fatality Rate	Outcome Rate
Total	**8437**	**813**	**7452**	**9.6%**	**9.8%**
China, Mainland	5327	348	4941	6.5%	6.6%
China, HKSAR	1755	298	1433	17.0%	17.2%
China, Taiwan	671	84	507	12.5%	14.2%
Canada	250	38	194	15.2%	16.4%
Singapore	206	32	172	15.5%	15.7%
United States	75	0	67	0.0%	0.0%
Viet Nam	63	5	58	7.9%	7.9%

the similar result in Vietnam suggests that a single-digit fatality rate is possible. Other factors such as treatment methods may have been responsible.

Some would argue that mainland China's data cannot be trusted either because its Government initially denied the seriousness of the outbreak or because obtaining accurate data from the provinces and cities was difficult, even for health authorities. However, in Vietnam, the WHO enjoyed the full cooperation of the Government from the start.

There are two other important issues to explore: why Hong Kong had the highest fatality rate at 17 percent, and what can be learned by comparing specific groups of SARS patients, in particular whether the fatality rates among the elderly and chronically ill were equally high across geographical areas. If the number of elderly patients was significantly higher in one place, that would raise questions.

Figure 4 plots the number of new cases over time as reported by the WHO for Canada, Singapore, mainland China and Taiwan. Similar to Figure 3b, all show an exponential decay. However, the time scale for each place is slightly different, indicating varying levels of success in controlling the disease.

In particular, the mainland had the shortest decay period, only lasting eight to nine days. Data available from China's Ministry of Health website[14] showed even shorter times for some cities and provinces.

Canada, Singapore and Taiwan, however, all had decay periods of 12 to 13 days, similar to Hong Kong. This suggests that China implemented more effective control measures, such as isolation and education. A study of the steps taken by mainland authorities would obviously be useful.

Finally, Figure 4 indicates that both Canada and Singapore experienced two distinct SARS outbreaks. This suggests that despite appropriate control measures, vigilance in tracking and containing the virus must be sustained. It takes only one unidentified case slipping through the cracks to begin another round of illness, fatalities and fear.

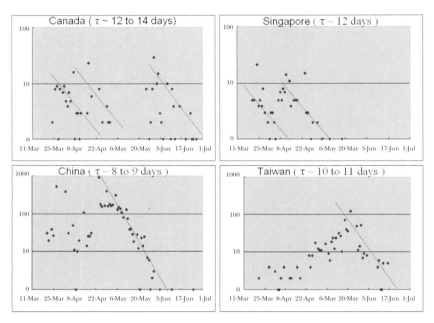

Figure 4 New SARS cases and decay time scales for Canada, Singapore, China and Taiwan

In need of data — and cooperation

To answer the many unanswered questions about the SARS outbreak, health authorities must release additional data to the public. Of the total SARS cases in Hong Kong, 22 percent were healthcare workers. While we assume that the majority of these infections took place within hospitals, this needs to be confirmed. Similarly, we still do not know how many of the other cases were hospital patients and visitors. This is likely to be a large number and would suggest that cross-infection within the healthcare system was the primary mode of infection. A thorough investigation of the infection dynamics and pathways and how to block them should be undertaken.

The importance of studying cross-contamination in Hong Kong's healthcare facilities should not be limited to SARS. Data from 1998 to 2001 indicates that in Hong Kong, typical pneumonia has a fatality rate of 13 to 14 percent and is responsible for about 3,000 deaths in each year.[15] Those affected are usually the elderly or chronically ill. Many are hospitalised for other conditions, but develop pneumonia once they are in a healthcare facility.[16]

It is possible that the transmission pathways for typical pneumonia are similar to those of SARS. While the meticulous collection of data and tracking done for SARS allows for a detailed investigation, this is not the case for other diseases. The widespread nature of typical pneumonia makes it much more difficult to track. But SARS can be a very good marker for identifying infection pathways. Should these be identified and minimised, the spread of many other diseases could be slowed as a result.

It is worth noting that the SARS infection rate in Hong Kong has not been determined. Questions surround the spread of the virus in the Amoy Gardens housing estate, a notorious SARS "hotspot," and how control measures implemented there had varying degrees of success (see Chapter 7). The infection rates within households, within linked sewage systems and through casual contact had not been released as of August 2003. The risks and modes of infection through the community deserve attention if we are to know how to minimise the spread of SARS should it recur.

Other questions surround the differing fatality rates for different geographical areas. Only a detailed breakdown of the ages, histories and treatments of the patients involved will reveal why Hong Kong had the highest death rate, while China had the lowest. The same-segmented data should be examined for different hospitals and different treatment methods in preparation for another outbreak. Compiling and analysing statistics take time, but because of the seasonal ebb and flow of viruses similar to SARS, it is important to do this work as quickly as possible.

Finally, the question of animal transmission of the virus has not been satisfactorily addressed.[17] If people originally contracted the SARS virus through animal contact, could future outbreaks begin the same way? Has the virus gone to ground temporarily in the animal population, poised to emerge again? Without doubt, further study of the SARS virus is necessary.

The experience gained from the outbreak, both locally and internationally, suggests that viruses can be controlled with strict vigilance. Complacency and denial lead to disaster. The lack of information can cause confusion and panic, while its timely release will help to arouse public awareness and enable the community to battle infectious diseases more effectively.

As Hong Kong aspires to be a modern, knowledge-based society, the open flow of information is critical. The lessons from SARS must not be forgotten. Decisions should be guided primarily by facts instead of by unsubstantiated beliefs or what the authorities think is best. Providing accurate news and data means that the community understands events better. This is important in the protection of public health.

Scientists have learned much even from the limited amount of information on SARS released to the public. Should more data be made available, our understanding of the disease will only increase. SARS offered an opportunity for collaboration among local and international health experts. The need to fight the outbreak led to enhanced cooperation among research laboratories around the world. We should seek to widen such interaction beyond medicine and microbiology to include other fields such as environmental science, engineering and statistics. These disciplines can all contribute to the discovery of many more aspects of an infectious disease such as SARS.

CHAPTER 7

The Mystery of Amoy Gardens[1]

Stephen Ng

Chronology of the Outbreak

When residents of Amoy Gardens woke up on 21 March 2003, they had no idea that their nightmare had just begun. In the next four weeks, Amoy Gardens would attain unprecedented notoriety, becoming Hong Kong's best known housing complex and a symbol of the mystery and terror associated with the new disease: Severe Acute Respiratory Syndrome, or SARS for short. By 25 April 2003, 329 residents had developed SARS, with 42 subsequent deaths.[2]

Amoy Gardens is a lower middle-class housing complex in Kowloon Bay, East Kowloon, built over 20 years ago. It consists of 19 33-storey high-rise blocks, with eight units on each floor. The buildings are located on top of a three-storey shopping mall, so the fourth floor is actually the ground floor. Hygiene at Amoy Gardens has always been substandard. Like the rest of East Kowloon, the area is overcrowded, with a high density in terms of human population. There were over 5,000 families and approximately 17,000 people living in Amoy Gardens at the beginning of the outbreak.

On 14 March, a 33-year-old patient with chronic kidney disease receiving hemodialysis treatment at the Prince of Wales Hospital (PWH) visited his brother at unit 7, on the 16/F of Block E of Amoy Gardens after being discharged from Ward 8A. The patient lived in Shenzhen and came to Hong Kong regularly for medical treatment, usually staying with his brother at Amoy Gardens. On 14 March, he developed fever, respiratory symptoms and diarrhoea and on 15 March was readmitted to PWH where he was treated as an influenza case. The patient then improved and was discharged on 19 March, when he visited his brother again. During a follow-up visit to PWH on 22 March, he was diagnosed as having SARS and readmitted to the hospital. He subsequently recovered and was discharged. This patient remains the most likely source of the SARS outbreak at Amoy Gardens.[3]

Three residents of Block E started feeling ill on 21 March. Strangely, these residents lived in the unit 8 apartments on the 29/F and 32/F, quite a distance from the unit 7, 16/F apartment visited by the index patient. On 22 March another four Block E residents developed SARS symptoms, three from unit 8 and one from unit 5. Residents of unit 7 did not become ill until 23 March, when four residents from unit 7 (including a relative of the index patient) and two from unit 8 developed symptoms. All of the cases in the first three days lived on or above the 16/F. On 24 and 25 March, a massive outbreak took place in Block E, with 36 and 20 residents falling ill on those two days, respectively.

Beginning 22 March, Amoy Gardens residents outside Block E also started to develop SARS symptoms. The first cases occurred in Blocks D and F, the two blocks located closest to Block E. On 23 March, residents in Block B were also affected. The disease eventually spread to 15 of the 19 blocks in the estate. In general, blocks located further from Block E had fewer cases and these also occurred later.

Due to the lag time in confirming SARS cases, the first media report on the Amoy Gardens outbreak did not appear until 26 March, when the Department of Health announced seven confirmed and seven suspected SARS cases at Amoy Gardens.[4] This caused widespread panic, with many residents packing up and moving out immediately. What they did not know was that the actual number of residents with SARS symptoms at that point was 144.

The number of SARS cases at Amoy Gardens continued to increase, and by 31 March the number of confirmed and suspected cases had risen to 213, 107 of which were in Block E. At 6 a.m. on 31 March the Department of Health issued an isolation order for Block E, preventing residents from leaving their homes for ten days. Food and other necessities would be brought to them. The order was issued very suddenly — staff from various Government departments showed up at 6 a.m. on

31 March to prevent people from leaving or entering Block E. Some residents who had left home for breakfast had to argue with Government staff in order to re-enter their homes. Similarly, people who returned home after a night shift at work found themselves barred from their own apartments. However, the isolation order was too little too late, since by that time more than half of the residents had already moved out of Block E. In addition, it did not cover the other blocks in the complex.

The number of SARS patients continued to grow at Amoy Gardens and by 1 April there were 267 confirmed cases. At 10 p.m. on 1 April, the Government decided to move all residents from Block E into isolation camps. A total of 250 residents from 110 apartments (out of a total of 264) were moved and put in isolation. The authorities suspected that the outbreak had been caused by contamination of the sewage system in Block E and ordered a massive clean up.

The mystery

The outbreak of SARS at Amoy Gardens was the primary motivation for the WHO travel advisory issued on 2 April. Prior to this outbreak, SARS was believed to be a disease transmitted by respiratory droplets through close person-to-person contact. Respiratory droplets are relatively large-sized particles (100 microns or above; one micron is one-thousandth of a millimetre) and thus cannot travel long distances through the air. The usual range of infectiousness is approximately three feet from the source. This mode of transmission cannot however account for the rapidity of spread and wide distribution of disease at Amoy Gardens.

An alternative possibility is airborne transmission. In airborne transmission infective agents are attached to smaller particles (considerably less than 100 microns) that can travel greater distances through the air. Transmission of airborne diseases can be far and wide and is not limited to high-risk places such as hospitals or households where there are infected patients. Airborne diseases can be contracted under many different circumstances. The suspicion that airborne transmission was responsible for the Amoy Gardens outbreak was what prompted the WHO to issue the travel advisory. However, with the exception of the cases at Amoy Gardens, SARS did not show any of the features of an airborne disease and most experts agreed that airborne transmission was unlikely.

Another known mode of transmission for SARS is contact with contaminated objects (known as fomites), such as doorknobs or elevator buttons. However, the speed, intensity and wide geographic distribution of the spread of SARS at Amoy Gardens cannot be explained by this mode of transmission either. Thus the mode of transmission at this housing estate remained a mystery. The WHO warned that one of the conditions for lifting the travel advisory was a satisfactory explanation of this outbreak.

Epidemiology of the outbreak

The initial outbreak, i.e. between 21 March and 1 April, was a classic "common source" epidemic. In this type of epidemic all cases are exposed to a common origin of infection within a relatively short period of time and patients come down with the disease in rapid succession. A typical example is food poisoning. Due to variability of the incubation period and different times of exposure of different individuals, not everybody becomes sick simultaneously and cases can spread out over several days or weeks. The source of infection is usually transient, such as contaminated food, and exposure time is usually limited to a few hours. In such transient common source epidemics the outbreak generally lasts as long as the incubation period for the disease, and there is one single peak at the height of the epidemic.

Common source exposure can, however, be more prolonged, as in the nineteenth century cholera epidemic in London, where residents were exposed to cholera-contaminated well water over a period of weeks; or in the first outbreak of Legionnaire's Disease in 1976, where many people were exposed to aerosols from contaminated air-conditioning water towers over several days. The longer the incubation period and the more prolonged the exposure, the harder it is to detect the characteristic features of the common source outbreak.

The SARS outbreak at Amoy Gardens fits the common source features very well: cases first appeared on 21 March, reached a peak on 24 and 25 March and declined steadily until 25 April. The majority of these cases, especially the 267 cases that occurred between 21 March and 2 April, must have been related to a common source exposure since all of the patients became sick within the range of the incubation period (2–10 days) and were very unlikely to have infected one another. The source of infection for cases after 2 April is less definite. These could have been secondary cases caused by person-to-person contact with primary cases rather than with the original common source.

Most epidemics of infectious disease are common source outbreaks and as such, usually pose little problem for the investigating epidemiologist. All that is required is identification of the commonality among patients, such as attendance at a church picnic and the food item most commonly consumed by the cases, and comparison of this information with the behaviour of those who did not fall ill (the controls). The larger the outbreak, the easier the investigation since the commonality tends to be quite obvious. In the Amoy Gardens outbreak, this was not the case. Despite identification of a possible common source, namely, the kidney patient, it was hard to explain how one person could have infected over 200 others in so many households within a matter of days. Common source infection usually occurs in a confined space where many people are gathered together, such as a restaurant or a hotel. There are however no communal facilities in Amoy Gardens, such as a clubhouse or swimming pool, where large numbers of residents congregate. Moreover, the index patient only spent two nights at Amoy Gardens. How could this short period of exposure lead to an outbreak involving more than 200 residents in 15 different blocks and covering an area of thousands of square metres?

Environmental findings

The sewage draining system at Amoy Gardens was repaired about seven years ago when the old iron pipes were replaced with PVC pipes. Each block has eight sewage pipes that connect the same unit on all floors. Each pipe is connected to the water closet, the basin, the bathtub and the bathroom floor drain. Each of these sanitary fixtures is fitted with a U-shaped trap (U-trap) to prevent backflow of effluent material. There are no connections between the sewage pipes of different units until they join the master sewage pipe underground.

The SARS coronavirus was isolated in samples taken from the sewage system of Block E, prompting the evacuation of residents.[5] However, as there were already many symptomatic patients by the time the samples were taken, the presence of virus in the sewage system may reflect the result rather than the cause of the outbreak. There was a cracked sewage vent pipe on 4/F of Block E that was repaired on 21 March. During the repair the toilet flushing system was shut down for 16 hours. However, by that time the epidemic had already started and the connection between the shut down and the outbreak is at most tenuous. Tests done by the Government revealed no leakage in any of the sewage pipes in Block E or in the other blocks.

The design and construction of the buildings at Amoy Gardens are fairly standard and typical of other housing estates in Hong Kong. There is a narrow light well about 1.5 metres in width between the adjoining units of each block of Amoy Gardens (Figure 1). For example, units 7 and 8 share a common light well into which the bathrooms of each unit open. The sewage pipes also run through this space. Clotheslines have been installed outside the bathroom windows and occupy almost the whole width of the light well.

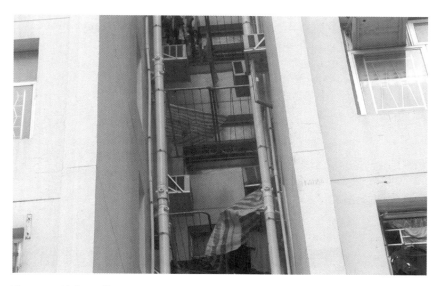

Figure 1 Light well at Amoy Gardens, Block E

Amoy Gardens is notorious for its poor hygiene and pest infestations. Because there are many restaurants in the shopping mall, rat infestation is a serious problem. It was estimated in the beginning of April that there were around 400 rats in the area. Cockroaches are also common, as is the case in other parts of Hong Kong.

Subsequent Government investigations revealed extensive SARS virus footprints in Block E.[6] Viral remnants were found on kitchen floors and sinks, and around the water closets. Viral presence was also found on cockroach legs and in rat droppings. Throat/rectal swabs from domestic cats and dogs as well as rats tested positive for the SARS virus. One cat also showed SARS antibodies. [7]

Prevailing hypotheses

Several hypotheses were advanced by the health authorities in Hong Kong to explain the massive outbreak at Amoy Gardens.[8]

Sewage contamination

The most popular hypothesis is sewage contamination. The index patient supposedly passed a large quantity of virus in his excreta during his visit to Amoy Gardens on 19 March that contaminated the sewage system in Block E. Virus-laden droplets were then sucked back into individual bathrooms via floor drains due to the negative pressure generated by bathroom fans, which is believed to have been too powerful for the size of the bathroom. Somehow the virus also found its way to other blocks, possibly through leakage of the sewage system and other unknown factors. This hypothesis can at best explain a few cases in units located below the index patient's household but cannot explain the wider epidemic for the following reasons:

1. **Fluid and air movements:** It would have been difficult for contaminated droplets to reach the sewage system at the top floors of the building where most of the infections occurred. One mechanism proposed was the upward flow of air and droplets due to negative pressure in the centre of the sewage pipe when sewage spiralled down the sidewall. But this upward negative pressure is rather weak and can only move droplets up a few floors, certainly not enough to travel all the way up to 36/F from the patient's apartment. Also, there are separate sewage drainage pipes for each of the units in the block, and there are no common connections until the pipes reach the bottom. There are therefore no routes or mechanisms of travel for contaminated sewage from a single point efflux to infect residents of a whole block.

2. **Dosage:** While we do not know the exact dosage of the virus that is needed for an infection, it is reasonable to believe that transfer from contaminated sewage to humans over a long distance is not that efficient and that wastage would occur. Therefore, it would take a huge amount of initial virus to contaminate enough sewage to infect over 200 people. Even if we had a system to deliver this contamination to each of these 150 households, it is doubtful that one single person could excrete enough of the virus to infect everyone in just two visits. One must also remember that infected excreta from this patient would be mixed with the excreta from other residents in unit 7 of Block E and this dilution would require an even larger initial amount of virus for effective transmission.

3. **Distribution:** Sewage contamination would affect lower floors more severely but that was not the case in Block E or in other blocks. In fact, there were very few cases below 9/F. The contaminated sewage theory also cannot explain the wide distribution of infection among different units of the 15 blocks unless a common water or food source or a place where everyone must pass by is contaminated. No such site of common exposure existed at Amoy Gardens.

4. **Timing:** Viral discharge from the index patient has a finite window of infectivity. Although some recent research has indicated that the SARS virus can live up to four days in diarrhoeal fluid,[9] this is under experimental condition and may not be applicable in real life, especially since flush water at Amoy Gardens is chlorinated sea water. It is highly unlikely that all residents of Block E, let alone all of the residents of the whole Amoy Gardens estate, visited the bathroom within a few hours after the index patient discharged the infectious material. The contaminated sewage would have lost its infectivity before everyone had a chance to be exposed.

The Plume theory

The distribution of many cases in units 7 and 8 of block E, especially on the upper floors, has led to the suggestion that the light well between the two units may have acted as a chimney and allowed virus-laden droplets to rise up quickly and contaminate the bathrooms of both units on the upper floors. There were three possible sources of virus-laden droplets: (a) a cracked sewer vent pipe on 4/F, (b) emission by the index patient while using his bathroom, either when taking a shower or passing excrement, and (c) influx of contaminated droplets from the sewage system into bathrooms due to the fan and subsequent release into the light well via bathroom windows.

The updraft of air in the light well is a real phenomenon and has been demonstrated by both the Health Department and the Department of Mechanical Engineering of the University of Hong Kong. This explanation, known as the Plume Theory, is physically possible but faces the following difficulties:

1. The theory can at most explain those cases in units 7 and 8 of Block E above the level of the index patient or the cracked sewer vent pipe on 4/F. It cannot readily explain cases in units 1 to 6 of Block E or cases in other blocks.

2. As the plume rises from its source, there is significant dilution so that the effective dose reaching households will be small. There were altogether 132 cases in Block E, the majority of them occurring between 21 March and 1 April. Neither the cracked vent pipe nor the index patient could have readily generated the astronomical amount of virus needed to infect so many people after rising up more than two dozen floors in the air.

Passive distribution of virus by pests

Passive distribution of the virus by insects or rodents, such as cockroaches or rats, is another hypothesis that has been advanced to explain the infection of residents in other blocks. According to this hypothesis, rats, cockroaches or both picked up the virus when they went into the contaminated sewer and transmitted it to various households throughout Amoy Gardens. Cockroaches and rats can and do carry diseases and they are certainly mobile enough to reach all of these households. There are however two problems with this theory: dose and timing.

1. **Dose:** As in the sewage hypothesis, it is difficult to imagine the index patient passing out a large enough quantity of contaminated excreta in his brief visits to Amoy Gardens, that even after dilution with excreta from other residents in the block, the concentration and dose remained high enough to allow contaminated pests to distribute the virus to over 200 people. A single cockroach or rat can only carry a finite amount of contaminated sewerage. It would have taken a huge army of pests to infect all of these households.

2. **Timing:** We do not know how long the SARS virus survives in moist

environments such as sewers, but the maximum lifespan on dry surfaces so far ascertained is 48 hours.[10] There was thus very little time for distribution to occur once the index patient had excreted the virus. The virus would have needed to be picked up quickly by the carriers and delivered to the 150 households, where it would have then had the opportunity to infect the unsuspecting residents. Rats are territorial animals that usually travel at night and only over short distances. Cockroaches travel a longer distance but are much slower than rats. It would have been quite impossible for either cockroaches or rats to reach all of the affected households within the time allowed by the lifespan of the virus.

Person-to-person transmission

The model of person-to-person transmission (by droplets or contact) was also used to explain the outbreak, especially for cases outside Block E, since most other hypotheses have difficulty explaining the rapid spread of SARS to so many blocks. The epidemic curve of the initial outbreak does not support this mode of transmission as the major cause of the outbreak, either within or outside of Block E (see the section below on Anatomy of the Epidemic Curves). In this case there are other factors that make the spread from person-to-person very unlikely.

1. **Insufficient time:** The second group of infections in Block E as well as the infections in other blocks, such as D and F, occurred within a few of days of the initial cases and are therefore unlikely to have been caused by person-to-person transmission from the first cases, since the mean serial interval (the time from the onset of symptoms in an index case to the onset of symptoms in a subsequent case infected by the index patient) is 8.4 days.[11] Timing of exposure to the index case is also problematic. If the patient contaminated the environment during his 14 March visit, then cases should have occurred earlier than 21 March. If he contaminated the environment during his 19 March visit, then the peak of the outbreak should have occurred later than 24–25 March. It would also be difficult to explain how he could have infected residents outside of Block E in such a short time.

2. **Lack of a corresponding outbreak in the community:** There is no reason why Amoy Gardens residents, if they are transmitting diseases person-to-person, should limit infectivity to their home environment.

Many Amoy residents worked and shopped in the general community, and before the enforced quarantine of Block E, had total freedom of movement. They would have been just as likely, if not more so, to infect their co-workers, people on the street, etc. through person-to-person transmission. However, there was no major outbreak of SARS among Amoy residents' co-workers or in fact in other parts of Hong Kong during this period (Amoy residents accounted for the majority of cases at the time).

3. **Watchmen at Amoy not particularly affected:** Amoy Gardens apartments have watchmen stationed at the entrance lobby of each building. They are the individuals with the highest frequency of contact with residents and therefore the most vulnerable to person-to-person transmission. With the exception of an unconfirmed report of illness in one watchman, none of the other watchmen were infected.

Oral-faecal transmission

To supplement what cannot be explained by these four hypotheses, oral-faecal transmission through contamination of door knobs, elevator buttons, etc. has been proposed to account for some of the cases at Amoy Gardens. Oral-faecal is an efficient mode of disease transmission and can cause common source outbreaks if a food or water source is contaminated with a large quantity of infectious material. But otherwise oral-faecal transmission is similar to person-to-person transmission and does not give rise to single-mode epidemic curves.

Anatomy of the epidemic curves[12]

Careful study of the epidemic curves for the initial outbreak between 21 March and 1 April revealed two very interesting features. First, the outbreak lasted longer than predicted by the conventionally accepted incubation period for SARS. Second, the outbreak actually started over a period of several days (Figure 2). These characteristics cannot be explained by a static common source of infection (such as a single discharge of contaminated material from the index patient that has a finite window of infectiousness).

The initial outbreak started on 21 March (this was the date of onset

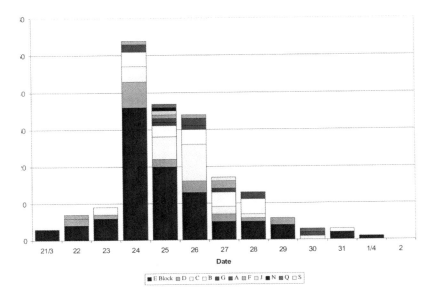

Figure 2 Epidemic Curve at Amoy Gardens as of 3 April 2003

of disease, not admission to hospital) with three cases from Block E. The number of cases continued to increase until 24 March, when it reached 54, before starting to decrease steadily until there was only one case on 1 April and no cases on 2 and 3 April. There was no secondary peak to suggest secondary infections during this time. The index patient visited his brother on 14 and 19 March, but the epidemic curve does not suggest two separate exposures so many days apart. There was only one peak and cases were closely packed within a 12-day period. The date of contamination must have been either 14 or 19 March. 14 March posed a problem for the static common source hypothesis (such as sewage contamination) since the first case did not appear until seven days later (21 March), already close to the upper limit of the incubation period for SARS (2 to 10 days). Subsequent cases (those later than 24 March) occurred outside of the known incubation period and therefore could not have been caused by exposure to the index patient. Therefore, 19 March seemed the more likely exposure date in this scenario. However, even if 19 March is used as the exposure date, the initial outbreak lasted too long to fit the conventionally accepted incubation period of 2 to 10 days, since the first and last cases were separated by 12 instead of 8 days.

When one looks at individual epidemic curves for the different blocks in Amoy Gardens, a very interesting picture emerges. The date of onset for the outbreak in different blocks was not the same, and progressed in an orderly way from Block E to the other neighbouring blocks (Figure 3). Cases first appeared in Block E on 21 March, followed by Blocks D and F (the two blocks closest to E) on 22 March, Block B on 23 March, Blocks C and G on 24 March and Blocks A, J, N and Q on 25 March. Block S did not have any cases until 27 March. Incubation periods, of course, vary among individuals. However, in those blocks where a large number of residents were infected (Blocks B, C, D and E all had total cases of 40 or more) one should still expect to see simultaneous onsets when the common exposure can last only hours. This is clearly not the case. Moreover, the staggering of onset dates in different blocks reflects their distance from Block E, the epicentre of the outbreak, with blocks closest to E having the earliest onset of disease. The intensity of infection in different blocks is in general also related to their distance from Block E, with blocks furthest from E, such as J, N, Q and S reporting only one or two cases.

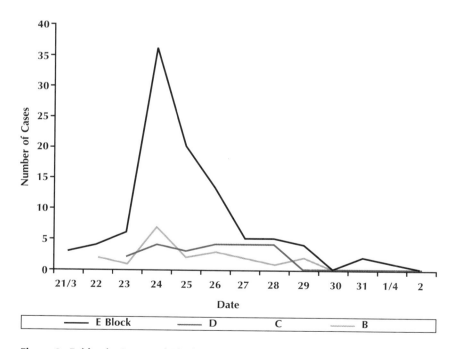

Figure 3 Epidemic Curves of Blocks B, C, D and E as of 3 April 2003

Dynamic common source

If the SARS outbreak at Amoy Gardens was indeed a common source epidemic, how can we explain the behaviour of the epidemic curves and the problems of dose, timing and geographic distribution?

Most of the problems can be resolved by replacing a static common source with a dynamic common source of infection. A dynamic common source is a living, continuous source of infectious material that can survive for days or weeks. It is not limited to a single spatial point but rather can move from place to place. A typical example of a dynamic common source infection is a disease that is zoonotic, i.e., a disease where an animal reservoir provides infectious material over space and time to a human population. Most zoonotic diseases, especially the more established ones, do not take on the form of an epidemic but rather exist as endemic diseases. A novel disease such as SARS, however, may take the form of an epidemic, as in the outbreak at Amoy Gardens. What is very likely to have happened at Amoy Gardens is a zoonotic spread, with roof rats as the most probable vector. Infected roof rats are highly mobile, can produce live virus for days and probably carry a form of the disease with a shorter incubation period, thus explaining the wide geographic distribution, the staggered dates of onset in different units and blocks as well as the explosive nature of the epidemic. This theory also removes the time constraint of the survival time of the virus since infections are the result of a continued supply of fresh virus.

The rat vector hypothesis

One or more roof rats from Block E went into the index patient's apartment on 14 March (this is the more likely date of contamination if rats were involved) looking for food and were infected by material (such as used tissue paper, left-over food or excreta) in the apartment. The incubation period in rats infected by naturally occurring coronaviruses is short (2–5 days) and the disease is benign.[13] Secretions from infected rats, such as urine, droppings or saliva, contain large amounts of virus and are highly contagious. Roof rats are aerial,[14] territorial and habitual animals that tend to follow the same pathways between their nest and food sources and make return visits time after time.[15] The first infected rats probably were used to visiting units 7 and 8 on the middle and upper floors of Block E, and subsequently made many returns to these units, which would explain the unusual concentration of cases on these floors. Roof rats seldom climb to the bottom of a building, thus lower floors were spared.

Two routes of transmission from rat to human are possible. Rats may have entered households, leaving infectious material in bathrooms and kitchens. Another possibility, quite unique to Amoy Gardens, is that clothes hanging on clothes lines outside of bathrooms and windows became contaminated. These clothes lines are installed next to the drainage pipes within easy reach of the rats. Besides infecting humans, one or more rats may have infected other rats in Block E, as well as rats in other blocks, starting an epidemic among rats that in turn caused the SARS epidemic among the human residents of Amoy Gardens. Since rats further away from Block E were less likely to be infected (rats are not very social), the human epidemic was earlier and more intense in blocks closest to E. The epidemic finally started to decline on 1 April when residents from Block E were evacuated, when rats recovered from their infection and when extensive rat trapping and baiting started at Amoy Gardens.

Compatibility with observations

The rat vector hypothesis provides a mechanism that would explain the sudden explosion of SARS in a large area. It also explains other features of the development of this epidemic, both in Amoy Gardens and in other parts of Hong Kong:

1. Amoy Gardens is known for its poor hygiene and rat infestation, especially since the recent clearing for redevelopment of a nearby hillock where many stray cats and rats used to live. The Pest Control Unit of Hong Kong estimated in the beginning of April 2003 that there were at least 400 rats in the housing estate. If rat infestation is common, an epidemic in rats could easily cause an epidemic in humans.

2. There is already a suspicion among virologists that the new SARS-coronavirus originated in animals and jumped species to infect humans. Recently, a virus virtually identical to the SARS-coronavirus was isolated from the droppings of six masked palm civets and one raccoon dog in Shenzhen, China.[16] Evidence of infection with the

virus was also found in the blood of a badger. If animals were the original hosts, the SARS virus would be able to pass easily from humans back to similar animals.

3. The presenting symptoms and clinical course of the Amoy Gardens cases differ substantially from that of other SARS patients.[17] Amoy patients present with diarrhoea much more often than other patients (60 percent of Amoy cases vs 10 percent of other cases). Amoy cases are also more seriously ill (20 percent required intensive care treatment vs 10 percent for other SARS patients) and respond less well to standard treatment with Ribavirin and steroids. The unusual symptoms and behaviour of the disease in Amoy cases suggests a different mode of transmission or a mutation of the causal virus.

4. Viral material was found around toilet bowls, kitchen sinks and on kitchen floors in households in Block E.[18] This could be due to contamination by infected residents. Contamination was however confined to kitchens and toilets and did not occur in bedrooms, an unlikely phenomenon if caused by humans. At Tung Tau Estate, where six SARS cases occurred in three families living in corresponding units on different floors in mid-April, the coronavirus was detected on the surface of a pipe on the roof of the affected building. In a more recent cluster in May in Lek Yuen Estate, where 11 people from five households in the same building fell ill, viral remnants were detected on the floor and windowsill of two apartments close to a SARS-affected household (one unit on the same floor and another unit directly above the affected household) where there were no SARS patients.[19] The residents of these two units could have brought in contaminants from the neighbourhood (the official explanation) but it is hard to explain how they could have contaminated their own windowsills. Windowsills, floors and roof pipes are however places frequently traversed by rats.

5. The outbreak at Amoy Gardens continued despite isolation (31 March) and subsequent evacuation (1 April) of all Block E residents for 10 days and rigorous cleaning by estate management. Another 59 new cases were identified between 1 April and 16 April (including several patients from Block E who were probably infected before evacuation and isolation). Secondary person-to-person infection via droplets from the primary patients is not a likely explanation for the persistence of the epidemic as most residents were aware of this mode of transmission and more than 80 percent of them were using

facemasks by this time. The continuance of the outbreak also does not show the peaks and valleys typically seen in secondary and tertiary infections but rather occurs in an endemic form with a steady number of new cases daily. Persistent household contamination by rats would provide a mechanism for the ongoing epidemic as residents were advised to keep their windows open for better ventilation, thus allowing easy entry for the rats.

6.   The progress of the epidemic outside of Amoy Gardens also points strongly to the presence of an infected animal vector. The disease has occurred in clusters in three other residential blocks adjacent to Amoy Gardens where between 8 and 49 SARS cases were reported, with those closest to Amoy being affected first and those with the worst hygiene being the most seriously affected.

7.   SARS spread widely in the community but areas around the four major hospitals where SARS patients were treated were the most heavily affected. This may be explained by hospital workers carrying infectious material to their communities or by visitors to hospitals spreading the disease. However, visits to all public hospitals were suspended on 3 April and hospital workers took all possible precautions not to bring the disease home. The possibility that rats were responsible for this spread as they became infected by garbage from the hospitals must be considered.

8.   Viral presence was detected in four out of eight rat droppings found around Amoy Gardens and in the throat and/or rectal swabs of five housecats, one dog and at least one rat.[6] Live SARS virus was cultured from the throat swab of at least one cat, which also was positive for SARS antibodies. These animals showed no clinical symptoms of the disease and became virus-free spontaneously. If cats (and possibly dogs) can be infected, it is very likely that rats can be too.

9.   Coronaviruses are ribonucleic acid (RNA) viruses with a great ability to reshuffle genes. The SARS virus has already shown differences in genome sequence in different reports.[20, 21] Recently, Haijema et al[22] successfully incorporated the coat protein gene from a mouse coronavirus into a feline coronavirus (feline infectious peritonitis virus, FIPV) by injecting cat cells with FIPV and adding a gene fragment from a mouse coronavirus. The exchange of the feline coat gene and the mouse coat gene took only several hours and made the new FIPV infectious to mouse cells. If rats at Amoy Gardens had naturally occurring rat coronaviruses and were exposed

simultaneously to the SARS virus, it is possible that gene reshuffling would produce a new SARS virus that is transmissible to both rats and humans.

Weaknesses of the hypothesis

Although the rat vector hypothesis seems capable of explaining many of the features of the SARS outbreak at Amoy Gardens, the following questions and problems still remain to be addressed:

1. So far no laboratory has been able to establish a rodent model for SARS. Autopsies performed on four rats caught around Amoy Gardens found no signs of active disease. A co-factor may be necessary for the infection of rats.[23]
2. Despite detection of the virus in rat droppings, the presence of a virus in rats may be transient and not a factor in human transmission.
3. For the hypothesis to work many rats need to be involved and they have to visit many households within a couple of days. Their movements must also be quite habitual to explain the pattern of infection, especially in Block E. Whether the rats in Amoy Gardens are really territorial and whether there are enough rats to cause the outbreak is still questionable.
4. Since many other buildings in Hong Kong are infested with rats, and there were many other SARS cases in the community, why did more outbreaks similar to that at Amoy Gardens not occur?
5. The original source of the infection, i.e., the renal patient, is a likely possibility but not a firm proof. If this patient did not cause the environmental contamination, another source must be identified. One of the construction workers working on a site across from Block E was diagnosed with SARS at about the same time and could be a second possible source of environmental contamination.
6. How the virus is transmitted from rats to humans is still not clear.

Further studies

The rat vector hypothesis is a strong possibility that needs to be studied rigorously. Urgent attention is needed especially in the following areas:

Human studies

1. **Case control studies:** Epidemiologic case-control studies need to be done at Amoy Gardens to identify behavioural risk factors for infection and establish possible mechanisms for rat-to-human infection. For example, if rat contamination occurs at night, people using kitchen and bathroom facilities early in the morning for activities such as cooking breakfast, taking showers, etc., will be more at risk. This might explain why housewives were affected more than husbands (the male/female ratio in Amoy cases was 45/55). Small children who crawl on the floor would also be at a higher risk. We have to establish the factors that account for the infection of some individuals but not others living in the same household.

2. **Comparison of clinical series:** There is strong suspicion that Amoy SARS patients have different presentation and clinical course than other SARS patients. Since there were over 300 Amoy cases, a detailed comparison of the incubation period, presenting symptoms, clinical course and outcome can be done between patient series. This would allow for exploration of the possible existence of multiple distinct types of SARS.

3. **Virology in humans:** To test the rat hypothesis, viral studies of Amoy patients should be carried out to determine if the virus has undergone mutation or incorporated rat genetic material into its genome when compared with samples from other patients. The viral genome from different series of patients should be mapped and compared. If the virus can still be recovered from the index patient (as is likely since his chronic medical condition means that his immune system is suppressed) it would be valuable to compare his viral genome with that of other Amoy patients to detect mutation or genetic reshuffling with rat genes.

Rat studies

Obviously rat studies are vital to test this hypothesis. Several lines should be pursued.

1. **Evidence of viral infection in rats:** Rats and droppings should be sampled in different blocks of Amoy Gardens and in neighbourhood estates. There are blocks within Amoy Gardens where no cases of SARS were ever reported. The rat population there may provide

clues as to why this was the case. Rats in areas around Amoy where no cases ever occurred should also be studied. Droppings should be assayed for viral presence by culture and polymerase chain reaction (PCR). Rats should be thoroughly autopsied to study for pathological changes and to determine the distribution of the virus and viral gene products in tissues, urine, saliva and faeces. Serological tests should be performed to detect for the presence of antibodies.

2. **Experimental infection of rats:** If the hypothesis is correct we must be able to establish either infection or tolerance in rats. Experimental rats, especially those locally found in Hong Kong, can be exposed to the virus by inhalation, ingestion and injection. Rats of different ages, young and old, can be tested. Pregnant rats should be exposed to determine intra-uterine infection. After exposure these rats should be studied for disease occurrence, antibody formation and ability to pass the virus to the environment. If the rats do not develop clinical symptoms, they should be studied for development of tolerance and a carrier state. The length of a carrier state, if any, is vital for future control of epidemics.

Environmental studies

We have to study the design and construction of Amoy Gardens and its water supply and sewage drainage systems to understand what factors are responsible for the easy spread of SARS through rats and humans in this housing complex. Other SARS patients must have discharged contaminated waste in their respective environments but before Amoy Gardens, no serious cluster outbreak took place. There must be lessons to be learned from detailed environmental studies of Amoy Gardens.

Conclusion

The SARS outbreak at Amoy Gardens puzzled epidemiologists worldwide and despite official reports from the Hong Kong Government and the WHO it has not been satisfactorily explained. The epidemic at Amoy Gardens has ended as it has in other parts of Hong Kong and mainland China. However, there is a high probability that SARS will come back. The possibility of an animal reservoir of the virus in the wild cannot be ruled out. In its short appearance the SARS-coronavirus has shown remarkable adaptability in its ability to attack the human population. In its second appearance, it may prove even more fatal. This is why we need to learn as much as possible from the first outbreak and determine the main route of transmission, especially outside the hospital setting. Community transmission in Hong Kong did not seem to be particularly virulent except at Amoy Gardens. As the building structure and facilities of Amoy Gardens are by no means unique in Hong Kong, it is surprising that similar outbreaks in other housing complexes did not occur. A unique set of circumstances may have resulted in this tragic outbreak and an important lesson is there to be learned. The sooner we learn it, the better for humankind.

CHAPTER 8

How the Stunning Outbreak of Disease Led to a Stunning Outbreak of Dissent

Michael E DeGolyer

The mystery disease

In late January 2003 stories swept through Hong Kong of a mysterious respiratory disease in Guangdong Province. Guangdong authorities finally admitted that an outbreak of unusual pneumonia had infected 305 and killed 5 people since November 2002, but said that the situation was under control and posed no threat to public health in Guangdong, much less Hong Kong. Under the "one country, two systems" policy Guangdong authorities had no power to even communicate with their counterparts across the border in Hong Kong. In fact, it was not until the end of January 2003 that 24-hour travel across land barriers was permitted, and then it was limited to the smallest of the three road crossings. Travel to Hong Kong by mainlanders required a special permit, and was allowed only in authorised groups. Though "the border" had become a boundary between municipal districts rather than a designation of separate sovereign territory on 1 July 1997, the demarcation between Hong Kong and the rest of China was regarded as a territorial division that required an especial act of the Central Government authorities to breach, even for the purpose of sharing of information.[1]

The SARS virus disregarded territorial markers, bureaucratic restrictions and other niceties. On 21 February 2003, a Guangdong resident and retired doctor, Liu Jianlun, visited the Metropole Hotel in

Hong Kong and ended up in Kwong Wah Hospital, where he died on 4 March. He became the index patient for an outbreak that would spread worldwide with Hong Kong as its epicentre. Upon admission to hospital, Liu warned healthcare workers that he had treated patients with a severe communicable disease and specifically requested that he be placed in isolation. However, the warning came too late. On 4 March, a 26-year-old man who had visited a friend at the Metropole between 12 February and 2 March was admitted to Prince of Wales Hospital (PWH) in Shatin with a high fever. Through this patient, the disease eventually spread to over 100 hospital staff at PWH.[2] But it was not until 11 March, after large numbers of staff at PWH began to fall severely ill and the disease received media coverage, that the Hong Kong Government first informed the public of an outbreak of disease in Hong Kong.[3]

The Government's initial reaction was to assure the public that the outbreak was isolated to PWH and that other hospitals had been put on alert. The call for the public to calm down and trust authorities to handle what they described as an isolated outbreak was repeated several times in the first two weeks of March. Other than issuing alerts to hospitals and calling on the public to behave as usual, the Government refused to implement further public health measures, such as the quarantine of those possibly exposed to the disease. The greatest danger, Hong Kong officials felt, was the possibility of undue panic.

On 15 March, the World Health Organisation (WHO), which had already released one health advisory regarding the outbreak of a "severe form of pneumonia," issued a second advisory cautioning travellers about travelling in SARS-affected areas. The Governments of Thailand, Singapore and Taiwan also issued travel warnings, advising their citizens not to travel to Hong Kong and to exercise unusual caution if doing so. The warnings triggered real anger among Hong Kong officials. They insisted, as Secretary of Health, Welfare and Food Dr. Yeoh Eng-kiong put it, "Hong Kong is very safe. It is no different from going to any big city in the world."[4]

On 17 March, Guangdong authorities claimed that the outbreak there was under control and stated that they could not cooperate directly with Hong Kong authorities because of the "one country, two systems" policy. Any exchange of information or cooperation with other provincial officials would require the direct approval of the central authorities, they said.[5] At the time, the central authorities were focused on the transfer of leadership from one generation to the next. They were not the only people whose attention was diverted.

Scandal diverts attention, as does a transfer of authority

During the first critical weeks of the SARS outbreak, two other events fought for public attention and the front pages of Hong Kong newspapers. Both concerned primary responsibilities of the Government, slowing, if not paralysing, its initial response to the health emergency. The first was Hong Kong's 2003 budget address, in which Financial Secretary Antony Leung had proposed many new taxes and massive cuts in a programme more stringent than any implemented in Hong Kong for at least a generation. Unveiling of the controversial budget programme was followed barely a week later by a scandal involving the self-same Financial Secretary. During the first two weeks of March, the budget and the scandal deflected attention from almost all other issues within Hong Kong.

The second event was the meeting of the National People's Congress and the transfer of the presidency from Jiang Zemin to Hu Jintao in the first peaceful transfer of power at that level of government in the history of the People's Republic of China. Officials on the mainland were under strict instructions to make sure that the month of March passed without any public embarrassments. All eyes in the first two weeks of March were fixed on these political events. The mainland media was under tight control in order to avoid any controversy or diversion of attention away from what was regarded as the most significant event in Chinese politics since the ascension of Deng Xiaoping to power in 1978.

The focus on political events, especially the scandal, and later the controls imposed on the mainland media served to heighten the sense of shock among Hong Kong people when they became aware of the outbreak of SARS. Few had paid much attention to the sickness of a small number of people when what seemed to be far more important and interesting events were taking place. The "sudden" breakout of the disease meant that the secrecy and lack of cooperation on the part of the mainland assumed particular importance for Hong Kong. Perceptions of mainland secretiveness were also to strongly affect views of another ongoing issue — the debate over the Article 23 legislation that had been presented to Hong Kong's Legislative Council (LegCo) on 13 February 2003.[6]

"Cargate"

The Antony Leung "cargate" scandal, which dominated public attention and paralysed the Government, especially at the top level, unfolded shortly after the Financial Secretary delivered a budget address on 5 March 2003, spelling out the steepest and most comprehensive increases in taxes in Hong Kong in a generation. Profits tax, income taxes, rates, a new border-crossing tax, a new tax on employing foreign domestic helpers and a list of fees and charges, including — in the end fatally for Leung — a steep hike in the first registration tax for new automobiles, were all proposed.[7] At first, although there was much grumbling about the overall fairness of the proposals, with the Democratic Party claiming that the middle class would be unfairly squeezed, the public appeared to accept that something had to be done about the increasing budget deficit. And while there was resistance to raising some fees and charges, the prospects for passing the bulk of the proposals appeared good until one of the Chinese language newspapers revealed that the Financial Secretary had bought a new car only weeks before announcing the tax raise. Estimations of the taxes he had escaped by doing so began at HK$50,000. Further investigation revealed that a huge price markdown had saved him some HK$190,000 in taxes.

In response to these revelations, Leung first pledged to donate three times the amount he had avoided in taxes to a charity. (He eventually did send a cheque for HK$380,000 to the Community Chest.) Then, when that failed to stem growing public and legislative anger, including considerable condemnation by the business community, he sent a letter of resignation to Chief Executive Tung Chee-hwa, which was promptly turned down.[8] After further controversy, the Chief Executive sent Leung a formal letter of reprimand, criticising his carelessness and "gross misconduct" in the performance of his office. Government critics in LegCo put forward a private member's motion of no-confidence in the Financial Secretary (as a private member's motion it was non-binding in effect). Leung "won" the motion on 7 May by a 20 to 5 vote in the functional constituencies, but "lost" in the directly elected portion of LegCo where a substantial majority supported the motion. In order to pass, private members bills must receive a majority vote from both functional constituency representatives and directly elected LegCo members.

LegCo did not launch a legislative inquiry into the matter, but the

Independent Commission Against Corruption (ICAC), which reports directly to Tung but has a reputation for being independent and thorough, released a report in mid-July 2003. By then, circumstances had changed utterly, due in no small part to the SARS crisis. Prior to the release of the ICAC findings, Leung gave the Chief Executive a second letter of resignation in the event that the report called for the Financial Secretary to be charged criminally. This time, Tung accepted Leung's resignation.[9] It is not public knowledge at the time of writing whether the report deemed Leung's behaviour worthy of criminal charges.

The ICAC investigation addressed the question of whether the Financial Secretary had deliberately avoided paying taxes on his new car. Leung had discussed a possible increase in taxes for new car purchases in July 2002, in October 2002 and again on 14 January 2003 before ordering his new car on 20 January and taking delivery of it on 25 January. He claimed he simply forgot about the purchase when the decision was made to increase taxes on 28 February. Other members of the Executive Council (ExCo) who had purchased new cars in the few months prior to the tax rise (none of whom was involved in the preliminary discussions over possible tax hikes) did ask if they should declare their purchases — in the presence of a silent Financial Secretary. Leung claimed his mind was elsewhere during these discussions, perhaps on his new baby. The Chief Executive accepted this explanation; public opinion and civil service associations rejected Leung's nominal punishment — a reprimand and an admonition to do better — as insufficient. When the Chief Executive put Leung in charge of a task force to re-launch Hong Kong's economy following the SARS crisis with the goal of targeting overseas investors, critics vehemently protested his choice of leadership.

Article 23

While concern regarding SARS was beginning to be evident in late February, attention was focused on the political events mentioned above and the controversy over Article 23 of the Basic Law, which instructs Hong Kong to "on its own" enact legislation against treason, secession, sedition, subversion and theft of state secrets. The article also directs the proscription of links between organisations in Hong Kong and foreign political bodies.

The debate over Article 23, which in December 2002 had prompted 60,000 protestors to take to the streets of Hong Kong, numbers not seen since the summer of 1989, died down substantially after 13 February 2003 when the Government introduced a legislative bill that dropped a number of the proposals in the initial consultation paper. Gone was the proposal that foreign permanent residents, wherever resident, could be charged with treason against China. Changed also were proposals for secret trials without a jury for charges of treason, secession or subversion. However, the tussle in LegCo over who would be the chair and vice-chair of the committee holding public hearings on the proposed bill resulted in a triumph by pro-Government forces. They promptly implemented rules limiting testimony by each group to five minutes, regardless of size or qualifications, meaning that ad hoc pro-Government groups with a few dozen members received the same amount of time as the Law Society and other long-established legal and human rights bodies. A number of critics continued to raise objections to the legislation, which proposed a series of amendments to three existing ordinances. Of primary concern to critics was providing a public interest defence for the press. At the time, the Government adamantly resisted amending the bill to allow such a defence. The bill would later be amended following the huge demonstration of over half a million people on 1 July in a last ditch attempt to pass Article 23 legislation on 9 July as originally scheduled.

This issue of a public interest defence for publishing "secret" Government information received new impetus with the SARS crisis, which was exacerbated by Beijing's instructions to the national press in March to maintain silence on SARS during the public transition in leadership at the National People's Congress. Reports on SARS were deemed "distractions" from the far more important business of seeing Hu Jintao assume power, or at least title, from Jiang Zemin, who retired to head the powerful central military commission. The secrecy surrounding SARS allowed Hong Kong to be blindsided by a single "super-spreader" who brought the virus into Hong Kong and infected scores, then hundreds, then thousands of people around the world until it was impossible for even Chinese authorities to ignore the outbreak.[10] In an article published in the South China Morning Post on 16 April, Bates Gill and Andrew Thompson made the connection between laws on state secrets and the spread of SARS explicit:

> The mainland's initial denial and slow response to the SARS outbreak characterises a political environment where individual initiative is

discouraged and social stability is protected above other interests. Additionally, the initial slow reaction by medical authorities can be explained by outdated laws that prevent effective communication about emerging epidemics. The State Secrets Law prevents local authorities from discussing an emerging outbreak until the Ministry of Health in Beijing has announced the existence of an epidemic. In the case of SARS, the silence of the bureaucracy, coupled with an increasingly mobile population, virtually guaranteed that an infectious disease would quickly spread well beyond Guangdong to the rest of the world.[11]

This lesson in the disasters that can result from Government secrecy prompted numerous calls for the Hong Kong Government not only to reconsider certain provisions of the Article 23 legislation but also to slow down the push to pass the bill by the end of the legislative year.[12]

SARS' contribution to the SAR's worst crisis

The crisis of the very survival of the Tung Government began with the turnout of over half a million people on the streets of Hong Kong in protest — a figure that stunned the Government, which had anticipated, and told Beijing to expect, from around 30,000 people to as many, possibly, as 80,000, but at most, 100,000. Organisers had told the police to plan for about 100,000 protestors.[13] But pent-up anger over the recent performance of the administration, particularly the Chief Executive's mishandling of economic and political affairs, triggered the largest anti-Government demonstrations in Hong Kong in almost half a century.[14] The turnout for the protest on 1 July, a public holiday intended to commemorate the 1997 establishment of the Hong Kong Special Administrative Region (SAR) and its reunification with the mainland, far surpassed everyone's expectations, forcing police to close roads and cordon off additional assembly areas. Despite the heat and lengthy wait, the crowd remained calm and orderly — so orderly that the Commissioner of Police praised participants for their model behaviour as they marched past the Hong Kong Government headquarters in Central.[15]

This orderliness was entirely unlike the social upheaval that characterised the violent protests of the 1920s and 1960s. Hong Kongers were therefore puzzled by the subsequent and repeated warnings by the

Central People's Government Liaison Office that the "chaos" and "turmoil" of the Cultural Revolution could be repeated in Hong Kong.[16] The use of the word "turmoil" is especially significant and ominous: under the terms of the Basic Law, which codifies relations between Hong Kong and the mainland, a declaration that Hong Kong is in turmoil is a signal for the PLA to step out of its barracks and onto the streets to restore order and protect mainland sovereignty over Hong Kong. While it is highly unlikely that the Central Government would issue such a declaration under almost any circumstances, the repeated use of the word indicates the extent to which Beijing was shocked by the demonstrations and the seriousness with which they were viewed, especially by the ultra-conservatives who dominate Beijing's Hong Kong information sources.

The warning was also double-edged, aimed as much at the Tung Government and its allies as at the general public and the anti-Tung camp. In 1997, Beijing envisioned that Hong Kong would prove to be economically active but politically quiescent following what it saw as the artificial politicisation of the Patten years. Beijing authorities have been stunned to see that despite — or perhaps in response to — the leadership of Tung Chee-hwa, who has attempted to minimise the role of politics in public affairs, Hong Kong has instead become economically quiescent and politically active. In large part, the 1 July demonstrations were an attempt by members of the public to take public affairs into their own hands and should be understood as a culmination of the leadership role forced on the public during the SARS crisis.

Members of the public, for example, pulled students by the thousands out of school and made the decision to close scores of schools voluntarily, even over Government threats, weeks before the Government closed all educational facilities until preventative measures could be put in place.[17] The media led a campaign to raise money for and purchase and distribute protective clothing to front line hospital staff — after the Government patently was failing to do so. Businesses launched informational campaigns to inform themselves and their overseas colleagues of the situation in Hong Kong, weeks before the Government could organise its own version.

The massive protest on 1 July also had roots in an unenviable record of mistakes and bad luck on the part of the Tung administration. However, the three most immediate contributors were the controversy over Article 23 described above, the mishandling of SARS and the perceived failure of the new "accountability system" to deliver the promised accountability and improvement in performance. The factors proved to be mutually reinforcing. For example, while Government mishandling of the SARS outbreak served to divert attention away from Article 23, SARS also highlighted the tremendous economic and personal costs that Government secrecy could have for Hong Kong.

The convergence of these two events transformed what had seemed like abstract issues of importance only to journalists, such as the publication of unofficial disclosures by official sources, into matters of vital public interest. Freedom of the press ceased to be abstract when it was measured in terms of the deaths of 299 people, the infection of over one thousand and the virtual collapse of key sectors of the Hong Kong economy, including the tourism and hospitality industry. The impact of SARS on Hong Kong was devastating because Hong Kong was not prepared — and this was due largely to secrecy on the part of Guangdong authorities, compounded by mainland censorship of the media. Nothing else could have driven home to the people of Hong Kong what was at stake when it came to protecting freedom of the press and freedom of information. Even the generally pro-Government and politically quiescent business and professional sectors mobilised, joining protests in numbers large enough to prompt the resignation of Liberal Party chairman James Tien from ExCo when Tung refused to reschedule the vote on Article 23 legislation. The Liberal Party holds eight seats in LegCo, representing a critical mass among LegCo's functional constituencies, which are dominated by business and professional groups.

Official accountability

The third factor that contributed directly to the massive 1 July protests was the conduct of the principal officials appointed under Hong Kong's new "accountability system." The system was put in place on 1 July 2002 and billed as a way of making the Government more responsive and accountable. However, as discussed above, the disclosure of the "cargate" scandal in mid-March generated widespread condemnation for the conduct of Financial Secretary Antony Leung. The Secretary for Security, Regina Ip, also stirred up huge controversy with her comments in defence of Article 23 legislation and her disdainful treatment of LegCo members in the run-up to the scheduled vote on Article 23 on 9 July.

A third principal official to face public censure was Dr. Yeoh Eng-kiong, Secretary for Health, Welfare and Food and head of Hong Kong's anti-SARS efforts, who became a lightening rod for criticism over Government handling of SARS, which was first hesitant and uncoordinated, then over-hasty and rough-shod, resulting in the virtual incarceration of suspected SARS cases. The Government's tardiness and stinginess in providing proper protective gear for hospital workers prompted local newspapers to take matters into their own hands by raising funds for, purchasing and distributing such items. These events underlined the Tung Government's ineffectiveness, or indifference, to the public. When Tung put Yeoh in charge of the group tasked with investigating and reporting on the Government's handling of SARS, critics from all sectors challenged Tung's sincerity in identifying and addressing mistakes that could have fatal repercussions if SARS returns later in 2003, as a number of experts predict.

The final straw in terms of Government performance came when Secretary for Justice Elsie Leung announced that she, and she alone, would decide whether Financial Secretary Antony Leung would be prosecuted once the ICAC investigation concluded in July. In 1998, Mrs. Leung decided not to prosecute Sally Aw, a publisher and friend of Tung Chee-hwa, on dubious grounds, prompting charges of favouritism that still dogged the Justice Department.[18] Regina Ip's comments that 1 July demonstrators were coming out because they had nothing better to do on a holiday merely reinforced what had become a cold determination to send Hong Kong's officials an unmistakable message that the Government's incompetence, indifference and stubborn unwillingness to listen to public opinion had to stop. The SARS crisis convinced many that it was literally a matter of life and death.

Contrasting Hong Kong's response to the SARS crisis with the response of mainland authorities only highlighted what was wrong, and what had to be changed, in Hong Kong. At the start of the SARS outbreak, mainland authorities delayed the entry of WHO investigators into China for days, while the mainland press either ignored or played down the crisis. Then, according to stories that came out first in the western press, SARS struck members of the communist party in Beijing. And as more details of the disease became known, communist party members truly panicked. Most SARS fatalities are among males aged 50 and above — the profile of the communist party leadership. At least 25 percent of males aged 60 and above died once infected with SARS. Almost no one under the age of 30 died of SARS.[19]

China's leaders, almost all males over 60, took drastic action — launching an informational press campaign; mobilising the army; quarantining whole sections of cities; shutting down airports, schools and public transport; establishing full cooperation with the WHO and other health authorities; and taking the unprecedented step of publishing daily updates and reports on the internet. President Hu, newly installed in office, took the reins of Government with alacrity and purpose.[20] When mainland authorities began firing officials by the score for maladministration during the SARS crisis at the same time that the Tung administration was refusing to fire anyone or even accept the resignation of officials, grumbling disaffection for the bumbling Tung regime turned to active opposition and even widespread disgust.[21]

District Council and LegCo elections

Hong Kong voters, who are scheduled to select District Council members in November 2003 and LegCo members in September 2004, focused their wrath on the political parties who were represented in ExCo. In July 2002, Tung Chee-hwa had appointed the heads of the Liberal Party, the Democratic Alliance for the Betterment of Hong Kong (DAB), the Hong Kong Progressive Alliance and the Federation of Trade Unions as members of ExCo.

As mentioned above, the Liberal Party, whose eight LegCo members are all elected by functional constituencies, cracked under the tide of public criticism and anger leading up to the 1 July demonstrations. Party chairman James Tien resigned from ExCo, overturning the Tung Government's effective majority control of LegCo. Desertion by a number of generally pro-Government independents on the issue of Article 23 forced Tung to postpone the scheduled 9 July vote, even after making several last-minute concessions. The 50,000 people who surrounded the LegCo building on 9 July 2003 in a previously arranged protest demanded improved accountability from the Government and, in particular, expansion of direct elections for LegCo and implementation of direct elections for the Chief Executive.[22]

Chief Executive Tung Chee-hwa was "elected" for a five-year term in 1996 by a 400-person Election Committee, the members of which were chosen by Beijing. In the 2002 "elections," for which Tung was the only candidate to stand, an 800-person Election Committee performed the ritual of re-election. Three-quarters of the committee members were returned by an electorate that consists of the fewer than 200,000 voters who also elect functional constituency representatives to LegCo. Of the 60 seats in LegCo, 24 are directly elected, with 30 seats (half the legislature) slated for direct election in 2004. The Basic Law provides that all LegCo members may be directly elected some time after 2007.

The resignations of the Financial Secretary and the Secretary for Security, announced shortly after Tien's resignation from ExCo, helped to placate public dissatisfaction with the Government, which reached record levels in mid-2003, with more than two-thirds of the public reporting dissatisfaction with the Government's performance.

The economic context and the financial impact of SARS

The three factors described above all took place within the context of, and also served to exacerbate, the economic difficulties that have plagued the SAR almost without pause since the autumn of 1997. Property prices are currently between 60 and 70 percent lower than their 1997 highs, leaving as many as 150,000 homeowners in a negative equity situation. Unemployment rose to a record 8.7 percent in the second quarter of 2003, while underemployment of more than 5 percent deeply affected a workforce accustomed to an underemployment rate of 3 percent or less.[23] Wages have fallen sharply across most of the workforce, with even the public sector experiencing thousands of job cuts and overall wage cuts for the first time since the Great Depression of the 1920s and 1930s. Between 1996 and 2002, the number of suicides skyrocketed from 11.3 per 100,000 to a record 16.4 per 100,000.[24] Morale among private and public sector workers, already poor, hit all-time lows during the SARS crisis.

During the outbreak, tourism fell to record lows not seen in Hong Kong since the events of Tiananmen Square in June 1989. Major hotels reported occupancy rates in the single digits in April 2003. Hundreds of restaurants closed while through traffic at the airport dropped to one-fifth of the usual flow of about 100,000 passengers daily. The Hang Seng Index lagged behind nearly all other regional stock exchanges in performance for months and fell to four-and-a-half year lows at the height of the epidemic. Nevertheless, as Stephen Brown indicates in Chapter 11 and as GDP figures for the second quarter of 2003 showed, the economy as a whole barely shrank while the export sector continued to grow. The unequal economic effects, however, aggravated people's feelings of unfairness in treatment or indifference on the part of Government to their plight.

The inability of the Chief Executive to determine the way forward, economically and politically, and to foster cooperation with Guangdong and Pearl River Delta authorities as well as the Central Government, brought criticism even from his pro-Beijing compatriots. Since his first Policy Address in October 1997, Tung had repeatedly mentioned the need to increase Hong Kong's ties to the Pearl River Delta. He claimed that the new political accountability system put in place in July 2002 would enhance the motivation of ministers in working with him to improve the economy and improve ties with mainland officials. However, the border was not even opened to 24-hour truck traffic until well into 2002 and to passenger traffic only at one small checkpoint in late January 2003. A decision to link the Hong Kong International Airport at Chek Lap Kok (located at the far end of an outlying island) to the western side of the Pearl River Delta via a bridge came only in late 2002 and ran into strong opposition from Shenzhen and Guangzhou authorities, as well as local Hong Kong tycoons such as Henry Fok and Li Ka-shing, who had their own ideas about delta development. Even mainland tourism, an area pushed hard by the Tung Government, lagged due to restrictions on mainlanders entering Hong Kong as individuals, as well as the absurd opening hours at the border.

All of these bottlenecks disappeared suddenly when Beijing intervened following the 1 July demonstrations. The bridge will be built by 2008; individuals and not just tour groups are being allowed to enter Hong Kong from the mainland; border crossing transport, facilities and personnel will be increased; and provincial and delta officials are scrambling to coordinate development plans and programmes. In addition, it appears that mainlanders and mainland firms will be governed by more liberal regulations when investing in Hong Kong properties and stocks. This programme of decisive action was the central authorities' response to what they saw as the underlying cause of discontent in Hong Kong — the economic downturn. The Hang Seng Index responded to mainland intervention and concessions, hitting record highs for 2003 in August, a time usually characterised by trading doldrums.

Three basic errors and the cure for Special Administrative Region Syndrome (SARS)

The central authorities also sent teams to Hong Kong to investigate what went wrong within the Government. From the beginning, the Tung administration has made a number of key mistakes, with each "reform" seeming to worsen the situation rather than improve it. These mistakes so weakened the "constitution" of the SAR that when SARS hit it nearly caused the Government to collapse.

Tung's performance as Chief Executive is shaped by his experience as the tycoon of a traditional Chinese family firm. His primary mistake lies in his attempt to re-mould Hong Kong's Government and society into a traditional Chinese family enterprise. But Hong Kong is too big, too diverse (40 percent of all employment is generated by foreign firms) and far too dynamic to fit into a traditional family firm framework. Tung's performance also reflects his tendency to be indecisive for long periods, conferring endlessly or simply gathering information without taking action. This is followed by abrupt "decisions" on policies without consultation or explanation. A case in point was his decision to announce, then abruptly rescind, a policy to build 85,000 home ownership scheme (HOS) flats a year. But it is not by any means the only, or even the worst example of this kind of behaviour. Tung's seeming inability to make decisions in an open and timely manner garnered sharp remarks from recently retired Chinese Premier Zhu Rongji and prompted Hong Kong civil servants to privately refer to the Chief Executive's office as "the Black Hole" into which information was poured, but which failed to generate either information or decisions.[25]

Error One: Organisational structure and management policy

Tung Chee-hwa took office in 1997, supposedly slated to work hand in hand with Chief Secretary for Administration Anson Chan, the veteran manager of reputedly Asia's most efficient, professional and clean civil service. This was, as the outgoing colonial administration put it at the time, the "dream team" combination most likely to succeed in achieving "stability and prosperity" for Hong Kong — the mantra and promise repeated ad infinitum by mainland officials.

But nearly from the beginning, Tung's pro-Beijing supporters poisoned relations between the Chief Executive and the Chief Secretary, finally persuading Tung that the failures of his first five-year term could be traced primarily to obstruction by British-trained civil servants and the powerful Mrs. Chan. Their solution? Abolish the old organisational structure in which the entire Government operated under the leadership of three non-political officials — the Chief Secretary for Administration, the Financial Secretary and the Secretary for Justice — and implement in its place a "principal officials accountability system." Each of the 14 principal officials or ministers would have responsibility for a particular portfolio and report to the Chief Executive, who would have sole power in coordinating Government policy and resolving conflicts in priorities and resources.[26]

Replacing the traditional pyramidal structure of Government with a hub-and-spoke structure puts a tremendous burden on the central figure. It also encourages infighting over decision-making and resource allocation and hinders cooperation between ministers. Organisational theorists universally condemn this kind of structure as unworkable, if not dangerous for the organisation itself. In practice, the worst effect of the new structure was to invite, if not force, Tung to intervene personally in almost every decision made at any time in any branch of Government, particularly on issues involving more than one department, which means, in practical terms, most Governmental issues. The Government response to SARS is a case in point, as it involved transport, mainland relations, home affairs, Government information services, the public health sector, hospitals, schools, urban and rural services involved in trash cleanup and so on.

Tung's personal and rather chaotic management style undercut ministers' confidence and actually reduced, rather than enhanced, their political responsiveness to the public. Since every public policy decision involves a personal decision by the Chief Executive, any change in policy requires changing the opinion of the Chief Executive, or getting him to admit to a mistake. To date, this has proved difficult unless the mistake has become overwhelmingly obvious and maddening to a large number of people outside of the now-cowed Government bureaucracy. Nevertheless, despite its signal and overwhelming failure to address one situation after another, the Government released a one-year report on the ministerial system in July 2003, deeming it a success. With "successes" like this, the Tung administration needed no enemies, much less one as powerful as the SARS virus.

Error Two: Political structure and policy-making

The Government's error in terms of organisation and management contributed to and exacerbated errors in political structure and policy-making. As a businessman with no political experience and an active disdain for politics, Tung assumed office with the assumption that efficiency in Government involved streamlining policy-making and involving as few people as possible in the process. He consequently abolished an entire layer of Government that dealt with local issues (the Urban and Regional Councils) and had the only independent policy-making powers outside of the executive office, though these concerned such local affairs as trash collection, management of neighbourhood sports and cultural venues, noise abatement and management of local wet markets. Rather than focusing policy-making and improving efficiency, the change succeeded in focusing public disgruntlement on Tung and his Government.

The Urban and Regional Councils were elected bodies whose officials were accountable for the kinds of local decisions most likely to prompt public dissatisfaction — thus their role in policy-making could have mitigated political pressure at a higher level of Government. In addition, the input of politicians active on a grassroots level would have provided the Government with an early warning that the SARS situation required urgent action. But without the Urban and Regional Councils, every decision about who uses which venue for what purpose and any failure to clean up trash or maintain drains or manage a wet market is the responsibility of the Chief Executive and his Government. When the Chief Executive is not elected by the people, dissatisfaction builds rather than dissipates, and focuses on the top level of Government.[27] And when the Chief Executive refuses to hold lower officials responsible for policy failures and demand their resignation, frustrations simply grow and grow until an event triggers an explosion. The SARS crisis added unbearable pressure to a system already under great stress.

The point in politics, as highlighted in beginning political science classes, is to provide safe outlets for public frustrations and to incorporate mechanisms for mitigating frustration into any political system. After Tung accepted the resignation of two ministers and made a number of the other changes demanded by the public, such as postponing the vote on Article 23 legislation and removing Dr. Yeoh as head of the post-SARS investigation, polls showed a sharp, immediate reduction in dissatisfaction with the Government.

Error Three: Separation of powers

Tung prides himself on policy-making, failing to realise that his personal style of policy-making is the very source of his troubles, not the basis of the solution.[28] A fundamental element of political economy is to separate the policy-making process from the policy implementation and evaluation processes. In practice, this concept involves the development of political parties to solicit and focus public participation in policy-making, and the development of a professional civil service that is deliberately separated from politics to implement and report on the feasibility of policies resulting from the political process. This division ensures that even when policy makers are deeply committed to a particular course of action, if the policy is not workable or does not work as expected, professionals will report the facts of the matter to politicians and the public without fear of retribution. The Government's post-SARS investigation was headed by two independent co-chairs, neither of whom was from Hong Kong or in any way beholden to the Tung Government, and as such, the investigation was a model of a separate, and hence credible, process of policy evaluation.[29] The co-chairs pledged in August that the investigation's report will be released simultaneously to the public and to the Government in October 2003, and could further impact policy-making in the SAR Government. There may be resignations by officials due to mishandling of SARS, following on from the resignation of Antony Leung and Regina Ip.

On a broader level, this point is reinforced by the current breach of the principle of separation by several western democracies. The politicising of intelligence services assessments of the Iraqi threat in both the UK and the US has put the political establishment of both countries in hot water, resulting in renewed support for the separation of policy-making from policy implementation and evaluation. Under Hong Kong's colonial administration, this separation was informal rather than formal. Non-local colonial officers developed policies with ad hoc feedback from local professionals on public reaction and policy implementation. It was in the interest of Hong Kong's British and local civil servants to maintain stability and prosperity as a bulwark against those who sought the overthrow of the colonial regime. Local civil servants were long regarded — and, at least in the eyes of die-hard leftists, are still regarded — as traitors to Communist China.

The prospects for reform

Tung has tried to de-politicise Hong Kong by ignoring politics, public opinion, political parties and even avoiding discussion of political reform.[30] This has instead convinced an increasing percentage of the public and local elites that political reform is the only solution to the economic and leadership problems now facing Hong Kong. Tung attempted to placate demands for reform by implementing the new accountability system, but then refused to hold ministers accountable for their actions, excusing even the "gross negligence" (his words) of former Financial Secretary Antony Leung. Tung and his business supporters also came to power convinced that Hong Kong wages and property prices were too high, but not convinced that profits were too concentrated and too high.[31] Tung has worked assiduously to drive wages lower, and even he now admits he drove property prices too low. But the Hong Kong Government continues to resist implementing comprehensive competition legislation despite repeated calls for enactment of such legislation by everyone from the European Union and the World Trade Organization to local legislators. The lack of competition, both in politics and in economics, has crippled Hong Kong and left its "constitution" weakened and vulnerable to crises such as SARS.

While Tung has gained a breathing space and benefited from significant cooperation on the part of regional and central authorities on the mainland, he now faces an invigorated and politically mobilised public and a number of opposition parties who are determined to make his supporters pay in the upcoming November elections. Currently, the opposition Democratic Party has the largest single grouping in the District Councils with 86 seats. Its rival, the pro-Tung Democratic Alliance for the Betterment of Hong Kong (DAB), holds 83 seats. Until the events of 1 July, the DAB was forecast to become the majority party in the District Councils, pushing the Democratic block to below 80 seats. This is now unlikely to occur, and if the Democrats raise their seat total to as high as 100 while the number of DAB seats drops below 75, Beijing may conclude that retaining Tung in office will threaten its power in LegCo, which will hold elections in September 2004.

Conversely, the DAB and other pro-Government parties that now have members on ExCo may conclude after the November elections that continued association with the Tung regime will be the kiss of death in the LegCo elections, and may consequently withdraw from ExCo and become much more vocal in criticising Tung and his ministers. The DAB and even Li Ka-shing, nominal leader of the big business interests that dominate Hong Kong's politics and economy, have stated, publicly, that more democracy and more public participation would be healthy for Hong Kong.[32] The SARS epidemic played a crucial role in convincing most people in Hong Kong, including traditionally pro-Government interests, that political reform is needed.

Conclusion

The SARS epidemic not only killed 299 people and hospitalised over a thousand in Hong Kong, affected thousands more elsewhere and resulted in worldwide panic; it also directly contributed to and was a major component of the frustration with Chief Executive Tung Chee-hwa's Government that drove over half a million people into the streets on 1 July 2003 in the largest demonstrations against a Hong Kong Government since the general strike of the 1920s and the Star Ferry riots of 1966. While major political upheavals occurred in Hong Kong in 1966–67 and 1989, in both cases, political unrest was driven mainly by events outside Hong Kong's borders. Unlike the demonstrations of 2003, the causes of these earlier upheavals were primarily national rather than local.

At the same time, although both the 1966–67 and 1989 movements were initiated by external events, they impacted local politics considerably. The events of 1966–67 helped push through major reforms during the 1970s, culminating in the 1982 District Board elections, the first elections based on universal suffrage in Hong Kong. The 1989 demonstrations, during which over a million people took to the streets, not once but twice, led to the establishment of the annual June 4 commemoration in Victoria Park, accelerated the introduction of direct elections for LegCo in 1991 and directly contributed to the decision by then UK Prime Minister John Major to appoint Chris Patten as Hong Kong's last governor in 1992. Under Patten's leadership, the colonial Government implemented a number of reforms, known as the ''Patten Reforms,'' intended to realise many of the political demands of the 1989 demonstrators. This was a reversal of the "through-train" approach to the 1997 handover set in place under Patten's predecessor, David Wilson.[33] Thus local reaction to the national events of 1989 laid the basis for the continued, and now, due largely to SARS, re-invigorated, demands for greater democracy and direct elections in Hong Kong.

In the long-term, the outbreak of SARS may prove as significant in changing the local political dynamic as the riots of 1966–67 and the mass demonstrations of 1989. The demonstrations of July 2003, which saw over half a million protestors fill the streets as they marched from Victoria Park to the Government offices in Central, marked a fundamental shift in local politics. For the first time, a major demonstration was motivated primarily by events inside Hong Kong and focused on the need for changes locally. The demonstrations resulted in the resignations of both the Financial Secretary and the Secretary for Security; the significant amendment, then postponement of Article 23 legislation; and the replacement of Dr. Yeoh as chair of the Government's post-SARS enquiry. As has been shown, the linkages between these events extend beyond their chronological proximity.

The mainland played a secondary, though crucial role in these political developments both as the source of SARS and by failing to provide information about the disease at an early stage, thereby contributing to its rapid spread. The SARS outbreak created a medical emergency and public health disaster that completely permeated Hong Kong's social consciousness at all levels of income and education. On the mainland and in Hong Kong, it played a key role in driving home the connection between freedom of the press and the need for transparency and accountability in Government. What had once been abstract and rather remote issues of interest to a small number of people suddenly became important matters of life and death for everyone.

Hong Kong people realised that passage of the proposed Article 23 legislation posed a direct threat to their personal health and well-being, not just a few of their freedoms or political rights. The myth that Hong Kongers are politically apathetic and politically uninformed was proven false yet again when hundreds of thousands of people took to the streets on 1 July. Public reactions to SARS and to Article 23 became linked not just in timing, but also in substance. The criticisms of the Government generated by one issue fed into, echoed and ultimately reinforced criticisms generated by the second. Taken together, SARS and Article 23 convinced a majority of the public that their health, safety and freedom could only be assured by reform of Hong Kong's political structure. The District Council elections in November 2003 and the LegCo elections in September 2004 will register in unmistakable terms the joint impact of SARS and Article 23 on attitudes toward the Tung Government and its political supporters.

Examining the interaction between the Government and people of Hong Kong during the SARS crisis provides valuable lessons in crisis management in and of itself, but understanding the SARS crisis in the context of its critical role as a contributor to a fundamental shift in relations between the Government and the public will reveal that SARS did far more than scare officials and administrators into implementing much-needed public health and health management reforms. SARS has triggered a series of far-reaching reactions and repercussions, the full impact of which remains unclear. In this sense, SARS is a case study of how structural problems within Government and structural weaknesses in the relations between Governments are disasters in waiting that need only the wrong circumstances to become manifest. SARS revealed weaknesses in the "one country, two systems" framework that are now leading to changes in the relationship between Hong Kong and its immediate hinterlands in the Pearl River Delta and Guangdong Province. The outbreak is thus a crucial episode in the ongoing transition of Hong Kong from its status as an isolated colonial enclave in 1982, when negotiations over its return to China began, to its ultimate, and as yet unrealised, destination as a Special Administrative Region ruled by Hong Kong people with a high degree of autonomy and with election of both LegCo and the Chief Executive based on universal suffrage.

SARS, a disease that struck down those with weak immune systems, also revealed the weaknesses and dangers within the SAR system. This chapter is thus a story of weak systems, one might say "poor constitutions," struck by a disease that threatened to be a massive disaster, but which, if experiences are taken to heart and the lessons learned lead to real reforms, may in the end prevent far worse disasters to both our personal and political constitutions.

Is SARS a crisis waiting to reappear? If so, what will the public reaction be? If Tung defends those who may be found guilty of neglect or maladministration by the now-independent Government enquiry, he will lose any political gains he has made in accepting the resignation of Leung and Ip and delaying the vote on Article 23. The problem of Tung's continued loyalty to those who cannot perform is not addressed by the current political structure and may not have been resolved in his own mind. The release of the SARS report will be a critical test of whether these structural and personality flaws can be corrected. SARS has left the Tung Government with a stark choice: reform now, or risk political death when the next disaster strikes, especially if, as with the SARS crisis, it does so when our attention is elsewhere and at a moment when our system is already under severe stress.

CHAPTER 9

The Politics of SARS:
The WHO, Hong Kong and Mainland China

Christine Loh

The lifting of the World Health Organisation (WHO) travel advisory for Hong Kong on 23 May 2003 caught everyone by surprise. Ever since late February the SARS outbreak had almost completely taken over daily life. There was a sense that although things might take on the appearance of normality again soon enough, in fact the ground had shifted under Hong Kong's feet. As SARS roared through Hong Kong, it forced the city to evaluate the readiness of its institutions to deal with infectious disease — an issue that had received little real attention despite recent warning signs. During the avian flu outbreak in 1997, over a million birds had to be slaughtered. What most people seemed to have forgotten was that the avian flu affected humans as well, although there were only 18 cases of the disease. The 1997 outbreak was caused by a new influenza virus that had jumped from chickens to humans. Fortunately, the virus (named "H5N1") was unable to transmit easily from person to person. Those who became inflected, however, became very ill, resulting in six deaths.[1] The avian flu returned in 1999, but the outbreak soon passed and Hong Kong lapsed back into complacency.

In 2003, SARS left a much more permanent mark on Hong Kong's consciousness. Next time — and there could well be a next time — the city will have to be more prepared to meet the assault. The WHO's Dr. Henk Bekedam warned that it is not enough to be 100% ready;

authorities "need to be 300% ready for SARS."[2] Experts have said that even if they find a vaccine for SARS, other new infectious diseases may be lurking.

But in the final analysis, the international community has much to be grateful for in Hong Kong's handling of SARS. The situation could have been much worse for both China and the world had Hong Kong been less open about the disease or the severity of the outbreak (see Chapter 10). One unexpected outcome of SARS is that Hong Kong now sees itself more clearly as part of the neighbourhood of Guangdong Province. Furthermore, it has also become more evident that Hong Kong is an integral part of China, although it functions as a Special Administrative Region (SAR). Indeed, the SARS experience indicated the extent of the difference between institutional instincts and habits in Hong Kong and on the mainland. Behavioural differences between Guangdong and Beijing were also apparent.

The challenge now is to ensure that Hong Kong's normal practice of transparency continues and is viewed in a positive and not a threatening light on the mainland, so that the authorities in both areas benefit. It should be blindingly clear to Beijing that its customary obsession with secrecy was the primary cause of the worldwide SARS crisis. As a member of the global community, Beijing is expected to abide by a standard of behaviour that does not condone hiding information.

Calm after the storm

When the WHO global alert regarding travel to Hong Kong was put in place on 2 April, Hong Kong was thrown into confusion. Hong Kong officials obviously failed to see it coming.[3] Only that morning the then Deputy Director of Health, Dr. PY Lam, had stated in a radio interview that: "The International Regulations of the WHO stipulate that an area would only be declared as infected in the case of discovery of cholera, yellow fever or plague…The regulations do not include atypical pneumonia, and Hong Kong therefore will not be declared as infected according to this mechanism."[4] As early as 16 March, the WHO did designate Hong Kong as a SARS "affected area."[5] The difference between an "affected" and an "infected" area was unclear, but the travel advisory was clear enough — don't go there.

Similarly, the Government did not know until the very last minute on 23 May that the WHO recommendation to avoid non-essential travel to Hong Kong would be lifted. The local media was sure of the news only after 4 p.m. Hong Kong time when the international news agency Reuters reported that the advisory had been lifted. Hong Kong's label as a SARS "affected" area was finally lifted on 23 June following the absence of any new cases for 20 consecutive days.[6]

The effect of the WHO label was to transform one of the world's favourite holiday destinations into a no man's land. Not only did the usual hordes of business travellers and holiday visitors stay away, people travelling from Hong Kong were unwelcome elsewhere. Hong Kong people felt as if they had become lepers overnight. Even at home, residents stopped doing what they were famous for — eating out and shopping. On 23 May, the happy news that the travel advisory had been lifted spread quickly through the community. People felt as though they could resume normal life again for the first time in almost two months. Hong Kong officials hastily put together a press conference to express relief at the lifting of the advisory and the continued vigilance of the Government against SARS. Then Financial Secretary Antony Leung even stage-managed a night out in the popular Lan Kwai Fong district that evening for drinks. It was smiles all round.

And yet only days before, Government sources indicated that the travel advisory was unlikely to be lifted before June, possibly as late as mid-June. This may not seem like a long time — but after schools had remained shut for weeks, restaurants were almost empty for days on end, inbound and outbound travel was cut back to a minimum, businesses closed down due to lack of custom and when people felt insecure about the risks involved in the most basic aspects of daily life — it felt like an eternity. It was unimaginable that the situation had gotten so out of hand.

The Hong Kong Government saw the travel advisory as a major setback because it damaged the city's international reputation. Authorities recognised that turning the situation around would require more effective control of the number of infections. The healthcare system was still trying desperately to cope with the rising number of cases, which finally peaked in Hong Kong on 17 April.

Pressure from the business community for Hong Kong authorities to do more about getting the advisory lifted began to mount. Four days after meeting with WHO officials on 3 May,[7] Secretary for Health, Welfare and Food Dr. Yeoh Eng-kiong spelled out the exact criteria for the lifting of the advisory: 1) the number of new SARS cases had to fall below five per day while the overall number of active cases could not exceed 60; 2) there should be no "export" of cases to other countries from Hong Kong; and 3) the mode of transmission for each case should be understood, meaning that there could be no "surprise" cases beyond the group of people who had already been traced as contacts of existing patients and their families.[8]

On 7 May, Hong Kong had already fulfilled the second criterion. However, the number of SARS patients in hospital was almost 500, 70 of whom were in intensive care — even though the number of new cases had fallen to single digits several days earlier. By the end of the second week in May, the number of new cases had fallen to below five a day for several days, and health authorities had a good understanding of the transmission mode for local SARS cases. Nevertheless, Hong Kong still had nearly 400 SARS patients in hospital.

Dr. Yeoh argued that Hong Kong might have over-counted the number of cases, noting that under the WHO's definition of SARS, anyone with atypical pneumonia who visited a SARS-affected area could be considered a SARS suspect. Since Hong Kong had already been designated as an affected area, he said, many atypical pneumonia cases that were not caused by the SARS-coronavirus might have been wrongly classified, simply on the basis of association. He emphasised that the Hospital Authority (HA), which manages all of Hong Kong's public hospitals, would do further laboratory tests to see how many of the reported cases were actually due to the coronavirus. On 13 May, he noted that the results of serology tests (used to detect the presence of antibodies or antigens) for cases that could not be linked to a known exposure source indicated that 52 percent of these cases were negative for the coronavirus, meaning that over half were not SARS cases. At the same time, Dr. Yeoh also highlighted the fact that Hong Kong was keeping its SARS patients in hospital for an additional week after recovery in order to minimise the risk of spreading the disease. He urged the WHO to take these factors into account in assessing whether to lift the travel advisory.

Dr. Yeoh also let it be known that the WHO was monitoring the situation in mainland China closely and made it clear that the WHO's decision regarding the travel advisory could not be divorced from events happening across the border, which were beyond the control of Hong Kong's health authorities. The advisory was ultimately lifted after vigorous lobbying by China during the first day of the WHO's fifty-sixth World

Health Assembly on 19 May in Geneva. The Chinese Government sent Vice Premier Wu Yi, China's new Minister of Health, to accompany Dr. Yeoh to Switzerland. Together, they were able to provide more technical information about the situation in Hong Kong and restate arguments for the lifting of the advisory in a high profile forum.[9]

SARS and the WHO

On 11 February 2003, the Chinese Ministry of Health officially informed the WHO of an outbreak of atypical pneumonia in Guangdong Province that had resulted in 305 cases and five deaths, affecting mainly healthcare workers and their families. On the following day, China informed the WHO that the outbreak in Guangdong had affected six municipalities. On 14 February, the Ministry of Health reported that similar cases had in fact been detected in Guangdong as far back as 16 November 2002. On 18 February, the WHO received a report from Hong Kong authorities that two people, a father and son, who had visited Fujian Province and travelled through Guangdong on their return to Hong Kong had contracted the H5N1 flu. The daughter of the family had also contracted the disease and died while in Fujian, where she was buried.[10] The WHO immediately demanded more information from the Ministry of Health about what was happening and whether there appeared to be any linkage between the Guangdong outbreak and the two cases in Hong Kong. The WHO also offered its help to China in combating the outbreak.

At the same time, the new disease was becoming an international cause célèbre. On 26 February, authorities in Vietnam informed the WHO of a case of an atypical pneumonia in Hanoi — within five days 22 hospital workers had come down with the same symptoms.[11] The WHO also began to receive reports from Hong Kong that similar outbreaks were occurring there. It was increasingly apparent that something new was taking place. On 12 March, the WHO issued a global alert to inform international health authorities that a new and unidentified disease had emerged in Asia.[12] The following day, Singapore reported three cases among people who had recently visited Hong Kong. Two days later, Singapore reported another 13 cases. On the same day, Thailand reported one case imported from Hanoi.

By 14 March it was clear that the disease had spread beyond Asia. Canada had reported seven cases, including two deaths. The cases occurred in two separate family clusters and in both clusters, at least one family member had visited Hong Kong within a week of developing symptoms. At 2 a.m. on 15 March, the Singapore Government notified the WHO urgently that a physician who had treated cases of atypical pneumonia in Singapore had travelled to New York for a conference with several colleagues and would be landing in Frankfurt on his way back to Singapore. After a series of discussions at the WHO, it was decided that these passengers should be removed from their flight upon landing and placed immediately in hospital isolation in Germany to minimise the risk of infection.[13] On 15 March, the WHO issued a general emergency travel advisory warning travellers to be aware of the new disease if they were leaving Asia and instructing them to seek medical care should they become sick with flu-like symptoms.[14]

The WHO feared that the world was facing a dangerous and unknown disease. The lack of any real information about it meant that the WHO had no idea of the potential health risks. It was also clear that healthcare workers were at particular risk. The concern was that the new disease could be caused by something that had breached the barrier from animals to humans and could move from human to human, creating the potential for a world pandemic. Virologists were already aware that high population densities, the close proximity of humans and animals and intensive animal husbandry in Guangdong may allow viruses to cross the barrier between beast and man more easily in this part of the world.[15] By putting out a second alert on 15 March — in which the name "severe acute respiratory syndrome" or "SARS" was used for the first time — the WHO wanted to ensure that governments understood that the disease was spreading quickly across national borders and that they needed to put in place procedures to prevent outbreaks in their own countries.

On 17 March, the WHO stepped up activities to strengthen the international response to SARS. Its Global Outbreak Alert and Response Network (GOARN), established in 1998, began coordination with the world's top microbiology research centres to identify the cause of SARS. GOARN works by sifting through credible reports of new disease outbreaks around the world to decide which require further investigation, by governments or by other agencies, and whether any are worrisome enough to warrant sending an investigation team. The network did pick up early signs that something was happening in Guangdong but believed it was just a bad flu epidemic.[16]

On 19 March, the WHO praised Hong Kong for its excellent

detective work in retracing the steps of seven people who contracted SARS — they had all recently stayed in or visited the Metropole Hotel between 12 February and 3 March. Extraordinarily, on the same day, China's then health minister, Zhang Wenkang, told the WHO that the outbreak in Hong Kong might have nothing to do with events in Guangdong.[17] By 25 March, 487 SARS cases had been reported in a dozen countries. A day later, Chinese authorities updated their figures for the Guangdong outbreak: between 16 November and 28 February, there had in fact been a total of 792 cases and 31 deaths.

On 27 March, the WHO urged the governments of the affected jurisdictions to screen passengers at their airports, using a series of questions to identify sick passengers. As of 29 March, the total number of reported cases worldwide had risen to 1,550, including 54 deaths in 13 countries. On the same day, a WHO communicable disease expert, Dr. Carlo Urbani, died in Thailand. Dr. Urbani was the first doctor to recognise the emergence of the new disease in Hanoi, where he treated Vietnam's first SARS case in February. On 1 April, the cumulative world total of SARS cases hit 1,804, with 62 deaths in 15 countries. The only comfort was that while the situation was serious, SARS was not the disease that virologists had feared — although highly infectious, it was much less so than the ordinary flu, indicating that the causative agent could not move easily from person to person. Perhaps the dreaded pandemic would not happen after all.

Still, air travel meant that SARS was spreading very quickly. The general travel alerts issued in March were effective in notifying governments to take precautions but did not stop international travel out of Asia. That was about to change. On 2 April, the WHO felt compelled to make a specific travel recommendation — something it had never done before:

> The SARS situation in Hong Kong has developed features of concern: a continuing and significant increase in cases with indications that SARS has spread beyond the initial focus in hospitals. These developments have suggested environmental routes of transmission from a SARS infected person which may be related to contamination of common systems that link rooms or flats together.[18]

The WHO recommended that people postpone non-essential travel to Hong Kong. This recommendation reflected what the WHO knew was happening in the city — that identified individuals who had travelled out of Hong Kong had carried and spread the disease to other places, and that the outbreak at Amoy Gardens indicated that some as yet unknown environmental factor beyond close personal contact might play a role in the transfer of the virus from person to person (see Chapter 7). The WHO also issued an advisory that travellers should avoid Guangdong, not because of what it knew but because of what it did not know.[19] Despite the reports provided by the Chinese authorities, the WHO felt that there was much more that China was not telling.

By May, the WHO listed Vietnam, Toronto, Singapore, Manila, Hong Kong, Guangdong, Beijing, Hebei, Inner Mongolia, Shanxi, Tianjin and Taiwan as SARS "affected areas" and had issued travel advisories for a number of these areas. This had the effect of limiting regional and international travel to and from Asia as a whole. Complaints began to surface that the WHO advisories reflected a poor sense of perspective. Critics noted that the travel recommendations turned entire cities and regions into a "no man's land." They highlighted the fact that SARS was not the epidemic that the WHO had feared, claiming that the way it had handled matters had contributed to a pandemic of unwarranted fear. Many regions were already suffering severe economic consequences as a result. Economically, SARS could not have come at a worse time, just as Asian economies were beginning to recover from the financial crisis of 1997–1999.

Did the WHO overdo it? The case against the WHO may be summarised thus:

> Several of the WHO travel warnings have bordered on the absurd. The warning on Vietnam was particularly bizarre given that there were just 63 reported cases and five deaths in a country of 81 million…The WHO doesn't seem to understand that it has the potential to do enormous damage to business and economies. The cavalier slapping-on of travel warnings by bureaucrats for little reason other than to be seen to be doing something dramatic is self-indulgent. Thousands of people in Asia will lose their jobs and many businesses will close, not because of SARS but because of SARS-induced hysteria…SARS itself has done little damage to Asia's economies. The same cannot be said of the hysteria that has accompanied the disease. For this, the WHO bears a good dose of the blame.[20]

The WHO is not new to controversy. In the 1990s, it was accused of being slow off the mark in responding to the global threat of HIV/AIDS, and for failing to stand up to the pharmaceutical industry to secure cheap drugs for the poor in the developing world. In 2000, the WHO was also accused of politicising its global rankings of health systems, where Colombia was the top-ranked country, with Canada in thirtieth place and the US coming thirty-seventh. Countries above this included Djibouti, Costa Rica, Oman, Morocco and Slovenia. These countries scored well because they spent a larger proportion of public funds on health — but critics argued that the WHO criteria failed to account for the actual state of health care in the country.[21]

In the case of SARS, it is hard to fault the WHO for leaning on the side of caution when there was a risk that the new virus might spread easily via air travel. The WHO regarded SARS as the first new disease of the twenty-first century to have international reach. Although other infectious diseases, such as the Ebola virus, created a demand for help on a national level in containing the disease, they did not pose a threat to the rest of the world. The WHO also felt that if it had not issued travel recommendations, countries around the world would have issued their own national advisories.[22]

However, there were two controversies that marred the otherwise solid performance record of the WHO during the SARS outbreak. In both instances, the WHO allowed political considerations to be placed ahead of public health considerations. The first concerned Toronto and the second Taiwan.

As the outbreak in Toronto continued to grow in magnitude and began to affect individuals outside of the initial risk group of hospital workers, their families and other close person-to-person contacts, the WHO issued a travel advisory for the city on 23 April. Although the WHO initially stated that it would review the travel advisory for Toronto in three weeks, it then lifted the advisory on 14 May after local and national political heavyweights, including prime minister Jean Chretien, pressured the WHO to withdrew the advisory on the basis that its decision had been factually unsound as the number of SARS cases in the city was subsiding. As part of their argument for the lifting of the travel advisory, Canadian officials gave assurances to the WHO that they would intensify screening of travellers to prevent the export of the disease from Toronto. In lifting the recommendation, the WHO's director general, Gro Harlem Brundtland, noted that the magnitude of probable cases had decreased, 20 days had passed since the last community transmission had occurred and that no new confirmed cases had been exported.[23] Furthermore, on 14 May, the WHO removed Toronto from the list of areas with recent local transmission altogether.[24] These decisions were controversial even within the WHO itself. Dr. Hitoshi Oshitani, the WHO representative in the Western Pacific Regional Office in Manila, indicated his concern.[25] The issue was rekindled on 23 May when Toronto reported new suspected cases.[26] On 26 May, Toronto was re-added to the list of areas with recent local SARS transmission[27] and by 4 June, more than 70 new cases had been reported.[28] On 10 June a SARS case was reported to have been exported to the United States.[29] During the second outbreak, 5,000 people were placed under "home quarantine" including 1,500 high school students. Despite extensive investigations by the Canadian authorities, the "exact chain of events leading to the second wave of the SARS outbreak remains a mystery."[30] Did the WHO's flip-flop decision-making encourage the Toronto authorities to ease up on preventative measures too soon?

The second WHO-related controversy during the SARS outbreak concerned Taiwan, which, since 1971, has made seven unsuccessful attempts to rejoin the WHO, even as an observer, over objections from Beijing. Beijing insists that Taiwan is an "inalienable" part of China and should therefore not be recognised as an individual entity. When SARS struck, Taiwan's 23 million people were effectively cut off from the WHO's information network, although much of the information was available on-line and Taiwan was able to work with the US Centers for Disease Control (CDC). When Taiwan asked the WHO for help during the outbreak, it did not respond. As Taiwan mounted yet another campaign to be allowed observer status at the WHO, China's Minister of Health Zhang Wenkang reiterated Beijing's longstanding position: "We hope that the leaders of the Taiwan authority no longer spread rumours with ulterior motives, or even use the disease as an excuse and in the name of human rights to try to enter the World Health Organization, which is only opened to sovereign nations."[31] When the WHO's executive director for communicable diseases, Dr. David Heymann, was asked at a press conference whether the WHO's avoidance of direct contact with Taiwan on SARS was due to "political factors," Dr. Heymann replied: "Your question is a reply in itself."[32]

After the number of infections in Taiwan surged in late April, the WHO finally sent a team of two experts on 3 May with the consent of Beijing but made no public statements regarding the visit, likely out of deference to Beijing's sensitivities.[33] On 8 May, the WHO placed a travel advisory on Taipei. Taiwan could not attend the WHO's fifty-sixth World

Health Assembly in Geneva in May where SARS was a prominent topic of discussion, although there was considerable international sympathy for Taiwan as the number of infections there continued to rise.[34] During the assembly, the WHO saw fit to extend the travel advisory to the whole of Taiwan. World sentiments were not lost on Beijing, which appeared to have softened its position sufficiently to enable the WHO to invite Taiwan to attend its Global Conference on SARS in Kuala Lumpur on 17 and 18 June — the first time in 30 years that Taiwan had been invited to a WHO event. Yet controversy arose again when the WHO invited a Taiwan legislator who was on good terms with Beijing but not nominated by the Taiwanese authorities. There is widespread belief that the invitation was issued at Beijing's behest.[35]

Beijing's response

After the WHO placed a travel advisory on Hong Kong and Guangdong on 2 April Beijing began to take the situation more seriously. Only then did Premier Wen Jiabao set up a working group led by Minister of Health Zhang Wenkang to control SARS. Up until the end of March, Beijing was preoccupied with the change in national leadership at the highest level of government, an event of extraordinary importance in the history of the People's Republic of China. It was only in November 2002 at the sixteenth Communist Party conference, a meeting held every five years, that the new Politburo, the Party's most senior decision-making body, was formed. The next major event on the political agenda was the tenth National People's Congress in March 2003, when the country's top government officials would be chosen. Thus, between November 2002 and March 2003, Beijing's attention was focused on preparing for the transfer of power to a new generation of leaders (see Chapters 8 and 10).

The mainland's political tradition is that nothing can go wrong during such sensitive times. As late as 27 March, Long Yongtu, the chief negotiator for China's accession to the World Trade Organization (WTO) and a well-known figure internationally, criticised the Hong Kong media for not providing "more balanced" coverage of SARS. He complained that the media showed a lack of social responsibility in publishing reports that could cause social panic and economic losses.[36] On the mainland, China's Propaganda Department prevented the state-run media from reporting on the SARS outbreak, even though WHO officials were already sitting in Beijing breathing down the necks of the authorities. Beijing could have used the National People's Congress to make information about SARS available to regional and municipal authorities — it would have been the perfect event to alert the entire nation. The lost opportunity was something Beijing would come to regret.

For the rest of the world, Long's remark was the final straw. It was a clear sign of China's irresponsibility at a time when many cities around the world were battling SARS. Beijing became the focus of an international uproar. The new Chinese Government suddenly found itself facing a crisis of global proportions. Beijing finally permitted WHO experts to visit Guangdong on 3 April. The WHO had made it clear for some time that it wanted to visit the southern province where SARS originated in order to examine conditions there.[37] President Hu Jintao visited Guangdong over the weekend of 12–14 April to be briefed directly about the situation in Guangdong and Hong Kong. He met Hong Kong's Chief Executive Tung Chee-hwa in Shenzhen on 12 April together with the director of the Hong Kong and Macau Affairs Office, Liao Hui; party secretaries for Guangdong and Shenzhen, Zhang Dejiang and Huang Liman; Guangdong's governor Huang Huahua as well as Shenzhen's mayor, Yu Youjun.

On 17 April, 22 weeks after the start of the SARS outbreak in Guangdong, the Politburo finally took a public stand on the issue, stating that "leaders and cadres at all levels should have an accurate account of the epidemic situation, faithfully reporting to the public on a regular basis…There should be no delay in reporting, and no cover-ups."[38] The day before, the WHO had publicly criticised China for failing to provide more accurate reporting on the SARS outbreak and questioned the validity of data on the reported number of cases. On 20 April, Beijing fired health minister Zhang for his poor handling of the SARS crisis, as well as Beijing city mayor Meng Xuenong,[39] as the number of cases in Beijing continued to rise. Meng's superior, Liu Qi, who is the party official in charge of the capital city and a Politburo member, also gave a public apology for his own failure to keep the public informed about the outbreak. Zhang's job went to Vice Premier Wu Yi, a highly popular official and the most senior woman in Chinese political circles.

Beijing clearly realised it also needed to do serious damage control on an international level. Premier Wen used the Special ASEAN-China Leaders' Meeting in Bangkok on 29 April as an opportunity to deliver

China's mea culpa. He stated that China would leave no stone unturned in preventing the spread of SARS, pledging that "the Chinese Government is here in a spirit of candour, responsibility, trust and cooperation."[40]

Central-provincial-Hong Kong relations

The administrative structure linking China's central and provincial authorities becomes evident when retracing the steps Guangdong took to inform Beijing about the SARS outbreak.

Doctors in Guangdong began to see increasing numbers of patients with flu-like symptoms in November 2002. Initially, authorities paid no special attention to the situation. In southern China many people tend to fall ill at this time of year due to the change in seasons. It was only as the condition of some patients continued to worsen that doctors realised they were dealing with something out of the ordinary. Local authorities set up an investigative team at the end of December after a case of unusual flu was reported in Heyuan. The deputy director of the Guangzhou Institute of Respiratory Diseases, Xiao Zhenglun, who headed the team, went to Heyuan to investigate. He noted that: "When we arrived in Heyuan, the city was already in chaos… the city leader was of the opinion that we should not report the case because it could spread more fear, but I said we had to inform the authorities in Beijing."[41]

The team also went to Zhongshan after a case surfaced there on 17 January. By then, team members had recognised that the isolation of patients was necessary to stop the spread of what appeared to be a highly infectious disease. They had also identified the likely index case: a cook specialising in exotic meat dishes, who fell ill on 16 November 2002 in Foshan. Xiao prepared a detailed report for the Guangdong Department of Health describing these findings, which he marked "top secret" and submitted on 23 January.[42] The report apparently remained unread for several days because there was no one with sufficient security clearance to open it. When it was finally opened, the information was supposedly sent to various regional authorities in Guangdong as well as to Beijing. Subsequently, the Guangdong Department of Health circulated guidelines urging hospitals to watch for patients with symptoms of the new disease and to treat these cases with extra caution.[43]

On 3 February, Guangdong health authorities issued another circular on the control and prevention of the disease, listing the criteria for clinical diagnosis, control and laboratory work.[44] A full report was prepared for Huang Huahua, the provincial governor, on 7 February. On 8 February, Guangdong made a formal report to Beijing on the outbreak of atypical pneumonia and asked the central authorities to visit Guangdong. A team from Beijing was dispatched on the same day.[45] Subsequently, scientists from the national Centre for Disease Control (CDC) in Beijing visited Guangdong several times to assess the situation. Thus, by the time that the Guangzhou Bureau of Health held a press conference on 10 February about the new disease, the fact of its existence was already known locally and had been brought to the attention of the Central People's Government and the Chinese Communist Party in Beijing.

China's Ministry of Health in turn reported the Guangdong outbreak to the WHO on 11, 12 and 14 February but then did little else for some time. The WHO flew a team to Beijing on 15 February, although Chinese officials prevented team members from reviewing data till 28 February,[46] by which time it was clear that the disease had spread not only to Hong Kong but also Hanoi. On 18 February, the CDC reported that it had identified *Chlamydia pneumoniae* as the probable cause of the atypical pneumonia outbreak in Guangdong.

On 9 March, the Guangdong Provincial Medical Bureau issued specific guidelines on the treatment of atypical pneumonia for all hospitals, setting out three sets of criteria for the diagnosis of the disease in adults, children and critically ill patients and outlining ten proposed therapies. On 27 March, more guidelines were issued for disease prevention and control in schools and kindergartens and in public places. Guangdong had a clear interest in controlling SARS as soon as possible in view of the fact that the annual Guangzhou Trade Fair was scheduled for mid-April 2003.

When a WHO expert team was finally permitted to visit Guangdong on 3 April, it found that "the health system in Guangdong responded well to the outbreak…The province had a health system in which every hospital at every level reports any new cases of SARS."[47] Dr. Robert F. Breiman noted that the number of local SARS cases was decreasing and that local doctors had gained much experience in treating patients.[48] In an interim report on 9 April, the WHO credited Guangdong authorities with realising early on that they were dealing with a new disease. Dr. Bekedam noted on 29 April that the WHO "really felt that in all aspects the Guangdong team was doing quite well and that they were getting to grips with the outbreak."[49]

The first SARS case in Beijing surfaced on 5 March — the first day of the National People's Congress. Had central authorities chosen to pay attention to the news from Guangdong and WHO warnings, they could have already been preparing to deal with SARS in the capital and in other provinces. The WHO's interim report of 9 April was critical of the handling of the disease in the capital and noted the overall ill-preparedness of municipal authorities. On the same day that the interim report was released, a retired military doctor, Jiang Yanyong, alerted international reporters that SARS cases being treated in Beijing's military hospitals had been excluded from the official count. He accused the Chinese Government of covering up the extent of the outbreak. Jiang was the former director of surgery at Army Hospital 301 where top officials were treated. He told the media that he could no longer keep silent after former colleagues had told him that they were treating 60 SARS patients, while seven had already died. He was upset that Minister of Health Zhang had underplayed the situation: "I couldn't believe what I was hearing. As a doctor who cares about people's lives and health, I have a responsibility to aid international and local efforts to prevent the spread of SARS."[50] Jiang turned out to be right — city officials had lied about the number of SARS cases in Beijing.

Hong Kong's reaction

In a report to the Legislative Council (LegCo) on 13 June, Hong Kong's Deputy Director of Health, Leung Pak-yin, stated that Hong Kong authorities were not provided with any direct information about the new disease by the mainland until the Guangdong press conference on 10 February. Secretary for Health, Welfare and Food Dr. Yeoh later added that: "The [Hong Kong] Government had been in contact with health authorities in Beijing and Guangdong province, but we have direct communication with Beijing only... we can only react to whatever information the mainland chooses to give us."[51] The SARS Expert Committee report released on 2 October 2003 makes it clear that the

Hong Kong Department of Health tried unsuccessfully to contact authorities in Guangzhou and Guangdong Province on 10 February to inquire about news reports of an outbreak of atypical pneumonia. Hong Kong authorities then sought assistance from the Ministry of Health in Beijing. On the same day, the Guangzhou Bureau of Health held a press conference to inform the public about the outbreak, but ignored Hong Kong's request for information.[52] This sequence of events is indicative of Hong Kong's passive approach to interaction with the mainland. Chief Executive Tung Chee-hwa did not comment on events across the border and from Dr. Yeoh's comments, it would appear that he failed to take a proactive stance in obtaining information about the Guangdong outbreak.

During his meeting with Tung in Shenzhen on 12 April, President Hu said that the Central People's Government would provide "full support" to Hong Kong by delivering medical supplies and backup. When Tung met Premier Wen in Bangkok at the end of April at the ASEAN meeting to discuss SARS, the offer was repeated. Upon his return to Hong Kong, Tung noted that: "After considering the situation and deliberating with my colleagues, I forwarded to the Central Government a request for the supply of protective outfits, facemasks and goggles and the deployment of medical workers. The Central Government promptly acceded, and Wen Jiabao specifically instructed that Hong Kong should be supplied with top quality medical supplies in the quantities required, and that all costs of such supplies and any future manpower support should be borne by the Central Government."[53]

While it would have made more sense for wealthy Hong Kong to source and provide protective gear for the mainland, this would have been politically incorrect, as largesse must flow from the politically powerful centre to the periphery, and not the reverse. When Tung went to Shenzhen to receive the first consignment of supplies on 8 May, he said that he had "mixed feelings" because the mainland also had an urgent demand for such products. However, he stated that: "These supplies also boost our spirits." That was precisely what the episode was intended to showcase — that the mainland cared about Hong Kong. Tung and his advisors may also have felt that this display of solidarity and support from mainland authorities was necessary in addressing local criticism for Beijing's initial cover-up of SARS, which contributed significantly to the outbreak in Hong Kong.

Hong Kong-mainland relations

The SARS epidemic provides an illustration of how Hong Kong and mainland authorities, especially those in Beijing and Guangdong, perceive and interpret their relationship. This issue remains the subject of considerable discussion and debate following on from the signing of the Sino-British Joint Declaration in 1984, when Britain agreed that sovereignty over Hong Kong would revert to China in 1997. The situation is indeed unique. In the 1984 declaration, China accepted that Hong Kong would continue to function as a separate system within the jurisdiction of the Chinese state and that a national policy of "one country, two systems" would be applied for 50 years after 1997. In addition to the treaty between Britain and China that codified this arrangement, Hong Kong also received its own constitution — the Basic Law — which fleshed out details of how Hong Kong would function with "a high degree of autonomy" from the Central People's Government in Beijing. As a measure of reassurance, the Central People's Government also made clear prior to 1997 that it would not allow provincial authorities to interfere in the affairs of Hong Kong. Thus, one function of the Hong Kong and Macau Affairs Office, an arm of China's cabinet, the State Council, was to prevent potential provincial meddling post-1997. This policy had the effect of limiting direct communication between Hong Kong and provincial authorities, most of which was funnelled through the medium of the central authorities in Beijing.

Four sets of issues related to this policy became apparent during the SARS crisis. First, by sheltering Hong Kong, the central authorities also prevented it from developing relations with the provinces, particularly its immediate neighbour Guangdong, meaning that ties between Hong Kong and other parts of China remain weak. This has not helped to create the bilateral conditions necessary for sorting out many issues of mutual interest, such as the development of the area connecting Hong Kong, Macau and the most urban parts of Guangdong, a region commonly referred to as the Pearl River Delta. Second, it has taken longer than expected for Hong Kong officials to understand how to deal with a variety of mainland institutions and issues since serious learning started only after 1997. The systemic separation of Hong Kong from the mainland has blocked a more open approach by all parties concerned. Third, and even more critically, Hong Kong officials were not hard-headed enough to understand that the culture of secrecy on the mainland meant that Hong Kong would have to develop its capacity for mainland-watching to a high level. Understanding how things operate on the mainland is crucial in enabling Hong Kong to find its own way of dealing with difficult situations and issues. Rather than ignoring such situations, or worse, to feel that addressing them is somehow "unpatriotic," Hong Kong needs to improve its own capacity for deciphering what is actually happening across the border. Fourth, despite efforts on the part of the Central People's Government to provide reassurance regarding Hong Kong's autonomous status, awkward questions remain — how does a capitalist, open and free society fit into a socialist state that does not have a free media and has no tradition of transparency or the rule of law? The fundamental differences between the two systems continue to prompt questions about whether Hong Kong really enjoys autonomy or whether Beijing in fact pulls the strings from behind the scenes.

Hong Kong had the capability to be better prepared for SARS as it has a good health system. When it became obvious that Hong Kong needed to operate at a higher level of preparedness, it was able to trace contacts quickly, implement isolation and quarantine arrangements, put health checks in place at border points and develop an on-line e-SARS database within a short time. However, despite these demonstrations of its capabilities, Hong Kong was slow to tackle SARS because health officials did not foresee that the city could be shut down by an infectious disease. The Hospital Authority (HA), the statutory body that manages Hong Kong's public hospitals, also failed to be more proactive in warning the hospitals and healthcare workers under its management to be on high alert. While a Working Group on Severe Community-acquired Pneumonia was set up as early as 11 February, not enough was done to inform hospitals and healthcare workers about the situation or how to deal with infectious diseases.

The SARS crisis created an urgent need for Hong Kong to work intensively with Guangdong authorities as well as with Beijing, providing valuable and much-needed opportunities for collaboration. Despite the many economic ties between Guangdong and Hong Kong, it took a disease to draw them closer together. SARS made it blindingly clear to authorities on both sides that they existed in the same neighbourhood and that it was important to be good neighbours if both were to flourish. Prior to SARS, relations between Guangdong and Hong Kong had a competitive edge.[54] Nearly six years after Hong Kong's reunification with China, there were still many gaps in developing lines of communication and cooperation with Guangdong and other mainland entities. On 11 April, Hong Kong and Guangdong reached a groundbreaking agreement to exchange information about disease, cooperate on medical issues, create a disease notification system and set up a border quarantine. No doubt agreement was made easier and quicker by President Hu Jintao's visit to Guangdong. After all, Guangdong is China's greatest export earner and Hong Kong is China's richest city — Hu knew that China needed to minimise the damage to trade and investments caused by SARS.

The case of Shanghai

During the peak of the mainland SARS outbreak, many questions were raised regarding the reasons for Shanghai's very low infection rate. The city had its first SARS case on 27 March, which was reported to the municipal authorities on 31 March. The WHO's Henk Bekedam noted that: "I think [Shanghai authorities] were lucky that their first case was not a super-spreader and...the Shanghai health system is most likely quite a lot stronger than Beijing and some of the other provinces."[55]

It would appear that in addition to having good luck, Shanghai authorities also worked hard on prevention. In mid-February, as SARS was causing public panic in Guangdong, health officials in Shanghai took note and started to develop a contingency plan for the city. By mid-March, when Hong Kong had already been badly hit by SARS, Shanghai had already established an Atypical Pneumonia Monitoring and Prevention Office under the auspices of the Shanghai Centre for Disease Control (CDC). Shanghai authorities were on high alert at a time when the rest of China was still in denial.

By 19 March, Shanghai had put out its own diagnostic criteria for SARS and by 25 March, more than 100 hospitals in the city were integrated into a monitoring network, which by 28 April had grown to 500 hospitals. City authorities also set up a well-functioning contact investigation and tracking team so that they could monitor and control those who were at high risk of developing SARS. In addition, authorities banned official travel outside Shanghai and also enforced a reporting and monitoring system that required all non-residents travelling from affected areas to Shanghai to report daily on their health status.[56]

Secrecy vs transparency

Retracing what happened within China during the SARS outbreak reveals much about provincial-central relations. The Chinese healthcare system is decentralised. Provincial authorities have a high level of authority to deal with health issues directly without reference to Beijing, as was evident in the case of Shanghai. This undoubtedly hindered the creation of a comprehensive, centralised database on SARS as the disease emerged. Dr. Bekedam noted that: "a new disease like SARS was officially a non-reportable disease for the provinces."[57] Additionally, there may well have been confusion among Chinese officials as to the "information status" of SARS. Although a 2001 regulation had amended a 1996 regulation that classified "highest level infectious diseases" as "highly secret," with the secrecy extending from the first occurrence of the disease until the day it was announced, it remains unclear whether the current law is widely known.[58] Furthermore, while reports were made to authorities in Beijing, information on the Guangdong outbreak was not provided to authorities in other parts of China, including Hong Kong. The lines of communication within the Chinese political and bureaucratic structures run vertically but not horizontally. Heads did not roll in Guangdong, which may well be due to the fact that provincial authorities did not hide information from Beijing, although they failed to inform residents of the province about the outbreak.

When the Chinese Government dismissed its health minister, followed four days later by the dismissal of Beijing's mayor, there should have been many more red faces at the top ranks of both the executive authorities and the ruling Chinese Communist Party as many officials held overlapping positions. The top party official, General Secretary Hu Jintao, was installed in November 2002. In March, following the sixteenth National People's Congress, Hu also became China's top executive, assuming the position of State President. Both Hu and Premier Wen Jiabao were members of the previous Politburo and State Council. During the Guangdong outbreak, the Minister of Public Security, Zhou Yongkang, also a Politburo member, reportedly directed Guangdong authorities to "maintain social stability,"[59] which in mainland political speak means that community panic is to be avoided.

While top leaders may have been preoccupied with proceedings of the National People's Congress during the month of March, it also appears that, astonishingly, they failed to fully appreciate the magnitude of the challenge presented by SARS. For weeks, as SARS rampaged through Beijing, the city authorities concealed the severity of the problem from the central authorities. Dr. Bekedam believed that although it seems implausible, "the centre really did not know" what was happening.[60] In any event, ignorance cannot be used as an excuse. There were many senior government as well as party officials who should have known, including Li Changchun, a Politburo Standing Committee member who was posted in Guangdong, where he was party secretary for the province, until after the sixteenth Party Congress. Moreover, Li's successor in Guangdong, Zhang Dejiang, also a Politburo member, was involved in efforts to contain the outbreak in Guangdong in late 2002 and early 2003. The price that China has had to pay for its delayed reaction to SARS has been high. Beijing lost more than a month, and by failing to inform provincial authorities about the Guangdong outbreak, it also denied them the chance to prepare.

In retrospect, Guangdong authorities acted more responsibly than Beijing officials. Bi Shengli, a leading virologist in Beijing, noted on 27 March that: "Once Guangdong realized that they had a problem, they began to take bold action...Guangdong moved quickly to tell its people how to protect themselves from SARS."[61]

SARS showed that the systemic culture of secrecy served China badly. The central authorities did not have the information they needed for decision-making in Beijing and thus the city was slowest to react. The initial denial that there was a serious problem destroyed China's international credibility. A second key observation is that China remains an introverted nation. The system was so obsessed with its own machinations between the November 2002 Party Congress and the March 2003 People's Congress that leaders were unable to deal with the looming crisis. Guangdong's greater openness and more aggressive stance on SARS starting in January 2003 helped to contain what could have been a national disaster. The fact that Shanghai was able to take early and effective precautions also showed that there was little excuse for Beijing's dithering.

The outbreak also highlighted the inadequacy of relations between Hong Kong and the mainland. Despite the intensity of economic and social contact between Hong Kong and Guangdong, somehow Hong Kong authorities failed to discover that something serious was happening across the border — and then to appreciate that it could affect Hong Kong. The lack of interest or the capacity to understand the systemic problems and inefficiencies on the mainland prevented Hong Kong from taking action without some official notification from either Guangdong or Beijing. Nevertheless, once Hong Kong officials recognised the severity of the situation, their instincts were not to hide information, as was the case in Beijing. Once Hong Kong's systems swung into high gear, they were able to handle SARS. The SARS episode shows that a more open attitude on the part of Hong Kong, and even Guangdong, is critical to China's drive for modernisation. If Guangdong and Hong Kong are able to interact and cooperate as residents of the same neighbourhood, they will have the opportunity to create the model for a new China.

As for the mainland, at present, it is only prepared for limited and selective openness. At the same time that it was telling the world that it would cooperate with the WHO and be open about infectious diseases, the authorities ordered the closure of a newspaper in Beijing after it ran an article criticising China's national legislature. Authorities also discouraged reporting on sensitive or embarrassing issues — for example, although Dr. Jiang was regarded as a folk hero for exposing the official cover-up of Beijing's SARS outbreak, he was eventually silenced by the authorities.[62]

For Hong Kong, the importance of Government transparency and access to information for the overall well-being of society was reconfirmed by the SARS experience. This may well have added to public discontent along with the national security legislation proposed by the Tung administration under Article 23 of the Basic Law, which requires Hong Kong to pass laws to prohibit sedition and the disclosure of state secrets, among other offences. A rally to oppose the legislation on 1 July 2003 drew half a million protesters. Although the vote on the legislation was originally scheduled for 9 July, the Chief Executive was pressured into delaying the process on 5 July to allow more time for consultation.[63] Tung was also forced to remove the Secretary for Health, Welfare and Food, Dr. Yeoh, as head of the SARS Expert Committee appointed by the Government to review its handling of SARS due to mounting controversy over how the central figure in the review could head an investigation against himself. On 5 September, the Chief Executive announced the withdrawal of Article 23 legislation from the legislative agenda altogether.

Acknowledgements

The author wishes to thank Peter TY Cheung for his general advice, Mitchell Kowalski for information on the outbreak in Toronto, Su Liu on her input for the situation in Shanghai and Alan Sargent for editing advice.

CHAPTER 10

SARS and China:
Old vs New Politics

Christine Loh and YIP Yan Yan

The 2003 SARS outbreak has already affected mainland China in significant ways and will likely continue to impact Chinese politics and society for some time in the future. While it was not a "Chinese Chernobyl," it was a transforming experience for the Chinese state.[1] The SARS crisis highlighted many of the contradictions inherent in the model of development applied since 1979, when China began its modernisation in earnest after the end of the Cultural Revolution. These contradictions, such as the lack of priority given to public health and social development vis-à-vis economic advancement and the continuation of an official culture of secrecy that actually prevents proper coordination of policy by the Chinese Communist Party (CCP) and the government, as well as hindering China's role as a global citizen, need to be resolved if development is to be sustainable.

While much remains to be done, China has nevertheless made important strides in acknowledging that the CCP is not all knowing and never failing. Chapter 9 describes how outside pressure, particularly pressure from Hong Kong and the World Health Organisation (WHO), played a critical role in prompting change within China. This chapter focuses on China's domestic power structure, key external relations issues arising from the SARS outbreak and the urgent need to improve the dilapidated mainland public health system.

The organisation of power

Between November 2002 and June 2003, the SARS virus emerged in Guangdong Province, spread to Hong Kong and from there was exported to many other cities around the world before subsiding. During this eight-month period, China underwent a crucial transition in leadership. The SARS outbreak proved to be the first domestic and foreign relations challenge faced by China's new leaders. To understand the impact of this challenge, it is useful to review how China is governed.

China's constitution confers on the CCP the exclusive right to control all national political organisations. Thus, the party in effect controls the nation's political, economic and social goals and policies. As an organisation, the CCP is "hierarchical, pyramidal, and centrist in nature."[2] The sixteenth National Party Congress, held from 8 to 15 November 2002, saw the most sweeping changes in Chinese leadership in more than five decades. A key task of the party congress, which is convened every five years, is to select the new Central Committee. Under the CCP constitution, the Central Committee governs party affairs and enacts party policies when the full congress is not in session.

The sixteenth National Party Congress was a landmark because it involved the first orderly transfer of power in the history of the People's Republic of China. In the past, leadership transitions have always been marked by ugly power struggles and even social turmoil. The new leadership, commonly referred to as "Generation IV," consists of younger and better-educated party members. The average age of the current Central Committee is 55, and nearly half of its members are first-timers.

The Central Committee elects the members of the Political Bureau (Politburo), which acts for the Central Committee. The Politburo Standing Committee takes care of the party's day-to-day affairs and represents the apex of political power in China. At the sixteenth National Party Congress, the Standing Committee was expanded from seven to nine members. Furthermore, with the exception of Hu Jintao, who succeeded Jiang Zemin as party general secretary, all the members of the previous Standing Committee stepped down.

A range of bodies that have responsibility for executing party policies and managing party affairs serve the Central Committee and the Politburo, one of the most important being the Central Secretariat. A key organ of the Secretariat is the Propaganda Department, which manages ideological, media, cultural and educational affairs.[3] Despite the fact that the environment on the mainland is now more free than in years past, the party still controls, albeit more subtly than before, the timing, frequency, level and content of public discussions. In understanding how SARS was explained and reported by the authorities and the domestic media, it should be recognised that ultimately the party set the agenda for how the subject would be presented and discussed.

The leadership transition initiated at the sixteenth National Party Congress in November 2002 was concluded at the tenth National People's Congress (NPC) in March 2003 when top CCP officials were installed as China's top government officials. The NPC is the highest government organ and also China's legislature. The full NPC is convened annually and when it is not in session, its Standing Committee serves as its executive arm. The State Council is China's highest executive body and manages government affairs through various ministries and commissions. In effect, it operates like a cabinet. The NPC appointed Wu Bangguo as the head of the legislature and elected Wen Jiabao as China's new premier, in addition to electing the other members of the State Council. It also selected Hu Jintao to replace Jiang Zemin as the new state president.

In China, the CCP controls and directs the government bureaucracy through an interlocking system of party personnel and organisational structures. The three most important positions are those of the party general secretary; the premier, who heads the State Council and therefore the government; and the head of the legislature. China's presidency is more a ceremonial post than a position of real power. The real political power is held by the party general secretary, currently Hu Jintao, who is also the state president, and the members of the Standing Committee of the Politburo. Politburo members usually hold cabinet posts as well. Thus, a tight inner circle of individuals oversees a vast country and makes all the key decisions on national policy.

Despite the centralised nature of the Chinese political system, where power flows from the central authorities in Beijing, actual authority is fragmented. The provincial and county systems are also part of the state super-structure, with numerous lines of reporting throughout the system. Separate lines flow to the party and to the government. For example, the Department of Health in the county of Zhongshan in Guangdong Province is subordinate to both the Zhongshan county government and the health bureau of the provincial government. The county government answers to both the Zhongshan Communist Party committee as well as the provincial government. County health officials must also obey party discipline, as most are likely to be party members of the party committee of the Department of Health. The point is that the officials in any given office have a number of bosses to whom they must answer – keeping in mind the relative importance of each one.[4]

China's complex and hierarchical bureaucratic system can create potential overload at the top "as lower-level officials avoid responsibility by pushing decisions 'up' the system," resulting in "*gridlock* from the fragmentation of power into different functional bureaucracies and territorial fiefdoms; *lack of accurate information* because of the distortion created by multiple layers of bureaucracy and because the CCP has not allowed any truly independent sources of information, such as a free press, to develop; and *corruption* and petty *dictatorship* as officials at each level have the opportunities and incentives to violate rules and cover up their transgression."[5] Thus, a serious problem inherent within the system is the difficulty of key decision-makers in obtaining timely and accurate information.

Culture of secrecy

Most information is reported level by level as it is passed up the bureaucratic chain of command, creating many opportunities to introduce distortions. This problem is exacerbated by the legacy of the long years when the central authorities forbade any criticism of the government, which resulted in the suppression of independent information sources. The primary agenda of China's media is still to serve politics.[6] Since the 1990s, China's media policy has shifted from disseminating political propaganda to setting the political agenda. The Chinese Government now seeks to influence what people think about rather than telling them what to think.

Despite some relaxation since the 1980s, the Chinese bureaucratic system is still characterised by an extraordinary degree of secrecy — much information remains confidential, including information about infectious diseases. The area of state secrets law in China is murky and difficult, as the scope of classified information remains vast and expandable.[7]

One of the best demonstrations of China's culture of secrecy occurred during the SARS outbreak when the report on the Guangdong outbreak commissioned by the provincial Department of Health sat in the departmental in-tray for several days before it was opened because no one had the security clearance to review such information. It was the impression of Dr. Henk Bekedam, the WHO's representative in Beijing, that up until the point when SARS became a full-blown crisis: "The centre really didn't know" about the outbreak. However, other observers doubt the validity of this conclusion because the decision by the Propaganda Department to suppress news coverage of SARS or the decision to avoid implementing preventative measures in the city of Beijing would have been made at the Politburo level and thus would have involved top leaders.[8] Whether the cover-up was deliberate or unintentional, the result was that China's habits in handling sensitive information cost valuable time in preventing the spread of the disease.[9]

The length of time that elapsed before Chinese authorities would permit greater information flow and cooperate with the WHO is indicative of how China dealt with the release of data during the crisis. This shows how slowly the system worked even at a moment when the world was losing patience with China and accusing it of covering up the disease.

China's Ministry of Health first reported the outbreak of the disease in Guangdong Province to the WHO on 11 February. Despite pressure from the WHO, it was not until 26 March, when SARS had already spread domestically and internationally, that China provided more information on the outbreak. Minister of Health Zhang Wenkang then reported that between 16 November 2002 and 9 February 2003, China had 305 SARS cases and five deaths. By 28 February the total number of cases had increased to 792 and the number of deaths to 31.[10] On 27 March, the Ministry of Health reported ten SARS cases in Beijing and three deaths.[11] The following day, minister Zhang agreed to improve cooperation with the WHO and provide reports on SARS cases throughout China, although he failed to follow through on this promise.[12] On 31 March, the WHO was still waiting for clearance to visit Guangdong.[13]

On 2 April, China reported that in the month of March, there had been 361 new SARS cases and nine deaths, bringing the cumulative total since November 2002 to 1,153 cases and 40 deaths.[14] On the same day, the WHO placed a travel advisory on Hong Kong and Guangdong, which finally prompted Beijing to allow the WHO investigators to travel to the southern province.

Up until 2 April, the central authorities were slow to grasp that they had a real crisis on their hands. It was only on 3 April that China's efforts to control the outbreak became more vigorous and better coordinated. A special task force headed by health minister Zhang was set up to fight SARS and a nationwide mechanism for outbreak alert and response was put in place shortly thereafter.[15] Zhang noted that at that point, the capital city had a dozen cases and three deaths. On April 4, China started to provide electronic reports to the WHO showing that there had been a cumulative total of 1,220 cases and 49 deaths.[16] Despite these numbers, it was not until 7 April that China announced that fighting SARS was "a high priority for the government."[17]

When Zhang provided an update on the number of SARS cases in the city of Beijing on 3 April, he did not know that a retired military doctor, Jiang Yanyong, would challenge his data – and that this would precipitate his own dismissal from office in a matter of days. Through the international media, Jiang revealed that Zhang's numbers did not include patients in the city's military hospitals. The real number of SARS cases in Beijing was in the hundreds.[18] Bekedam had this to say about China's system of data reporting: "…there were some [institutional problems]…the military…have a different kind of reporting system and normally don't report anywhere else than through their own headquarters."[19]

Once the figures for SARS cases in Beijing were proved wrong, questions were raised about the veracity of data on the Guangdong outbreak given to the WHO. However, it was quickly concluded that Guangdong's numbers had always included cases in military hospitals. The differences in practice between Beijing and Guangdong showed that the Chinese system is neither uniform nor helpful for those in power. The initial cover-up could well have been the result of institutional instincts and reflexes at the various levels of the Chinese state structure.

While it cannot be confirmed if minister Zhang deliberately gave out incorrect information on the number of SARS cases in Beijing, as his numbers were proved wrong, the Chinese Government suffered an enormous loss of credibility, both nationally and internationally. This was a heavy price to pay for a nation seeking to be accepted as a world leader. It did not help that the WHO was also openly critical of China's handling of the outbreak. Bekedam went on record to say that: "We have clearly told the government the international community doesn't trust your figures … Now it's time to start building some trust."[20] The sense of international outrage was expressed by US Secretary for Health and Human Services Tommy Thompson: "We've been very upset with the transparency of the Chinese Government — we think lives could have been saved, we could have controlled it...If we had this information in November or December, we might have been able to control the spread of [SARS] to other countries."[21] China's poor handling of SARS also gave Taiwan an opportunity to argue that mainland authorities could not be trusted. The Taiwan authorities were quick to urge Taiwanese not to visit the mainland.[22]

As Chapter 9 shows, events in China then began to move quickly. On 17 April, the Politburo Standing Committee held an urgent meeting at which it agreed to acknowledge that the government had failed to provide the correct information and affirm the commitment of the authorities to fighting the disease. President Hu Jintao called for the "accurate, timely and honest reporting" of SARS cases.[23] On 20 April, the Chinese Government announced the removal of Zhang from office, as well as the removal of Meng Xuenong, the mayor of Beijing. Liu Qing, the top party official in Beijing, also apologised to the Chinese people for supplying late and incorrect information. These public admissions of fault at the top level of leadership were significant within the context of Chinese domestic politics because they acknowledged that the CCP was not all knowing or always right — a significant departure from past behaviour. Only by admitting to its fault could the leadership improve the accountability of its decisions and actions. Eventually, the authorities also fired many lower ranking officials throughout the country for not having provided accurate information on the SARS outbreak.[24]

On 20 April, China's deputy health minister, Gao Qiang, held a press conference to announce that Beijing had 339 SARS cases and that the situation there was serious and worrying. At the same time, the government said that the traditional May Day holiday would be cancelled in order to prevent people from Beijing from travelling back to their hometowns in the countryside, potentially taking SARS with them. The following day, Beijing reported to the WHO that it had another 109 cases.[25] On 23 April, the State Council announced that it had set up the "SARS Control and Prevention Headquarters of the State Council" to combat the disease with vice premier Wu Yi at the helm. A fund was also created to help with prevention and control of the disease as well as pay for medical treatment of those with SARS who could not afford it.[26] In addition, the government allocated more money for the China Centre of Disease Control and Prevention (CDC).[27] Amazingly, the Chinese Government was able to build a dedicated hospital for the treatment of SARS in the suburbs of Beijing within a week.[28]

Beginning of openness?

A key issue following the leadership change was how "Generation IV" would govern China, particularly with so many new faces in top positions. The SARS outbreak presented these leaders with their first major test, which spanned economic, social and political issues on both a national and an international level. On 17 April, the Politburo realised that China's international reputation had been severely damaged by its handling of SARS. China was regarded as being unreliable and irresponsible. Top leaders likely also examined the possible impact on the economy if SARS was not contained.

Economic performance is critical to the party's continued claim to legitimacy, which is based on performance-based improvements determined to a large extent by the government's ability to sustain economic growth. SARS had the capacity to dent this growth significantly. Early casualties included China's booming tourism, retail, entertainment and transport sectors. Economists predicted that if the outbreak could be brought under control within one economic quarter, then the impact on China's Gross Domestic Product (GDP) would be limited to a 0.5% drop for the year 2003.[29] (On 17 July 2003, China's National Bureau of Statistics estimated that the GDP growth rate for the second quarter would be 6.7%, a reduction of 3.2% when compared to the first quarter.[30]) What was hard to predict at the time was whether the disease would impact other sectors, such as the manufacturing centres in the Pearl River Delta in Guangdong and the Yangzi (Chang Jiang) Delta near Shanghai. In view of the unfolding possible consequences, the Politburo decided that it needed to take resolute action to win back trust and prestige internationally and at the same time show citizens that the new government could act decisively.

In order to be regarded as trustworthy, leaders knew that they needed to provide information to the WHO and cooperate more fully in the fight against SARS. Leaders also recognised that demonstrating their ability to control the outbreak was critical in minimising panic among citizens. Their first act was to fire two top officials — a move designed to show that "Generation IV" expected accountability, which would go down well internationally and domestically. The appointment of vice premier Wu Yi as the new health minister was unusual, as vice premiers do not normally take on ministerial roles, but it was a calculated step. Wu has always been highly regarded in Chinese politics as a no-nonsense person and is well known to the international community because of her past role as a trade negotiator. The appointment of Wang Qishan, the young party secretary for Hainan Island, as the new mayor of Beijing was also calculated. His more open personal style in dealing with the media provided the contrast needed to show a departure from past behaviour.

In addition, Liu Qing's public mea culpa was likely also calculated to minimise international questioning as to whether Beijing remained a suitable site for the 2008 Olympics. The building of the Xiaotangshan Hospital for SARS cases and the transfer of more than 1,200 medical staff from all over China to the hospital was meant to demonstrate China's capacity to mobilise resources quickly to get things done. No doubt Chinese leaders were pleased that the WHO described the building of the hospital as "tantamount to a miracle."[31]

The SARS experience showed what could happen in a society rooted in secrecy when it was suddenly flooded with information about a public emergency such as the outbreak of a new infectious disease. Now that the government was telling people how serious the situation was, did it mean that things were no longer under control? The residents of Beijing found out that the number of SARS cases in the city was ten times higher than previously acknowledged by the authorities. Premier Wen Jiabao's visit to Beijing University and various areas in the neighbourhood was intended to urge people to remain calm and help the government fight the disease.

Fighting SARS had to be transformed into a test of the nation's spirit. To counteract doubts about its ability to manage the situation, the government not only imposed quarantine and closed schools, entertainment centres and other public places — its draconian instincts also resulted in threats to execute "intentional transmitters" of SARS and arrest people who sent short text messages (SMS) "spreading rumours" about the epidemic. An unfortunate doctor who accidentally infected his family with the disease was imprisoned.[32] At the same time, whistle-blower Jiang Yanyong, while not punished, was pressured into not speaking out further.[33]

What Chinese leaders sought to do was to "manage openness" as a part of their strategy in fighting SARS. An example of the extent to which authorities sought to create the impression of genuine openness was the setting up of the Chinese Medical and Biological Information website, hosted by Peking University's Institute of Cardiovascular Sciences. The website had the latest figures for SARS infections and deaths, their distribution by province, recommended preventative measures, latest information about the virus, statements from medical specialists, utterances from Chinese leaders as well as various news reports from the domestic and foreign media, such as *The Washington Post* (usually not available in China due to censorship). Media articles were carefully selected to include only those that reported on the scientific aspects of SARS. Furthermore, "the links to be clicked on in order to read the article [were]...hosted on the same site, but...in order to be authentic, the presentation and the logos have been faithfully reproduced to give the impression that a door to the outside had been opened."[34]

Becoming a responsible power

The new leadership's external priorities are to deal with cross-strait issues, build a better and more stable relationship with the US and continue to improve relations with the countries of the Association of Southeast Asian Nations (ASEAN). One aspect of China's international relations strategy is to behave responsibly as a world power as the country becomes increasingly integrated into the international economic and political fabric. China's international prestige is therefore vital to the pursuit of its external goals. The early handling of SARS hindered China's attempts to be regarded as a responsible world power. A responsible power plays its role in international affairs not only according to its own national interests, but also with the goal of promoting global stability, development and progress. A world power needs to take its international obligations seriously, and participate in the formulation of international rules of conduct.[35]

China's international prestige is heavily dependent on its handling of the issue of Taiwan, which China regards as an internal matter even though Taiwan issues invariably have external ramifications, particularly in terms of Sino-US relations. Beijing's ultimate goal is the reunification of Taiwan with the Chinese state. A key aspect of China's foreign relations with other nations vis-à-vis Taiwan is to deny international space to Taipei and punish those who are prepared to maintain formal relations with Taiwan. Officially, the US recognises the People's Republic [of China] and maintains only informal relations with Taipei; US policy favours voluntary reunification but at the same time would extend to providing military support to Taiwan in the event of force or threat of force by the mainland. Sino-US relations have become more complex with the victory of the pro-independence Democratic Progressive Party's Chen Shui-bian in Taiwan's 2000 presidential election.

The SARS experience provided Taiwan with fresh evidence that Beijing could not be trusted, the sub-text being that the international community should look with sympathy on Taiwan's struggle to define its relationship with mainland China. Chapter 9 notes that international opinion was an important factor in persuading Beijing not to object to Taiwan's participation in the WHO Global Conference on SARS in Malaysia on 17–18 June 2003. Thus, at least in the area of infectious disease, Taiwan has gained a measure of space to manoeuvre on the international stage. In return, by not objecting to Taiwan's participation in the conference, Beijing was able to play a more humanitarian role at a time of crisis. However, it remains uncertain whether Beijing will eventually resume its objections to Taiwan's participation in the WHO as an observer, something Taiwan has been trying to achieve for years.

China's initial behaviour of denial of the SARS crisis and non-cooperation with the WHO created tension not only with the West but also with the ASEAN countries. Although only Singapore and Vietnam had high numbers of SARS cases, other ASEAN countries were also concerned about the rapid spread of the disease. In any event, the sharp drop in international travel in and out of Asia after 2 April, when the WHO recommended that people postpone non-essential travel to Hong Kong and Guangdong, had a severe impact on many Asian countries. Thus, everyone suffered. Furthermore, the SARS outbreak created an additional obstacle to Sino-ASEAN relations. In addition to the existing concerns arising from China's military and economic aspirations, infectious disease became a new issue with the potential to destabilise the region.

ASEAN's serious interest in SARS was evident in the decision to arrange three high-level meetings on SARS in close succession. The first urgent meeting on SARS was a Ministers of Health Special Meeting held on 26 April in Kuala Lumpur, Malaysia. Following this meeting, a joint statement was released highlighting the need to undertake practical measures to contain the spread of SARS. Three days later, a special ASEAN-China Leaders' Meeting followed in Bangkok, Thailand to explore possibilities for greater cooperation to fight the disease. A third ASEAN meeting was held from 10–11 June 2003 in Cambodia. To show that China attached great importance to this matter, it sent Premier Wen Jiabao to the Bangkok meeting on 29 April, whereas it would normally have sent a vice premier. It was Wen's first overseas mission since becoming head of the Chinese Government. At that meeting he did not attempt to excuse China's handling of SARS to date, emphasising instead that China would be candid and cooperative in the future. Wen talked about human suffering in China, its inadequate public health system and the daunting task faced by the new leadership. China also pledged RMB10 million to launch a fund to support bilateral programmes for fighting SARS.[36]

The more open style Wen adopted in Bangkok was echoed by deputy premier and health minister Wu Yi at the Asia Pacific Economic Cooperation (APEC) forum at the end of June 2003. Wu stated that: "When the epidemic first struck, we were unaware of its gravity. Moreover, our public health system was weak and flawed and there was neither unified chain of command nor smooth flow of information. Having overcome the SARS epidemic…Chinese society is more mature and open."[37]

Improving public health

Despite China's solid advances in agricultural and industrial reform since 1979, the creation of a more market-sensitive economic system, entry into the World Trade Organization (WTO) and establishment of the financial architecture for the nation, China is still struggling with the social transformation that needs to accompany economic transition. With rapid development occurring all over China, the natural environment has deteriorated significantly during the last 20 years, leading to a rise in morbidity as a result of pollution as well as poor sanitation. Respiratory, waterborne, digestive and infectious diseases are, as a consequence, prevalent in many areas.[38] For example, a recent study showed that more than 33 percent of children in the urban areas of China suffer from lead poisoning as a result of polluted water sources.[39]

China's ability to deal with public health problems, particularly in rural areas, has been compromised due to the abandonment of communal farming in the 1980s, with the result that the rural co-operative health systems, which provided basic healthcare to 85 percent of the population, have disintegrated. A pillar of these systems was a corps of "barefoot doctors," which has since been disbanded. Experts note that: "China used to be regarded as one of the great success stories in public health."[40] However, the programme of economic reforms involved administrative decentralisation of public health funding and responsibility from Beijing to the provinces, cities and townships. As a result, the portion of total health care funding from the central authorities fell from 36 percent to less than 20 percent in 20 years. While China's total spending on health has increased more than ten times, 25 percent of the expenditure is focused on the wealthy areas of the country, mainly the big cities and the richest provinces. Moreover, health care costs have soared 500–600 percent in the last decade because of the high costs for medicine.[41] While fees for hospitals and clinics remain modest, drugs are very expensive because this is where healthcare providers recoup costs. Furthermore, China's immature health insurance system, put in place since 1999, does not as yet cover the vast majority of Chinese citizens.

The SARS outbreak has refocused attention on three aspects of disease control in China. First, SARS provided a reminder of the unique circumstances existing in southern China, which has a history as a "viral incubator" for epidemics. This is largely due to the close proximity of crowded urban populations to animals and intensive animal husbandry.[42] Following the discovery that civet cats and other wild animals carry the SARS coronavirus, the Guangdong authorities ordered an end to the wildlife trade at the end of May 2003. The trade had been supplying increasing quantities of wild animals to restaurants to feed the appetite for "exotic" dishes, which is linked to growing prosperity and to traditional beliefs about the ability of such dishes to boost virility and strengthen immunity to disease.[43] The ban was subsequently lifted in July 2003, indicating that more permanent restrictions must be put in place before there is any change in the behaviour of poachers, traders and diners.

Second, the authorities need to see China's health problems within the context of the government's development model so that public health is not sacrificed for the sake of economic advancement. One glaring issue is China's inadequate response to HIV/AIDS, which the authorities consistently refused to acknowledge as a major public health issue up until very recently. There are an estimated one million people with HIV/AIDS in China and this number could soar to 10 million or even 20 million by 2010.[44]

Third, China has to create a public health infrastructure that focuses on professionalism and not party politics. News reports have indicated that the government pledged US$55 million for prevention and control of SARS.[45] However, in addition to giving top level attention to health policy issues and allocating funds to upgrade the public health architecture, the party needs to allow health professionals to become autonomous in the sense that they can be relied upon to maintain and enforce healthcare standards rather than being directed by party goals. In other words, the party has to create an environment for China's health workers that encourage true professionalism.

Conclusion

While China's economic efforts to date have created "a picture of dynamism" for the outside world because of its potential market size, consistently high growth rates and ability to attract substantial amounts of foreign direct investment (over US$80 billion in 2002[46]), making "multinational corporations salivate at the thought of its future growth,"[47] what the SARS outbreak showed is a China that has neglected the social transformation that must accompany economic transition, most glaringly in the public health sector. Indeed, economic and social development must go hand in hand. A positive outcome is that the leadership has been forced to review its policies and will hopefully reorder its priorities in considering how China should continue to develop. Only time will tell, however, whether "Generation IV" will put China's development plan on a more sustainable path.

On 24 June, when the WHO declared that Beijing had been removed from its list of SARS-affected areas, Chinese leaders could declare that the campaign against the disease had been victorious. Deputy health minister Gao Qiang credited this achievement to the leadership of Hu Jintao and Wen Jiabao: "The lesson of SARS is that as long as we struggle together and follow the leadership of the Central Committee, no problem will be insurmountable for us."[48]

Perhaps the most significant contribution of the new leaders was to make a series of public apologies for their official handling of SARS. In 2001, when former premier Zhu Rongji apologised to the nation for the many deaths caused by an explosion in a primary school in Jiangxi Province, believed to be a site where students were forced to make fireworks, it paved the way for a new style of leadership that incorporated the potential to admit fault on the part of individual leaders and the CCP.[49] Another important development in this regard was the level of detail released in May 2003 when 70 sailors on board a Chinese submarine died as a result of an accident. Chinese leaders were also seen consoling family members of the deceased.[50]

"Generation IV" still needs to review why it took so long to focus on SARS so that a better crisis management system can be devised for the future. However, while China continues to operate within a culture of secrecy, its response ability will be negatively affected as information flows too slowly to allow prompt decision-making. New and old styles of leadership have been shown to be visibly in conflict. While on the one hand, top leaders called on officials to be accurate in reporting SARS, the system still prohibits others from speaking out. Hence, whistle-blower Jiang Yanyong was silenced and the media remained under tight controls.

The fact is that once China's top leaders focused on the disease, they were able to move quickly and decisively to control its spread. But it does not compensate for the reality that it was China's initial systemic denial of the issue that caused a higher number of deaths and greater suffering than would otherwise have been the case had China's political system been designed to behave differently. Herein lies the inherent contradiction — China's own ability to be better informed about facts and react appropriately in a crisis is compromised by a political system that puts the CCP at the core of decision-making. When the party is slow or wrong, there is no alternative mechanism for others to step in to avert problems.

CHAPTER 11

The Economic Impact of SARS

Stephen Brown

Writing about the impact of SARS on the Hong Kong economy involves a great deal of crystal ball gazing. However, the outlook for the Hong Kong economy post-SARS does not look to be dramatically different from pre-SARS trends. In trying to assess the longer-term impact of the disease on Hong Kong, it is important to understand what the Hong Kong economy actually consists of, what drives it and where it fits in the international chains of connectivity that are increasingly important. In addition to exploring future development of the economy, it is important to understand how we got where we are in the first place.

When it comes to the local economy, one thing is certain — the Hong Kong economy is a highly complex beast. Most of the commentaries that readers will have come across on the topic, even in purportedly serious press reports, will simply have been wrong. There is probably no other economy in the world that has been more often misunderstood by commentators, both local and foreign, and even by some specialist economists.

Apparently, it is what is seen on the streets within Hong Kong's 400 square miles of landmass that determines the opinions that are published in the newspapers and seen in the media. But the fact is that domestic economic activity here is, in many ways, only a small part of our economy, the health of which is a result of Hong Kong's activities in the rest of

179

the world. If you want to understand the Hong Kong economy, home is not the place to look. Misunderstanding of this fact is nothing new. In recent decades, Hong Kong has often been used by those who advocate the benefits of free markets as the shining example of how the policies they espouse can bring enormous benefits. Even the most revered gurus of the free market have loudly proclaimed this view. While it may be perfectly tenable to hold the view that Hong Kong has been a relatively free economy, especially in its external sector when it comes to trade, some of the excessive praise for its free market "miracle" has been based on a highly distorted interpretation of reality.

The recurrent problem that people always seem to have when addressing the issue of Hong Kong's economy is that they are overwhelmed by the physical presence and sheer density of our developments, the tall buildings and the general hustle and bustle. Postcards and television commentaries highlight the Central waterfront with its array of glass and concrete monuments to money. It is this spectacle that seems to stop people from looking any further into the machinery behind the physical manifestation of our wealth. The wealth comes from hard work, our deepwater port and a nose for making money out of buying and selling anything that is profitable. In particular, in recent times, it has been fashionable to characterise early Hong Kong as a barren economy until the post-war miracle, the occurrence of which, according to these pundits, was entirely due to its free market working in juxtaposition to the generally highly restricted economies in the region.

As with all good stories, the truth is somewhat different. Hong Kong has been a trading centre ever since the British gained accession almost a century before World War II. It was struck by devastating typhoons, the plague, cholera, dysentery and trade spats of all sorts over the ensuing hundred years. By 1938, Hong Kong was home to a population of over one million. Essentially, for the first hundred years, Hong Kong went through booms and busts dependent almost entirely on the trade cycle, especially with China, and the status of political relations with the Chinese mainland. The British decanted their international trading activities to the new colony; it was never a barren rock awaiting the magic of post-Keynesian liberalism.

The ebb and flow of economic life in Hong Kong is recorded in the excellent reports that were filed annually by the colonial Governors. The report of 1910, for instance, states that a reported 547,164 vessels had called at the port, exceeding all previous records. The carrying capacity of the ships had also doubled over the previous 20 years and tonnage had risen by a factor of 4 to 12 million tonnes. Opium imports were down again to only 31,743 cases, and exports also fell to 28,333 cases. The major onshore industries in Hong Kong at the time were cotton spinning, sugar refining and cement. The hot sectors "under Chinese management" were the manufacture of rattan furniture, tobacco and local spirits. By 1910, Hong Kong was a bustling port that saw over fifteen hundred ships come and go a day, importing and exporting like fury and making money by trading with all and sundry. 1910 was a good year, with properties changing hands at increasing prices in increasing numbers, and the Government coffers were doing well, despite the fact that the colony had seen 100,000 people leave to work on the burgeoning plantations in the Malay Peninsula.[1]

The 1934 report records the continued growth of the colony. The then Governor could not foresee that the colony was about to face a terrible decade. Already the first signs of the global depression were noticeable, not helped by the fact that China had just put up tariff barriers, severely affecting Hong Kong's trade with Guangdong. Both imports and exports fell that year by 20 percent in local currency terms, with China being Hong Kong's biggest trading partner, accounting for 30 percent of the import trade and 50 percent of our exports. Local economic activity was also dull and the 550 factories in the colony experienced difficult times. The key hosiery and knitting trades saw several high profile bankruptcies, shipbuilding was slack and prices, including rents, were falling sharply. Unemployment was rising, alleviated somewhat by the return of locals to the mainland if they could not find work in Hong Kong.[2]

After the war, the problems would have appeared insurmountable. The Chinese Communist Party gained control of China, the market upon which Hong Kong's economy had always depended. Then famine caused an enormous influx of refugees to the colony and the war in the Korean Peninsula broke out. Any one of these events could have toppled Hong Kong. The actual outcome of post-war events could never have been predicted. The influx of knowledgeable business people from cities such as Shanghai who had expertise in manufacturing proved to be of great benefit. Capital flowed into the colony as it had safe haven status. These factors were fortuitously combined with a huge supply of immigrant refugee labourers, then living in temporary huts on Hong Kong's hillsides. The final ingredient in this heady cocktail was the fact that the colony was governed by the rule of law, while even the newly introduced income tax was modest and did not apply to earnings from overseas.

In addition, and not least of all, Hong Kong possessed a large allocation of textile quota that ensured that its textile exports had a market. These ingredients were randomly mixed to produce the foundations for the modern Hong Kong, under the auspices of a succession of colonial civil servants who generally believed that market forces and economic matters were best left alone. Controls over imports were relaxed as much as was permitted by international obligations, and industry blossomed, despite the fact that many pundits of the day held to the belief that industry was inappropriate for a city that had only ever been a centre for trade and not manufacturing.

Manufacturing grew and grew. In every quarter from 1947 until 1971, the zenith of Hong Kong's manufacturing industry, employment in the sector rose, reaching 613,000.[3] Despite the banking crisis of 1965 and the riots of 1967, economic growth — during an admittedly highly inflationary period — was 50 percent in the three years prior to 1971.[4] By the time of the first oil crisis, manufacturing accounted for 43 percent of GDP and domestic exports were growing by 25 percent per annum.[5] With the benefit of hindsight, it is patently obvious that just as the door closed on Maoist China, another door had opened up for Hong Kong. In the thirty years since the peak of the manufacturing industry, which ended in the collapse of the equity market in 1973, the story of Hong Kong's economy has really been the story of a city returning to its traditional role as the key trade centre for China, now allied to a much greater global influence than was previously the case. The glorious days of manufacturing that some in Hong Kong still think we should hanker after were merely an aberration, the result of a unique set of circumstances. In the century prior to World War II, Hong Kong experienced the normal relationship that it should naturally enjoy with China — a relationship that was based on trade and trading.

China very gradually opened up its economy after 1976, the year that saw the demise of The Gang of Four and the end of the Cultural Revolution. Hong Kong spent the next few decades shedding the manufacturing sector that had grown up during China's hibernation from the world. The loss of industry and manufacturing jobs in Hong Kong, which has paralleled the opening up of the mainland and is now being replicated in the loss of some poorly paid clerical jobs across the border, is not a sign of a lack of competitiveness on Hong Kong's part. Rather these changes reflect the normal progression of an advancing economy. In fact, it would appear that this supposed "hollowing out" merely represents the continued rebalancing of our economy. It is not a sign of terminal decline, as the more dramatic commentaries would like us to believe.

These trends reflect a return to the normal division of labour between the two economies: a division that utilises the complementary resources of each; a division of activities that existed for the first century of the colony's existence. The winding down of the domestic manufacturing industry in Hong Kong looks likely to be completed in the next few years as Hong Kong's beneficial position as a large holder of textile quota finally disappears when quotas are abolished in 2005.[6]

However, in the best Hong Kong tradition, another even bigger opportunity arose as China opened up. We have not lost our manufacturing; instead, we have moved it across the border. Some 63,000 Hong Kong companies now employ 12 million people in Hong Kong-connected factories in Guangdong Province.[7] This figure is very much larger when compared with the maximum number of people ever employed by Hong Kong companies — 800,000 — when they were based in the city. In addition, all of the significant ports in the Pearl River Delta are managed and controlled by Hong Kong firms. Nearly 500,000 people are employed domestically in Hong Kong to provide direct support for these activities. When indirect activities are included, this figure represents 43 percent of our total workforce.[8]

In fact, Hong Kong is now the world's most externally oriented economy and controls more manufacturing than ever before. It has never been so influential in managing global trade flows, and profiting from them, at any other time in its history. In addition, this time around, and in contrast to its position in the nineteenth century, Hong Kong has acquired the capital to be able to fund many activities at either end of the trade pipeline. Hong Kong companies, both private and public, rarely have their businesses entirely contained within the SAR. Hong Kong's broad interests span retailing companies operating in the West, mile after mile of factories across the border, major shipping lines and the world's leading sourcing and procurement companies.

Today, the overseas investments of Hong Kong entities are equal to almost twice the GDP. In per capita terms, this equates to every man, woman and child in Hong Kong holding US$50,000 in investments outside Hong Kong. Seventy-one percent of all foreign direct investment (FDI) in Guangdong is from Hong Kong companies.[9] The value of the physical exports handled directly through Hong Kong is 1.2 times its GDP. The value of Hong Kong services sold overseas every year is equal to almost US$40 billion (HK$311 billion), running a trade surplus on services exports that was well over 10 percent of GDP in 2001, and has risen since.[10] It is this very international emphasis that is the unique feature of our overall economy.

To give some idea of the overall relative scale of Hong Kong, it is not sufficient to talk in mere numbers. It is best to establish some sort of benchmark that reflects the standing and importance of Hong Kong in the hierarchy of global cities. While no one would claim that Hong Kong ranks alongside New York and London in terms of the arts, global media presence or educational institutions, Hong Kong stacks up fairly well on the activities that reflect purely economic criteria. This is especially true when one bears in mind that the city was decimated by World War II and received no special help in establishing itself in the aftermath. Essentially, in all the statistical measures of physical economic activity, Hong Kong ranks alongside the world's greatest cities, including Greater London and Metropolitan New York. Hong Kong's gross domestic output per capita is nearly identical to that of these two cities at somewhere around the US$25,000 (HK$194,000) mark.[11] Its population of 6.8 million people is about 5 percent less than that of London and some 15 percent less than New York's, but the size of the employable population is very similar.[12] Like London and New York, Hong Kong has also now lost its local manufacturing base. Twenty years ago the manufacturing sector here employed nearly 900,000 people, representing the largest single source of employment and generating over 25 percent of GDP.[13] By 2001, employment in the sector had fallen to less than 200,000 people, or less than 6 percent of the workforce, and its contribution to the city's GDP had fallen to under 6 percent.[14] The monuments to the decline in domestic manufacturing are scattered throughout the former industrial area of South Kowloon in the form of dilapidated industrial buildings from the 1960s, which still occupy a total of nearly 200 hectares of land.

On a purely statistical basis, there are also many other similarities between Hong Kong and New York and London. In terms of the myriad activities that make up these economies, it is the services sector that dominates in all three. Actually, Hong Kong is the most service sector-oriented city in the world. Almost 85 percent of our economic activity is generated by the service sector, slightly ahead of the contribution of this sector in both New York and London.[15] Moreover, and strangely enough for those who see the crowded streets of Causeway Bay as a testimony to our craze for shopping, the majority of the average household's income in Hong Kong every month goes towards buying services and not goods.[16] However, there are two surprising differences in the comparison of Hong Kong with London and New York. The first involves the skyscrapers that characterise Hong Kong in the minds of so many people. Despite its dramatic cityscape, Hong Kong has a much smaller property sector than either London or New York. Hong Kong has significantly less housing, both in terms of built floor area and the number of units available, as well as having much less office space than either of the other two cities. Hong Kong only has a little over two million residential units, as opposed to the over three million units in both London and New York and, of course, has much smaller floor area per unit, with a third less space being available to the average Hong Kong family in the typical high rise flat.[17] And when it comes to office space, despite the imposing harbour front high rises, Hong Kong is dwarfed by New York, a city that has over three times as much office space and also by London, which boasts more than double the office space of Hong Kong.[18]

The other major difference between the three cities will be apparent to anyone who manages to travel five miles north from Central; Hong Kong has the world's largest container port. It is the presence of the container port that gives you the first clue of how Hong Kong makes, and has always made, money. At this moment in time, Hong Kong is in fact returning to its roots and making its money through trade again, a fact that also explains why our economy has so much less modern office space than either London or New York. Hong Kong's 300,000 small firms — the Small and Medium-sized Enterprises (SMEs) — are not keen on big overheads or flashy addresses.

Turn left on the expressway a few miles further up and there is Chek Lap Kok, the site of the new airport that opened for business in 1998. Most passengers standing in the cavernous arrivals hall probably cannot imagine that the airport where they have landed is also the world's leading airport for international airfreight cargo.[19]

One way or another, trade and its related activities make up over one-third of Hong Kong's GDP, a figure far in excess of the relative contribution of this sector in London and New York. In their economies, this gap is taken up by their large media, advertising and much larger financial services sectors. Hong Kong's emphasis on trade may just be considered a matter of its immaturity, as both London and New York have, in their time, also been major global ports. Indeed it was only 35 years ago that New York was the world's busiest container port, although the number of containers it handled then was only 10 percent of the current annual throughput at Hong Kong's terminals. Nevertheless, this prognosis is probably too simple. It is not merely the handling of goods that constitutes trade and, despite the fact that Hong Kong's airport handles two million tonnes of cargo every year, a figure that is growing very sharply, while some 18 million containers pass through Hong Kong waters annually, our real business now is in sourcing, organising and controlling trade flows. In fashionable terms, we are the world leaders in what is described as supply chain management between many parts of Asia, in particular China, and the rest of the world.

When it comes to these critical activities Hong Kong, with its rule of law, lack of offshore income tax, free and tariff-free trade policy and completely convertible currency, is without peer. The story of the Hong Kong economy pre- and post-SARS is still that of the city's role as the world's leading centre for trade. This story also has to be framed in terms of Hong Kong's relationship with China and China's development, and Hong Kong's role as the key catalyst, facilitator and beneficiary of this development, especially now that China has entered the World Trade Organisation. Therefore, as so often happens, when it comes to the economy what you see is not what matters. Those buildings on the waterfront are merely a red herring for those seeking the root of Hong Kong's wealth. Hong Kong's most prominent and famous feature, its tall skyscrapers, is in fact no more than a repository for the money that has been made in trade over the last 150 years. Moreover, the financial and legal services firms that occupy them would not be there if it were not for the trade machine that underlies Hong Kong's economic prowess.

Many recent commentaries on SARS, including some near hysterical warnings, used words like "disaster." Phrases such as "profound long term impact on our economy" were not uncommon. The "damage" to tourism has also been a particular point of focus. As with London and New York, tourism is a highly noticeable contributor to economic activity in Hong Kong. It is a high profile industry everywhere in the world with the hotels in all three cities occupying a prominence in the local consciousness that is out of all proportion to the more economically valuable office buildings nearby. The political clout of the lobby groups involved in tourism is also out of proportion to the absolute importance of tourism to each city. Tourism is undoubtedly useful; but it is not vital. In fact in cities such as Hong Kong, where there are no local sales taxes to boost local Government revenue from visitors' purchases, the overall benefit to the economy is undoubtedly less than is normally claimed.

The gross contribution of tourism to GDP in major world cities is normally estimated as being between 8 percent (New York) and 12 percent (London).[20] However, this figure does not include the leakage that occurs from outbound tourism by the city's own residents. In Hong Kong's case, residents actually spend more overseas than the city receives from visitors and the overall tourism account is, at best, in balance. A word of caution is needed at this stage, however. Claims for the absolute level of the importance of tourism to these cities have to be treated cautiously as the calculation of this sector's contribution cuts across many different categories of activity as analysed by GDP numbers. Indeed, different official bodies in London attribute contemporary tourism's contribution to the city's economy as being 12 percent (according to the Mayor of London's Report) or 8 percent (according to the London Tourist Board). This divergence illustrates just how difficult it is to precisely assess the importance of tourism in a vibrant urban economy. The figure that does seem to carry some authority is the employment created by tourism, which is equal to about 250,000 jobs in London and New York.[21] New York had 5.7 million international tourists in 2001 and almost 30 million domestic tourists. London had 17 million domestic tourists in 2001 and over 11 million international tourists. Hong Kong had a comparatively modest 16.5 million tourists in total in 2001 and a lower per capita spend with visitors staying a shorter time.[22]

The fact that Hong Kong is the little brother of New York and London in the tourist stakes is reflected by the disparity in the number of hotel rooms; with 70,000 hotel rooms, New York has nearly twice as many hotel rooms as Hong Kong.[23] On balance, and possibly in the face of some claims to the contrary by local tourism lobby groups, tourism is substantially less important to Hong Kong than to the other two cities. In March 2003 the World Travel and Tourism Council forecast that: "In Hong Kong, 41 percent of industry GDP will be lost, as well as 27,000 industry jobs, representing 38 percent of total industry jobs."[24] The comparatively small number of estimated job losses due to SARS seemed to emphasise that Hong Kong is comparatively small fry by the standards of cities like New York and London when it comes to tourism.

However, from a political perspective, there is another reason why tourism is seen as being important in all three cities. High impact urban conurbations tend to experience relatively higher rates of unemployment than their hinterlands. The elderly retire elsewhere to access lower living costs while the city attracts the young and new immigrants. The workforce is typically made up of highly qualified professionals at one end of the spectrum, with over 30 percent of the workforce being graduates. At the other end of the spectrum, the unskilled and young have to find work in the low-end service sector, providing services to the well off and the tourist.

In short, having looked at some aspects of Hong Kong's economic history and the current structure of its economy, we are in a position to assess whether or not the impact of SARS is going to be highly detrimental. From the foregoing thumbnail sketch of Hong Kong's economic role historically and the challenges it has previously surmounted, it should be apparent that SARS is most unlikely to have been the killer blow to the economy that some have had us believe. Similarly, the comparisons with London and New York enable us to surmise that if New York can survive as an economic entity after the horrendous terrorist attacks of 11 September 2001, it is highly unlikely that SARS will bring us to our knees. But what about all the gloom and doom one hears about Hong Kong? Yes, it is true that the domestic economy has been weak since 1997. Much of the ensuing softness in the domestic economy, as opposed to the vitality of our external trade and services economy, has been the result of an unfortunate confluence of factors.

The Asian Financial Crisis started just as Tung Chee-hwa took office as the Chief Executive of the Hong Kong Special Administrative Region (HKSAR). The crisis occurred after a frenetic 12 months of speculative activity in an exuberant property market. The collapse in regional liquidity, combined with the strengthening of the US dollar, against which the Hong Kong dollar maintains a linked fixed exchange rate, further compounded Hong Kong's problems and those of other countries in the region. Unfortunately, a weak external trade environment further exacerbated the downswing. And while many of the detrimental influences on Hong Kong's economy were not of its own making, the Hong Kong Government did inadvertently emphasise these negative influences by massively increasing the supply of residential property with the explicit intent of lowering prices. The drive to lower prices was a stated policy target of the post-1997 administration in response to the doubling in residential prices that occurred in the 12 months prior to the change of sovereignty in 1997. Eighty-five thousand flats a year were to be produced for a decade, with the target of improving homeownership to 70 percent. The supply target was derived from a model that took no account of external economic factors and, as such, was fundamentally flawed if monetary and external conditions altered. The new supply was to be met by extra land supply to the private sector and also a massive expansion in public housing for rent and sale.

Unfortunately, the external conditions did change, and they changed dramatically with the onset of the Asian Financial Crisis. Liquidity drained out of Asia and just as classic monetary policy would have called for a weakening of our currency, the US dollar to which the Hong Kong dollar is linked strengthened and investment demand for housing collapsed just as supply soared. At the time of writing, residential property prices have fallen for the last six years and are now down some 70 percent from their artificial peak in the summer of 1997. Quite obviously, such a contraction in domestic balance sheets has resulted in a dramatic decline in private sector domestic demand, which the Tung administration has attempted to offset somewhat by an expansionary fiscal stance since its 1998 budget.[25] Households continue to try to pay down their debt. Although nominal interest rates are low, they remain high in real terms. Inflation indicators that contain a large housing cost component have fallen and have now actually turned into mild, if fairly consistent, deflation for the last few years. This is of itself a problem insofar as it is impossible to lower interest rates sufficiently for them to also become negative. Thus, while borrowing costs are low now, with mortgage rates of 2.5 percent, they are still too high when adjusted for deflation.

This process has been further exacerbated by the fact that there has been a significant increase in the labour supply since 1997. Although there are near record levels of people working, Hong Kong has not been able to create enough lower paying jobs to take up the slack in this segment of the job market. Unemployment has just touched 8 percent, a very high level by Hong Kong standards. Yet banks are awash with money and the financial system has not exhibited any signs of stress during this period, a sign of the underlying solidity of the economy, and absolute verification of the premise that Hong Kong relies on trade, and now offshore manufacturing, and not real estate for making its money.

With the US dollar weakening, a move which infers an easier monetary regime for Hong Kong because of its link to that currency and with the impact of the 2003 Iraq war fading, there were signs that a recovery in the domestic economy could slowly kick in. Just released figures for the first quarter showed that the Hong Kong economy grew by 4.5 percent in real terms at that time, just prior to the height of the SARS outbreak. Initial optimism was somewhat justified, although this growth was still being generated largely by handling Hong Kong and Taiwanese factories' exports from the Pearl River Delta and from supplying services to them, as services sector exports. But there was one other sector that had continued to help offset the very depressed domestic demand picture: tourism. In particular, efforts by the administration to facilitate mainland tourism had been successful, and while tourism is never going to be the driver of our economy, it was a source of new external spending power for our hoteliers, retailers and restaurants.

In many ways SARS could not have hit Hong Kong at a worse time. In late spring 2003, exports from China were picking up very strongly, the majority of which come from Hong Kong manufacturers operating across the border, with growth in exports from foreign invested enterprises up 50 percent. The main ports in Guangdong controlled by Hong Kong were full and the Hong Kong ports were showing good growth, as was air cargo traffic. Retained imports were rising, as were retail sales. These factors were surely all precursors of a recovery in domestic demand against a weak US dollar and further cuts in interest rates. But all of sudden, the hint of optimism was shattered. Passenger arrivals by air and land collapsed and tourism dried up. Hotels were reporting lettings in the single digits. Domestic economic activity ground to a near halt as restaurants and shops were deserted.

This was bad enough but was then followed by the final straw. It quickly became apparent that the mainland SARS outbreak could be worse than had previously been imagined — and this was followed by the revelation that Taiwan was also similarly affected. A startled Hong Kong administration reacted initially in a shocked manner, re-enforcing the dramatic reporting of the outbreak by the international news media. As more and more flights were cancelled, the lifeblood seemed to be draining out of the virtuous economic triangle that ties together Hong Kong, Taiwan and mainland China.

Cathay Pacific, which was buoyed by its excellent air cargo business, cut its scheduled passenger flights by over 60 percent and throughput at the Hong Kong airport fell 80 percent. Some hotels had less than ten rooms occupied at the height of the crisis. Restaurants closed, but in surprisingly small numbers, and generally it was the weak that went to the wall. Shortening of working hours in the most affected industries was normal and forced unpaid holiday was used as a means to defray costs. The administration was in a difficult position, as it was obvious that some help was needed, if only for political reasons. But bailing out shareholders in companies that were in any case marginal was obviously not the way forward.

On 23 April 2003, the HKSAR Government announced a package of measures that offered a little over HK$11 billion (US$1.4 billion) in aid. It did not just give the money away and attempted to target workers, rather than shareholders, in a package that consisted of the following measures:

1. Rates, water and sewage charges and trade effluent charges were to be waived for one quarter, or four months, to help reduce business costs. Rent concessions were offered for one quarter to most commercial tenants in public housing estates and certain tenants in Government-managed properties. These rent reductions ranged from 30 to 50 percent. The total concessions were worth approximately US$139.74 million (HK$1.09 billion).

2. License fees for tourism-related businesses, caterers, retailers, taxis, school buses and tourist coaches were also to be waived for one year. The total concession was worth US$35.89 million (HK$280 million).

3. The general public received rates, water and sewage rate concessions for one quarter, worth an estimated US$226.92 million (HK$1.77 billion). Hong Kong taxpayers also enjoyed a partial rebate of their salaries tax, amounting to US$294.87 million (HK$2.3 billion).

4. The four hardest hit business sectors — retail, tourism, entertainment and catering — became eligible to apply to a US$448.71 million (HK$3.5 billion) loan-guarantee programme with the Government acting as guarantor for loans from authorised financial institutions to allow these businesses to pay staff salaries.

5. The Government created 21,500 training places and short-term jobs to strengthen service training in the most affected areas. These jobs were intended to provide home cleaning services for the elderly and boost environmental hygiene, at a cost of about US$55.12 million (HK$430 million).

6. About US$128.2 million (HK$1 billion) was set aside for a large-

scale publicity campaign to promote Hong Kong and encourage the return of exhibitions to get trade activities back to normal. The publicity event was launched after the spread of the disease was brought under control.

7. The Government allocated US$166.66 million (HK$1.3 billion) for disease control, medical research and strengthening of public-hygiene measures. An additional US$25.64 million (HK$200 million) was earmarked to provide assistance and professional training for health care workers.

8. The Government pledged to not propose any adjustment to Government fees and charges for the ensuing six months.

Looking back, this was not the first time that Hong Kong has had to undertake a package of financial support for its businesses. This also happened in 1925, under much more dire circumstances,[26] when a Chinese embargo of trade with Hong Kong brought the colony to a near halt for nine months, and the stock exchange was shut. The administration set aside three million pounds to help businesses survive, comparatively, a much larger amount than the sum dedicated to that purpose this time around.

Moreover, despite the SARS-induced slump, the trade machine did not stop and Hong Kong continued to make money. Now that SARS is at least in remission, it will hopefully be possible for people in Hong Kong to reflect on the real impact of the disease and reconsider the validity of some of the more hysterical forecasts.

Tourism has been hurt, but is starting to recover more rapidly than was the case for New York after the 9/11 incident. The shops are busy and there are queues outside the restaurants once more. The first tour groups from the mainland have come across the border and Hong Kong people are travelling across the border for vacation once more.

Perhaps I am being rather too sanguine, but I have lived in Hong Kong long enough to have experienced the uncertainties over the resumption of sovereignty 20 years ago. I remember well how dark Hong Kong's future looked after the Tiananmen Square crackdown, as stories of impending civil war swirled around the city. Those events were much more life threatening for Hong Kong than SARS. In fact, it is likely that SARS will come to be seen as a blessing in disguise in due course. Its occurrence has dramatically emphasised the importance of the liberal values that Hong Kong was fortunate enough to inherit from its former colonial masters. It is all too easy to mouth the expression "freedom of the press," but it is much more rare to see such an explicit illustration of why this freedom is so important.

The comparison between the freedoms that we take for granted here and the systems and inherited mindsets that still persist on the mainland will not be readily forgotten. A Hong Kong population that had been dispirited by constant media chatter about the emergence of China may well realise in future that it takes much more than raw GDP numbers to enter the realms of the first world. If we are really lucky, people in Hong Kong may even realise that China is only developing because of the expertise and capital that market-hardened Hong Kong business people are providing.

Ultimately, SARS proved to be deceiving, rather like those dramatic buildings on the waterfront in Hong Kong whose physical presence has caused even experienced local commentators and policy makers to blandly conclude that all that matters in Hong Kong is property. The future of Hong Kong will be dictated, as always, by what happens on the mainland. In that context, SARS could well help to speed the opening of China as the experience showed the leadership there that GDP numbers are built on the very fragile basis of international confidence. And further opening will mean that Hong Kong's role in China's development will be enhanced. Just as the beneficial outcome that arose from the apparently dire confluence of factors after World War II could not have been foreseen, so it may be with SARS. It may not be too far fetched to say that SARS may turn out to have been the best thing that has happened to Hong Kong and China for a very long time.

CHAPTER 12

The Media and SARS

Christine Loh, Veronica Galbraith and William Chiu

For the international media, the SARS virus was the next big story after the Iraq War. As SARS spread quickly around the world via Hong Kong, the medical, social, economic and political aspects of the disease were the subjects of extensive media coverage. At the outset, the lack of information about the virus led to some highly sensational reporting. This situation was compounded by the fact that SARS originated in China, where the government's penchant for secrecy made it hard to get at the facts. Early reports were often incomplete and raised many worrisome questions. However, despite criticisms that the media was fear mongering, intense and highly critical international reporting helped pressure the Chinese Government to be more transparent about the outbreak.

For the Hong Kong media, SARS was one of the biggest news stories ever. The local media played a special role in the reporting of the outbreak worldwide, as it was only when SARS hit Hong Kong in late February 2003 that it received international attention. Unlike mainland China, Hong Kong enjoys freedom of expression and freedom of the press, factors that enabled both the local and the international media to report on the domestic situation as Hong Kong emerged as the epicentre of the worldwide SARS outbreak and provide the global community with information about the new disease.

The SARS outbreak showed that a free media is vital in a crisis situation and in keeping the authorities honest. While there have been criticisms that the media "hyped" the outbreak and exaggerated its effect, it should remembered that the initial sensational reporting had much to do with the novelty of the disease and the lack of information from mainland authorities.

This chapter starts by examining how the international media reported the outbreak in Hong Kong, which in turn shaped public perceptions worldwide. It goes on to discuss the HKSAR Government's shortcomings in handling communication with the media and takes a look at the various roles played by the local media during the crisis. It notes, for example, how the Hong Kong media defended press freedom when it saw this being threatened by the government's attempt to pass new national security legislation under Article 23 of the Basic Law. It continues by comparing how SARS was reported in Hong Kong and Toronto in order to draw insights about the differences between the two societies. Finally, the media's situation in mainland China is discussed.

International media coverage of Hong Kong

At the start of the outbreak, the international media suspected that the HKSAR Government was attempting to cover up the number of infections. This was probably not the case, but as the Hong Kong authorities and the World Health Organisation (WHO) used different criteria in diagnosing SARS, it created the impression that Hong Kong was trying to conceal the actual number of cases.[1] While mistakes were made in the government's handling of the situation, as recounted in some of the other chapters in this book, WHO officials in fact commended Hong Kong on its transparency and cooperation. However, early reports that raised doubts about the honesty and effectiveness of Hong Kong authorities had already done damage to the city's international reputation.[2]

Hong Kong was portrayed internationally as "death city." The Canadian news magazine *Maclean's* featured a picture of a mask-wearing woman riding on the Star Ferry.[3] Behind her, emerging from the pale-green waters of Victoria Harbour, was the grey Hong Kong skyline, barely visible under a low-lying cloud. The immediate impression conveyed by the photo was ominous and sickly: an infected city smothered by fog, surrounded by stagnant water. Other pictures of the now infamous

Metropole Hotel, where Hong Kong's first known SARS "super-spreader" stayed briefly before checking into hospital, and Amoy Gardens, the site of the most serious community outbreak, depicted large and ugly structures against a darkened sky.

The most widely publicised image of the SARS outbreak in Hong Kong was the facemask. Photographers captured it everywhere — on couples at weddings, people attending religious services, in business meetings, classrooms and restaurants and on the streets. The young and old, humans and animals, even images of Madonna and Buddha, all sported facemasks. The N95 mask, reported to be the most effective type of protective mask, became an icon of the outbreak in Hong Kong, but images of Hello Kitty, Doraemon and knock-off "Louis Vuitton" and "Burberry's" masks drew media attention as well. Cartoonists from around the world also provided many poignant images of the impact of SARS on Hong Kong.

International media reporting on SARS frequently used emotive language, which influenced story slants. Newspapers and news shows described SARS as a "serial killer" or a "killer virus," contributing to worldwide fear and panic. Other dangerous diseases have not been given such strongly worded names. Malaria, for instance, is generally not referred to by the media as a "deadly parasitic killer," even though one million people die from the disease every year.[4] Some newspapers, such as Spain's *El Mundo,* referred to SARS as *"neumonia asiatica,"* or the "Asian pneumonia,"[5] a throwback to stereotypes of Asians as the "yellow peril."[6] The fears raised by the association of the disease with Asian communities helped to empty restaurants in Chinatowns around the world. The de facto boycott of Chinese restaurants in the US and Canada was a good example of how media sensationalism led to an unnecessary level of public anxiety. In an editorial in the *Asian Wall Street Journal,* Nobel laureate virologist David Baltimore took the US media to task for what he saw as alarmist coverage of SARS.[7]

On 16 March 2003, the WHO began to compile a list of the cities and countries that were "SARS-affected areas." Updates were provided regularly and available on its website. Given the fear of SARS worldwide, once a place had been added to the SARS "affected area" list, few wanted to travel there. The WHO travel advisories for Hong Kong and Guangdong Province, issued on 2 April 2003, made headline news, locally, nationally and internationally. While the travel advisories recommended the postponement of non-essential travel, they had the effect of stopping international travel to and from these areas almost completely. The WHO's explanation that the goal was only to alert travellers to take greater care while travelling and *not* to suggest that they should cancel all trips, was lost on the international public.[8] The impact of the travel advisory on Hong Kong, particularly in terms of the travel and tourism sectors and discrimination against Hong Kong residents, is discussed in greater detail in Chapters 9 and 13.[9] The good news was that as the outbreak eased, the economic impact on affected countries, while severe in the short term, appeared to be not nearly as great as the media had originally anticipated for the medium term (see Chapter 11).

Once it was reported that the new virus was likely to have come from animals, media reports began referring to Guangdong Province, where SARS originated, as "China's Petri Dish to the World."[10] Descriptions of humans and animals living "cheek by jowl" were common in the press.[11] The media questioned mainland hygiene practices, citing the "Chinese" habit of spitting.[12] Images of billboards in China condemning spitting, stories about volunteers distributing plastic spitting bags and increased spitting fines, combined to draw an unpleasant picture of Chinese hygiene habits.[13]

An article in the Swiss magazine *L'illustré* that portrayed Hong Kong as a ghost town, whose leaders were out of touch with reality and whose citizens were trying to be optimistic in a desperate situation, was typical of the tone of international reporting.[14] The sub-heading "*veritable psychosis*" implied that in addition to physical illness, SARS had also induced a state of mental illness in the city. The impression was that citizens were not coping, while leaders were overwhelmed. The international media did become more balanced in its reporting over time as more information about SARS became available, but the initial tone and style of reporting helped to create an undeservedly negative perception of Hong Kong.

Lack of a communication strategy

The HKSAR Government was an important source of information for the international media. However, the initial decision by Hong Kong officials to downplay the danger of the virus and the uncertain manner in which they dealt with such issues as quarantine arrangements and closing schools created the impression that Hong Kong authorities were less competent than those in Singapore or other affected areas.[15] Hong Kong was hit hard by the SARS outbreak — but none of its officials proved equal to playing the kind of leadership role demonstrated by former New York City mayor Rudy Giuliani after the terrorist attacks on 11 September 2001. Without strong leadership, Hong Kong appeared rudderless, and this did nothing to improve its international image.

Media calls for more official information on the SARS outbreak resulted in daily press briefings that were usually conducted by the Director of Health Dr. Margaret Chan, and a representative from the Hospital Authority (HA), which manages the city's public hospitals. These briefings, which focused on the Chinese-language media, were useful in terms of informing the local population about the status of the outbreak but were not designed to communicate information to an international audience. For example, simultaneous translation from Cantonese to English was seldom provided, and questions asked and answered in Cantonese were often not repeated in English for the benefit of international reporters.[16] Furthermore, there were few press briefings and interviews by top officials in English, indicating that they did not have a focused strategy for communicating with the international media.[17] The lack of attention to the international media was curious because Hong Kong promotes itself as being "Asia's World City," a title that implies an outward orientation. How the authorities communicated with the world on SARS indicated that they have become much more inward looking in recent years. Officials were apparently more concerned about how their actions and decisions were seen locally via the domestic media than internationally. Otherwise it would be difficult to explain why so little attention was paid to engaging the international media during the SARS outbreak.

For example, one event that could have generated positive international coverage of Hong Kong in terms of cooperation with the mainland was the meeting that took place in Shenzhen on 12 April between Hong Kong's Chief Executive, Tung Chee-hwa, and the Chinese President, Hu Jintao.[18] However, the meeting was kept secret until after the event. It should be noted that in this instance, the decision for confidentiality would have been made by Beijing. As Chapters 9 and 10 highlight, it was only after Hu returned to Beijing that a Politburo meeting was held to discuss SARS at the highest level of the Chinese Community Party, after which Hu called for open and honest reporting of SARS on the mainland.

In addition to its apparent lack of sophistication in handling the international media, the HKSAR Government was also slow to develop effective public relations strategies for informing people in Hong Kong about the situation. The SARS outbreak showed that the HKSAR Government was poor at handling crisis situations. A crisis, by definition, happens quickly but is usually preceded by warning signals that something is wrong. This was certainly the case with SARS, as media reports had already indicated that there was an infectious disease outbreak in Guangdong. There can be no excuse for the failure of Hong Kong authorities to pay attention to the press conference held by Guangdong authorities on 10 February 2003 regarding the outbreak of atypical pneumonia in the province. When authorities are confronted by a crisis, there is often an urgent need to make decisions quickly. Both the Department of Health and the HA appear to have been slow in several instances in acknowledging the problem and taking necessary action, as other chapters show. In order to manage a crisis, decision-makers need to be able to rapidly assess events and take action, as well as devise a communication strategy to inform the public and the media about the situation and the government response.

No doubt one of the lessons of the SARS experience for Hong Kong is that it needs to respond better to crisis situations, whether the threat is posed by SARS or another illness, and at the same time ensure that an effective communication strategy is in place. One way to counter negative international press would have been to draw media attention to Hong Kong's strengths and abilities, many of which were highlighted by the SARS outbreak. For example, Hong Kong's long and distinguished tradition in medicine was hardly mentioned in the international media. Although Hong Kong has a world-class healthcare system, media reports focused on the death of patients and portrayed the system as being "on the verge of collapse."[19] The reality was that local hospitals and healthcare professionals were coping well, albeit under very difficult circumstances. Apart from stories about the courage of individual healthcare workers in treating SARS patients, there was little other positive reporting on Hong Kong's healthcare system, the one exception being coverage of the excellent detective work of Hong Kong's virologists in identifying the coronavirus as the SARS culprit.

Other positive developments that the HKSAR Government could have highlighted were the signification advances in public health management and interdepartmental cooperation during the crisis. These included the development of a specialised, standardised and centralised internal registry with the capacity to register probable SARS cases accurately and quickly. Without this SARS system, it would have been extremely difficult to track and manage cases. The system linked into the police information network, enabling the authorities to trace contacts and monitor location alerts in an extremely efficient way. A multi-disciplinary team made up of members from the Department of Health, the Environmental Protection Department and the Hong Kong Police Force used information gathered through the system to work together in fighting SARS. A WHO official commented that this was the first time the Internet had been used to assist in the management of a public health problem.[20] The new systems were developed under pressure, and the fact that they were rapidly and successfully implemented indicated that Hong Kong had the capacity to cope. The HKSAR Government could have played on these strengths much more effectively in its dealings with the media and the public.

Local reporting in Hong Kong

The SARS outbreak received more coverage than any other story in recent Hong Kong history. Experienced journalists have noted that SARS occupied headlines for a longer period of time than any other news story since the Gulf War in 1991. It was also the story that had the most substantial and direct impact on Hong Kong society during this period.[21] The local media pieced together the SARS story as it developed and made it understandable to the public, a task made more difficult when there was so much that even experts did not know about the disease.[22] The outbreak showcased the Hong Kong media's greatest strength — its speed and timeliness in getting information to the public.[23] Media efficiency helped to raise public awareness of the seriousness of the crisis and publicise measures to minimise the risk of contracting the virus.[24]

The Hong Kong media's role in reporting SARS helped to salvage its sagging reputation. Over the last few years, the local Chinese-language press in particular has been continuously criticised for its poor ethics and sensationalism in providing too much explicit "sex and blood."[25] In their reporting of SARS, publications that were well known for "embellishing" stories, such as *Apple Daily* and *Next Magazine*, were careful in the way that they handled facts.[26] More serious publications, such as the *Hong Kong Economic Journal*, maintained their more cautious style of reporting. In many ways, there was no need for the media to be sensational in its reporting because the SARS outbreak was sensational enough. Dramatic moments included the press conference held by whistle-blower Dr. Sydney Chung (see below), the Dean of Medicine at the Chinese University of Hong Kong (CUHK), and the Amoy Gardens outbreak. Another emotionally charged story was that of Dr. Joanna Tse Yuen-Man, a young doctor who died after being infected while treating SARS patients. She became a symbol of the courage and professionalism of Hong Kong healthcare workers and a local heroine. Her death and funeral received extensive coverage.

In general, Chinese-language publications devoted more space to SARS-related stories than their English-language counterparts, although at the height of the crisis, there was also extensive coverage in the *South China Morning Post* (*SCMP*), Hong Kong's major English-language newspaper, and *The Standard*, Hong Kong's English-language financial paper. The popular *Apple Daily*, for example, devoted special sections to SARS every day throughout the crisis.

In addition to differences in the number of pages allocated to SARS coverage, there were differences in the way that the English- and Chinese-language press in Hong Kong reported on the disease. This contrast was largely in terms of sensibilities rather than information, reflecting cultural differences more than anything else. For example, during a public discussion on when schools would re-open, Westerners were generally keen for classes to resume as they saw the risk of their children catching SARS at school to be very low, whereas Chinese parents preferred to wait until they felt more assured that the environment was safe.[27] Readers of the English press in Hong Kong include the city's foreign community and Chinese residents who read English as a matter of habit, even though many also read Chinese newspapers. A longstanding subject of discussion in Hong Kong is the fact that those who only read the English newspapers get a very different sense of local affairs than those who only read the Chinese newspapers.

Challenging official views

By early March 2003, the atmosphere in hospitals, particularly at the Prince of Wales and Princess Margaret hospitals, had become extremely tense as staff continued to fall ill. Those within the healthcare system used the media as a platform to communicate directly with the public about what was happening. A watershed event was Dr. Sydney Chung's press conference on 17 March. As the head of CUHK's medical school, which uses the Prince of Wales Hospital (PWH) as its teaching facility, Dr. Chung witnessed the SARS outbreak firsthand. As a healthcare professional, he felt the need to inform the public about the virus and the extent of the outbreak, which, contrary to statements by the Secretary for Health, Welfare and Food Dr. EK Yeoh, and the Director of Health Dr. Margaret Chan, had spread to the general community.[28] Dr. Chung wanted to close hospital wards to prevent the spread of the virus.[29] He felt that his superiors at the HA and government officials were not listening, and that he had to take matters into his own hands by going public with his concerns.

After Dr. Chung's emotional statement to reporters, Hong Kong people finally realised how serious the new virus was. The local media also became convinced that the SARS story was important and began devoting more resources to cover it. The media noted that as SARS spread to other countries, authorities overseas immediately put in place isolation and quarantine measures and demanded to know why the HKSAR Government was not doing the same. The authorities eventually did implement similar measures.[30] Dr. Chung's own assessment was that Hong Kong's free media had nudged the HKSAR Government into action. He described the overall reporting of the outbreak by the media as being of a high standard.[31]

Monitoring the authorities

The media is often termed the "Fourth Estate" because of its role in checking the power of the three branches of government — the executive, the legislature and the judiciary. Its agenda is to be alert for anything out of the ordinary and keep those in power honest. The existence of a free and aggressive media may be particularly important in Hong Kong because of the unusual nature of its polity, under which people enjoy a high degree of personal freedoms, including freedom of speech, but do not participate in the creation of the government through democratic elections. The local media therefore plays a vital part in monitoring the authorities and providing a space for people to articulate public opinion as a way of holding decision-makers to account.[32] During the SARS outbreak, the local media was clearly proactive in carrying out this role.[33] Its aggressive stance towards the government stemmed both from its distrust of the authorities in general and the particular concerns raised by Dr. Chung's press conference.[34]

The media was also a channel for members of the public to vent their dissatisfaction and anxiety, providing them with a measure of psychological release. Although the Letter to the Editor and editorial sections of newspapers were important channels for expressing public sentiment, the most significant outlet was phone-in radio programmes. One of Hong Kong's most popular radio shows is *Teacup in a Storm*, a morning programme on Commercial Radio hosted by the outspoken commentator Albert Cheng, well-known for his tough questions, and his partner Peter Lam.[35] Programme listeners make up 80 percent of all Hong Kong listeners between 7:30 a.m. and 10:00 a.m. Given its wide audience, *Teacup in a Storm* is an important forum for shaping public opinion on all kinds of issues. During the SARS outbreak, Cheng demanded information and answers from ministers and senior officials and provided airtime for doctors, nurses and politicians to put their views across. In turn, government and health officials also used the programme to make public statements. A regular caller into *Teacup in a Storm* was Dr. Ko Wing-Man, Director of Professional Services and Public Affairs for the HA. As the outbreak raised many questions about medical management of SARS, distressed frontline doctors and nurses called into the programme to confront Dr. Ko on air. The programme became a daily enquiry into how Hong Kong's hospitals were dealing with SARS, with Cheng passing judgment on official decisions and initiatives. As a result, the HA was forced to change course or amend its policies on some issues.[36] Since the print media closely monitors *Teacup in a Storm*, key issues brought up during the programme were often echoed in newspapers and news magazines, shaping public discussion for several days. Similarly, when the government-appointed SARS Expert Committee released its report on the government's handling of the outbreak on 2 October 2003, phone-in radio programmes provided an immediate interactive platform for members of the public to respond.[37]

During the outbreak, the influence of media figures like Albert Cheng reinforced the impression that the government was under siege, as officials no longer seemed to be taking the lead in providing guidance to the public. In a number of instances, Cheng's position on an issue prompted a knee-jerk reaction from the government, highlighting the lack of an official policy on the issue. For example, after Cheng promoted the wearing of facemasks, the government also endorsed facemasks, but did not give clear directions as to how and when they should be used. Government officials began wearing masks during television interviews, which not only muffled their voices but also suggested that facemasks should be worn at all times. Once officials started wearing facemasks, government offices expected staff to wear masks at meetings, which then led public utility companies and universities to encourage staff and students to wear facemasks. The issue of personal protection was brought to a new height when the Chief Executive's wife, Mrs. Betty Tung, paid a visit to Lower Ngau Tau Kok Estate to hand out hygiene kits. Mrs. Tung wore not only a facemask but also a plastic protective gown, gloves and shoes guards, in addition to a protective cap. Her protective gear was even more elaborate than those worn by healthcare workers in intensive care units (ICU) and had the effect of increasing the alarm of local residents about the public health situation. While her visit was well meaning, the media reported the event as a misguided attempt to fight SARS.[38]

Media pressure also affected how officials handled the demand for information about the extent of the outbreak in the community. Initially citing legal privacy concerns, the government refused to release information about which residential buildings had suspected and confirmed SARS patients. This information was of particular interest to the public given the high population densities in Hong Kong. Because they live in such close proximity to each other, people worried that they would easily become infected. The Internet proved to be an invaluable tool for concerned citizens to use in challenging government secrecy on this issue. A small group of "techies" — Edwin Chan, Nelson Kwan, Bernard Chung and John Lau — joined forces to provide information to the public via their website, www.sosick.org. The website provided lists of buildings where tenants had been diagnosed with or were suspected of having SARS, which were updated daily. Once the site was available, members of the public also began contributing information. Between 2 and 21 April, the site reported five million hits. The print media caught on and used data from the site in its own daily reporting. On 12 April the government finally began providing official information on the outbreak to the public via its own website. On 15 April, the www.sosick.org webmasters decided to stop updating the list of SARS-affected buildings, as the government was now providing this information.[39]

Creating a network of care and support

Hong Kong people have often been portrayed as being materialistic and more interested in making money than anything else. However, the SARS outbreak demonstrated that they were also capable of great generosity and compassion. There was a massive outpouring of sympathy and support for doctors and nurses, who, through their bravery and professionalism, won the respect of the public. During the crisis, ordinary people performed extraordinary acts of courage. The media played a critical role in documenting the human stories of these heroes and making the public aware of their contribution.

The words and images of weeping healthcare workers and their emotional reunion with family members after quarantine were captured in media reports. The tears of fear and joy were real and Hong Kong people could identify with these emotions. Media stories presented a human side of Hong Kong that went beyond wealth or professional life and touched people's hearts. This positive aspect of the SARS crisis created solidarity between medical workers and the public and provided medical workers with much needed support. The deaths of eight medical staff received extensive coverage from the media and elicited widespread sympathy from the public.[40]

The unfortunate residents of Block E of Amoy Gardens were also in the media spotlight. The spread of SARS to this private housing estate was quite sudden, and resulted in the infection of over 200 people in a period of ten days. Residents were eventually moved to quarantine camps. Anxious about the possibility that similar outbreaks would occur in other housing estates in Hong Kong, the public followed every development. Television cameras captured scenes of tearful and terrified residents wrapping themselves in homemade protective suits and being herded out of the housing complex.

Through the media, members of the public and in many cases, media organisations themselves, initiated campaigns and projects to raise money for those directly affected by SARS, including healthcare workers and children of SARS victims. Many media organisations assumed an activist role, going beyond their usual job of reporting objectively on events to become high-profile "enablers"[41] or "campaign facilitators," in the fight against SARS. One of the first media projects was the "One Person, One Facemask" fundraising campaign initiated by Commercial Radio and phone-in talk show hosts Albert Cheng and Peter Lam. The campaign aimed to supply N95 facemasks to all healthcare workers in contact with SARS patients, a direct response to criticisms of healthcare workers regarding the apparent uneven distribution of N95 masks by hospital management. As the campaign evolved, funds were also raised to provide surgical masks, protective gear, vitamins, oranges and bird's nest soup, a traditional Chinese food that strengthens the immune system. In addition, "One Person, One Facemask" mounted billboards all over Hong Kong as a tribute to the hard work and dedication of healthcare workers.

Another prominent example of media activism was the *SCMP*'s "Project Shield." Newspaper readers were invited to contribute to a fund to buy protective gear for hospital workers. The paper was concerned that the HA did not have enough equipment for its staff. In one month, over HK$20 million was raised, to be used in buying equipment and providing funds for the HA to purchase additional equipment. Contributors to the campaign extended well beyond the *SCMP*'s usual readership, clearly reflecting the widespread community desire to help health workers.

The media and SARS in Toronto

Having examined how both the international and Hong Kong media handled SARS, it is useful to compare the domestic media coverage of SARS in Hong Kong with that in Toronto. Differences in the tone and content of reporting reflect important cultural differences, as well as differences in the circumstances of the SARS outbreak in each city.

The WHO placed a travel advisory on Toronto on 23 April, seven weeks after the city's first SARS patient died. On that day, Toronto's cumulative SARS cases totalled 136. Toronto's mayor, Mel Lastman, was furious about the advisory, arguing that Toronto was still safe to visit and accusing the WHO of being uninformed.[42] While Lastman used strong and aggressive language, his anger reflected the feelings of the people of Toronto at the time: SARS was dangerous but it was not a major threat and their city had a good healthcare system that could cope with the situation.[43]

The SARS outbreak was a major media story in Toronto. It even knocked Iraq War reports off the front page. *The Globe and Mail* put five journalists onto the SARS story, a large number given the newspaper's size. Toronto reporters used the Hong Kong media as their source in initial reports about SARS in Hong Kong.[44] Once SARS became an important story in Toronto, reports focused on the situation in local hospitals. Between 20 and 26 April, most of the stories on SARS centred on the economic impact of the outbreak, the need for stronger leadership and how residents were coping. The media noted that unlike Hong Kong, few people in Toronto wore masks as they went about their daily routines. Some businesses did suffer. Hotels experienced a drop in customers, which showed that people were not travelling to Toronto. Diners also avoided Chinese restaurants, which they obviously associated with the risk of catching SARS.

Why were there far fewer facemask wearers in Toronto than in Hong Kong? The answer may well lie in differences between Hong Kong Chinese and Westerners in terms of how their respective cultures assess risk and social etiquette. Whereas Westerners appeared to have focused more on the actual risk of catching the disease in deciding whether to wear a facemask, Hong Kong residents felt safer wearing facemasks.[45] As more and more people wore facemasks, it seemed to encourage even more people to follow suit. At the height of the SARS outbreak, as many as a quarter of the people on Hong Kong's streets wore facemasks. Hong Kong people also felt that it was courteous to wear facemasks in order to reassure others that precautions were being taken, whereas in the West, the facemask represented undue panic.

While many people in Toronto felt that the media there was sensational in covering the outbreak, the coverage was tame when compared to that in Hong Kong. The differences in domestic media coverage reflect cultural differences between the two cities and the circumstances of the outbreak in each. First, Hong Kong people were already used to a more sensational style of journalism. The city has more newspapers and magazines per capita than any other city in the world. Reporting styles span the spectrum from conservative to "infotainment." Second, Hong Kong people were aware that they were at the epicentre of the new disease as they were just across the border from Guangdong, where SARS originated. The border is busy and porous, factors that enabled the initial transfer of SARS to Hong Kong. Third, Hong Kong people knew that the risk of catching infectious diseases increases with population density; Hong Kong's population density is eight times that of Toronto. Indeed, Hong Kong has one of the highest population densities in the world with 6,300 people per square kilometre.[46] Fourth, after the Amoy Gardens outbreak in mid-March, during which more than 40 residents of a Kowloon housing estate died from SARS, Hong Kong people had good reason to be alarmed about the spread of SARS in the community. Many other apartment blocks in the city are similar to the ill-fated estate in terms of construction and design. Moreover, it took some weeks before the authorities could begin to explain what caused the outbreak. As of this writing, no definitive conclusions about what happened at Amoy Gardens have been put forward (see Chapter 7).

Thus, the situation in Hong Kong was more alarming and the tone and style of local media reporting reflected the intense and totally absorbing experience of the outbreak in Hong Kong. By contrast, while the media in Toronto treated SARS as a major story, the disease never overwhelmed daily life as it did in Hong Kong. In addition, it should be noted that Canada, unlike Hong Kong, is a representative democracy. The fact that citizens participate directly in the formation of the government may reduce the importance of the "Fourth Estate" role played by the media. Another obvious difference between Hong Kong and Toronto is the fact that Hong Kong operates within the context of the "one country, two systems" framework. The impact of this policy is discussed in greater detail below.

Reporting on the mainland

Mainland media organisations in Hong Kong supported the HKSAR Government's efforts to fight and contain SARS and maintain social and economic stability.[47] Reporting about SARS in Hong Kong was limited to the number of cases, recoveries and deaths in the territory.[48] This restrained stance echoed the reporting on the mainland SARS outbreak by the domestic media. Until 17 April, when the Politburo permitted more extensive coverage of SARS, the mainland media was highly constrained in what it could say (see Chapters 8, 9 and 10). Media reports echoed the official line that the situation was under control. In a nation where there is a strong culture of official secrecy, even the government-run Chinese Centre for Disease Control (CDC) had to be careful about what information it put out. By mid-April, the CDC website did include links to various press reports on SARS.[49] One possible explanation for this shift is that reports that had already been published were considered "safe." Although the reporting of SARS in China was novel in terms of its frankness and detail, the newfound "transparency" was limited.[50]

The inability of official institutions to discuss SARS in an open and transparent way forced whistle-blowers like Dr. Jiang Yanyong to use the international media as a forum to counter the official line. After China's health minister, Zhang Wenkang, gave a press conference on 3 April saying that China was "safe" and the SARS epidemic there was "effectively under control," Jiang, a retired military doctor, sent an e-mail to China's Central Television and the Hong Kong-based television station, Phoenix, accusing the minister of covering up the truth. He alerted the media to the hundreds of SARS cases in Beijing's military hospitals, which had not been included in official reports on the number of cases in the city. Initially, his e-mail was not acted upon. Jiang then sent his message to the foreign press. On 8 April, the story was reported by the German weekly *Der Spiegel*, and the following day, on the *Time* magazine website.[51] Once the truth was out, Jiang became a folk hero in China for exposing the official cover-up. His message was widely circulated nationally by e-mail and posted on university internal e-bulletins. Although the Chinese Government subsequently admitted that SARS cases in military hospitals had not been included in previous reports on the situation in Beijing, Jiang was put under a gag order not to say any more in public.[52] Even after China was removed from the WHO "affected area" list, signalling an "end" to SARS, domestic media organisations and academics were cautioned not to analyse the government's handling of the SARS crisis.[53]

Some of the most important stories about SARS in mainland China came from the international media organisations based there, as foreign correspondents had more latitude than the domestic media to investigate what was happening. In late March, the Atlanta-based television network *CNN* produced a report on the situation in Guangdong. The report helped the WHO pressure the Chinese Government to begin an investigation into the outbreak.[54] In another instance, the *Boston Globe* pieced together what had happened on Air China Flight 112 on 15 March from Hong Kong to Beijing, during which 21 people contracted SARS. The report highlighted the attempt by Chinese authorities to hide information that might have saved lives and stopped the chain of infections across Asia.[55]

Hong Kong reporting of mainland news

Since 1997, Hong Kong has been a Special Administrative Region of China. Its immediate hinterland is Guangdong Province. Some 350,000 people travel across the Hong Kong-Guangdong border every day, and this number continues to grow.[56] While the Hong Kong media pursued the SARS story aggressively once the virus hit Hong Kong, it did not investigate early signs that something unusual was happening across the border. Hong Kong's mainland-controlled newspapers, such as *Wen Wei Po*, took the official line that the situation in Guangdong was under control. However, even the non mainland-controlled media failed to probe what was really happening. It was not until 24 March 2003 that an investigative report was published by *Ming Pao*, which teamed up with Dr. Leung Ping Chung of CUHK to visit five Guangzhou hospitals. The report cast doubt on the validity of China's official line by noting that the investigative team had found more than 100 SARS patients as well as health care workers still wearing heavy protective gear.[57] A *Ming Pao* editorial criticised the lack of cooperation between Guangdong officials in dealing with the disease, but this was the extent of critical reporting in the Hong Kong media.[58] Even after SARS became a major news story in Hong Kong, the local media did not produce detailed investigative reports comparable to those produced by international media organisations such as *CNN*, the *Boston Globe* and *The Washington Post*.[59]

It is possible that media stories contradicting the official party line are too politically sensitive and politically risky for Hong Kong journalists to report. For instance, the existence of additional SARS cases in Beijing's military hospitals might have been considered a state secret, meaning that risks would have been involved in covering those stories for Hong Kong reporters and media organisations. Hong Kong journalists and academics have already found themselves in serious trouble for reporting on mainland issues. For example, in 1994, *Ming Pao* reporter Xi Yang was sentenced to 12 years in prison for disclosing an alleged financial secret that involved plans by the People's Bank of China to sell off part of its gold reserves.[60] In 2001, academic Li Xiaomin was detained on the mainland and charged with spying although the circumstances of his case were never made clear.[61]

An encouraging sign that the Hong Kong media is now taking a more proactive stance in covering mainland issues was the fact that an outbreak of encephalitis B in Guangdong in mid-June 2003 was reported by the Hong Kong media before the mainland media picked up the story. Although this was a mild, seasonal outbreak, given the post-SARS climate and the demands for improved Guangdong-Hong Kong cooperation in terms of information sharing and prevention and control of infectious diseases, Guangdong authorities should have alerted Hong Kong authorities of the outbreak as soon as it occurred. [62]

Conclusion

A post-SARS survey showed that the Hong Kong public approved of local media coverage of the outbreak both in terms of information provided and monitoring of the authorities.[63] The public also acknowledged the courage and professionalism of frontline reporters, who faced personal danger when reporting from high-infection risk locations, such as hospitals, Amoy Gardens and Lower Ngau Tau Kok Estate. Indeed, reporters have been hailed as the people's heroes for their role in helping to save lives by keeping the public informed about disease transmission and prevention.[64] This encouragement should inspire confidence among Hong Kong's frontline reporters, many of whom are young, that their work is appreciated and that the public is interested in reporting that is accurate and informative. For media owners, the SARS experience may also provide an opportunity to reflect on how they can invest in developing the skills and careers of journalists and editors to improve the quality of reporting.

Exploring how the Hong Kong media could do better in developing its skills to report on mainland stories is also important as more and more Hong Kong people become interested in national and provincial affairs. However, being able to report accurately and critically while negotiating the mainland's culture of secrecy and without falling foul of China's state secrecy laws is a daunting task. Striking this balance has been a longstanding challenge for the Hong Kong media. The media was especially concerned that reporting on mainland stories would be further complicated by the proposed Article 23 legislation, which addresses, among other issues, the reporting of state secrets. Concern about the impact of the legislation on press freedom prompted the media sector to come out in force to object to the government's push for hasty passage of the legislation by 9 July 2003.[65]

There is, however, controversy over whether the media should have played such an activist role during the SARS outbreak and on the Article 23 issue. During the outbreak, media personalities such as Albert Cheng actively promoted certain courses of action. Newspapers used their publications to raise funds to buy protective gear and equipment for hospital workers when hospital management appeared unwilling or unable to do so. They were therefore promoting their own campaigns and reporting on the supply of protective gear and equipment at the same time. In a positive way, the media helped to bridge the communication gap between the public and the authorities when official institutions appeared unable to do so. On the other hand, questions have been raised as to whether "advocacy journalism" is professional and ethical. Some commentators believe that the large showing at the Article 23 rally on 1 July 2003, which drew half a million protestors, was partly influenced by the advocacy journalism of some publications, most notably *Apple Daily*, which produced special pull-outs and stickers opposing the draft law.

The reality may well be that given Hong Kong's current political situation, where the Tung Chee-hwa administration has failed to win the trust of the public over the past six years, the media has a special role to play "to connect and respond to the aspirations and needs of the people."[66] It can only play this role effectively if Hong Kong continues to enjoy freedom of expression. Thus, both the SARS outbreak and Article 23 saga held special significance for the local media. In the case of SARS, the ability of the Hong Kong media to hold local authorities to account for their management of the outbreak contrasted with the strict controls on the role of the mainland media vis-à-vis the provincial and central authorities. Hong Kong's media organisations value their freedom to report on issues fully and critically. The proposed national security legislation would directly impact their ability to do so. It is therefore unsurprising that reporters and media organisations saw the SARS outbreak and Article 23 as being not only critical for the Hong Kong community but also fundamental to their role within the community. The local media proved willing to overstep the traditional boundaries of this role in the interests of safeguarding media freedoms.

Acknowledgements

The authors wish to thank David Armstrong, Richard Cullen, Bob Dietz, Anthony Fung, Clement So and Jan Wong for their advice.

CHAPTER **13**

SARS and the Hong Kong Community

Christine Loh and Jennifer Welker

T he SARS experience in Hong Kong left residents with a sense of pride in their community. Despite the fear associated with the outbreak of an unknown disease that took many lives and affected thousands more throughout the city between the end of February and June 2003, the overall community response was mature, professional, generous and compassionate.

By mid-April, people knew that they could no longer hide at home to escape SARS. There was a strong surge of civic energy to promote disease prevention and help each other get through difficult times. New civic networks and alliances were formed. Healthcare professionals overcame their own anxiety about catching the disease to care for the sick. Doctors and nurses provided comfort to the dying when their families were not allowed into isolation wards. The local media, often accused of sensational reporting, provided extensive daily reports to the public in a responsible manner. As Hong Kong was forced to slow down, individuals found time to reassess their personal priorities. Companies realised that they had social responsibilities above and beyond maximising profits.

SARS provided Hong Kong with an opportunity to see its own strengths more clearly. What was left in the devastating trail of SARS was a strong sense of civic pride among Hong Kong people. The experience had renewed their sense of love and commitment for their city. They found that they desperately needed to feel strong and confident again as the years since 1997 had not only been tough economically, but also seemed to have sapped some of Hong Kong's vital spirit and energy.

This chapter tells the story of how fear turned to action and eventually to pride for the people of Hong Kong during the SARS outbreak. Its heroes were ordinary people who found themselves capable of extraordinary things under pressure. Their efforts embodied the Hong Kong spirit and helped the community to understand itself better. SARS provided a defining experience that left a sense of pride and also a feeling of self-empowerment among Hong Kong citizens. Whether or not SARS re-emerges in Hong Kong, the SARS spirit is likely to have a long-term impact on Hong Kong's future development.

The longest day

While the first SARS case hit Hong Kong on 21 February, it took some time before the government realised and acknowledged the seriousness of the new disease and for the community to understand its full impact. Hong Kong's first SARS hero, from the community's point of view, was Professor Sydney Chung, dean of medicine at the Chinese University of Hong Kong (CUHK), who took things into his own hands on 17 March by holding a press conference to speak out about the high number of infections at the Prince of Wales Hospital (PWH) and the spread of the disease into the community. He went public because he could not get the speedy response that was needed to control the spread of the disease by working within the system of the Hospital Authority (HA), which manages Hong Kong's public hospitals, and the Department of Health — and because he was frustrated by the lack of official transparency regarding the actual extent of the outbreak. While Hong Kong authorities subsequently released more complete and accurate information on the SARS crisis to the public, including a SARS Expert Committee report[1] on government handling of the outbreak, released on 2 October 2003, it was Chung who helped Hong Kong to begin asking questions and demanding answers from the authorities.

By the weekend of 22 and 23 March, Hong Kong was still able to welcome thousands of overseas visitors for the annual Rugby Sevens, one of its most popular international sporting events. However, a week later, events started to spiral out of control. On 1 April 2003, residents of Block E of Amoy Gardens, a private residential estate in urban Kowloon, were placed in isolation camps following an outbreak of SARS in the building. Within a matter of days, the number of infected residents had grown rapidly — a situation made even more frightening because of the lack of understanding about how transmission was occurring. SARS seemed to be taking over the community. On the same day, the US Department of State authorised non-emergency employees at the US Consulate and their families to leave Hong Kong on a voluntary basis as a result of the mysterious disease. In a tragedy unconnected to SARS, Leslie Cheung, one of Hong Kong's most beloved singer-actors, jumped to his death that evening, causing deep mourning among his tens of thousands of fans. The mood in Hong Kong was becoming eerie.

The events of April Fool's Day were sobering enough, but the joke that played on the fears of Hong Kong residents came from a 14-year-old boy who sparked a major panic by posting a fake message on what appeared to be the website of the local *Ming Pao* newspaper. The bogus message stated that Hong Kong would be declared an "infected port" imminently and be cut off from the rest of the world, that the Hang Seng Index had collapsed and that Chief Executive Tung Chee-hwa had resigned. Terrified, people rushed to supermarkets and grocery stores to stock up on rice and other essential goods. Tens of thousands of telephone calls were made that afternoon as residents warned each other about the impending disaster. The following day, the WHO placed a travel advisory on Hong Kong, and the US Centers for Disease Control (CDC) followed with another warning. The advisory recommended that people postpone non-essential travel to Hong Kong — a message that convinced international travellers to stay away altogether. The emergency press conference held by Director of Health Dr. Margaret Chan in order to quell rumours fuelled by the April Fool's Day prank did little to calm public anxiety when so many signs were pointing to a crisis.

International reporting about what was happening portrayed Hong Kong as a devastated community — an image that coloured international perceptions of the outbreak and, in turn, impacted how Hong Kong saw itself. Tales of public panic and images of people in masks spread like wildfire through major international news channels. Here are two examples of how Hong Kong was characterised overseas on March 31 and April 1:

A Deadly Virus on its Mind, Hong Kong Covers its Face

Health officials in Hong Kong announced 60 more cases of SARS, bringing a total for the last four days to 204; this is more than the rest of the world combined not counting mainland China … In Hong Kong, some expatriates and affluent citizens are beginning to flee the city. For those who stay, common surgical masks have become the obsession…the health news is getting scarier by the day.[2]

— *The New York Times*, 31 March

Mystery Bug Sets Tongues Wagging

More than a month into the outbreak of a mysterious and deadly pneumonia virus, Hong Kong is a city gripped by fear…a place that markets itself as "The City of Life" and whose lifeblood is travel, trade and international business, is acquiring a reputation as a place of disease.[3]

— *CNN*, aired 1 April

Hong Kong: Forsaken

Hong Kong's economic lifeblood is the constant flow of people, cargo, services and capital. When people started to avoid Hong Kong, the perception of residents was that they had been forsaken. Multinational companies around the world stopped employees from travelling into and out of much of Asia. Travellers avoided Asia for fear of catching the disease and the sheer inconvenience of potential quarantine on their return home. It was clear that until the WHO's travel advisory was lifted, the world would continue to stay away from Hong Kong.[4] The message was clear: "Hong Kong, you are on your own."

Prior to 2 April 2003, the Hong Kong International Airport received 90,000 to 100,000 inbound passengers every day and was one of the world's busiest air hubs. In the month of April, passenger numbers fell 68 percent. While the normal number of passengers for the month would have been around 2.9 million, the actual number was only 909,000. Things worsened in May with only 565,000 arrivals, down nearly 80 percent from the same time a year earlier. During the height of the crisis, the airport had a mere 15,000 arrivals a day.[5] Even the number of visitors from mainland China fell by 40 percent as China, too, was caught up in its own efforts to fight SARS.[6]

The situation was equally dire for Hong Kong people going overseas. Malaysia was the first country to impose stricter entry requirements. Swiss health officials barred Hong Kong participants from the World Jewellery and Watch Fair in Zurich, resulting in the exclusion of more than 300 Hong Kong representatives from one of the industry's most important trade fairs. A *New York Times* report captured the despair and defiance of Hong Kong traders who could not attend the show: "In an empty case at the booth of a Hong Kong company, [a sign] said, apparently in bitter jest, 'Due to our fear of Swiss Aggravated Respiratory Syndrome we are going home.'"[7]

Other unhappy experiences reinforced Hong Kong's sense of being a pariah. Hong Kong youngsters attending boarding schools in Britain had to be quarantined on the Isle of Wight after the Easter vacation.[8] A number of US universities, the most high-profile being the University of California at Berkeley, took decisions either to ban Hong Kong students or to ask them and their relatives to stay away from graduation ceremonies.[9] In mid-May, the Irish Government asked athletes from SARS-affected regions not to attend the Special Olympics being held in June in Dublin.[10] Many Hong Kong residents stopped travelling overseas since they felt unwelcome in so many places.

With travellers staying away from Hong Kong and in the absence of outbound travel, almost overnight, airline seats and hotel beds became empty. Hotel occupancy rates dipped into the single digits and stayed there for weeks, in sharp contrast to average monthly occupancies of 80 to 90 percent, citywide.[11] Travel operators had little to do. Even Hong Kong residents did not feel like going out or eating in restaurants. They were in no mood to shop either. Restaurants, cinemas and shopping malls were empty.

Fear of the unknown

The fear of the unknown can be a powerful stimulant for all kinds of atypical behaviour. In the early days, it was hard to come to grips with SARS because no one knew what it was, where it had originated or how it was being transmitted. Medical experts could not be certain about most aspects of the new disease — but knew that there was no cure. It was clear that some of those who became infected had the capability to spread SARS to a large number of people — these cases became known as "super-spreaders." Even more frightening, some SARS carriers displayed mild symptoms but could be highly contagious. It remains a mystery why some people were infected while others were not, even in instances when both were in the vicinity of a SARS carrier at the same time. Equally mysterious was the low infectivity of SARS for children.

People in Hong Kong would have appreciated official guidance on how to handle the situation, but this was not forthcoming. When so much was unknown, people had to make decisions based on myth, opinion and a limited number of facts. From early April onwards, not only were meetings and large gatherings involving overseas attendance postponed or cancelled, Hong Kong residents began to rearrange their activities as well. Many people avoided meetings, not only in their business lives but also with family and friends. The eventual closure of schools on 27 March, and later universities, meant that SARS affected the lives of everyone in the community, even the very young. Hong Kong people could not recall another experience that had been so pervasive and so invasive. The widespread usage of facemasks in Hong Kong was a symbol of the underlying panic. It was the one easy thing everyone could do to give themselves a small sense of control.

Overseas coverage of the situation in Hong Kong continued to prey on public uncertainty and fear:

In Hong Kong, SARS Fears Infect Hearts and Minds

Hong Kong is under siege. Each day brings government announcements of more deaths and an average of 40 new infections. Ordinary life is on hold...and even some Catholic churches [are] refusing to give communion. An advice columnist in the *South China Morning Post* told a worried mother not to attend the ballet with her children "to be on the safe side."[12]

— *USA Today*, 15 April

Hong Kong's guardian angels

On 26 March, Professor Sydney Chung described SARS and what was happening at PWH as "a holocaust." He told reporters that: "It is a war with an unknown enemy... It is the worse medical disaster I have ever seen."[13] Chung has remained a key figure in memories of Hong Kong's fight against SARS due to his principled stance against the Hong Kong authorities, which on 17 March denied that the disease had spread to the community. CUHK's faculty of medicine weighed the fine balance between warning the public and causing unnecessary panic and leaned on the side of truth. Chung noted that: "I have never in my life wished so much that I was wrong," and said that the faculty "felt a social and ethical responsibility" to speak out "whatever the cost to the Faculty and whomever might be annoyed."[14]

As Chapter 2 describes, hospital workers and medical students started to fall ill in large numbers at PWH starting in the first week of March. Chapter 3 tells the personal story of Dr. Gregory Cheng, one of the doctors who became ill. Yet healthcare professionals continued to battle on. The PWH team that cared for SARS patients called themselves the "Dirty Team." Their daily work became treacherous and potentially deadly. The team's first moment of triumph came on 29 March when the first group of recovered SARS patients were discharged from the hospital, although there was still a long way to go before SARS would eventually run its course.

During the first four weeks of the outbreak, Hong Kong had 1,190 SARS cases, including 287 healthcare workers and medical students, and 47 deaths. It was heartbreaking for the city's medical professionals to see colleagues and students coming down with the disease. During the first month, there were two fatalities among healthcare workers and doctors knew there would be more. Even the head of the HA, Dr. William Ho, was infected; during his illness, he attended to hospital affairs from the Queen Mary Hospital's isolation ward.

There were many other stories of commitment and professionalism among Hong Kong's medical workers. The foresight of Dr. York Chow, the head of Queen Mary Hospital, in quickly introducing infectious disease prevention refresher courses helped healthcare workers there to operate with extra care. The team at the Princess Margaret Hospital, which took in the largest number of SARS patients during the height of the Amoy Gardens outbreak, had to work against extraordinary odds, dealing with 510 cases at one stage. Dr. Chow noted on 13 April that: "Health care workers are yearning for support and relief, but they have to fight on."[15]

The frustration with officialdom felt by some of Hong Kong's most senior and experienced medical professionals was intense. CUHK's faculty of medicine, which uses PWH as its teaching facility, found it hard to excuse public officials for not alerting them "to earlier SARS cases in other hospitals in Hong Kong — a lapse that remains a mystery...."[16] Dr. Chow, who chaired the Anti-SARS Task Force, described the situation for the medical profession in mid-April thus: "[SARS] resembles a scenario where people are washed by floodwaters into a river, with the downstream lifesavers frantically trying to save everyone, with many drowning in the process. Is there really no way to stop the flood, or to equip everyone with floating devices?"[17]

Many public sector and even some private sector doctors volunteered to help SARS patients even though they knew they were putting themselves in danger. Nurses and other hospital staff also showed dedication and commitment to their jobs. They did not ask to be paid more for taking risks, and continued to put their professionalism above all else. Many of the doctors said that the reason they had chosen to study medicine was to save lives — SARS gave meaning to their vocation. The death of a young doctor, Joanna Tse Yuen-man, on 13 May touched Hong Kong deeply. Tse graduated from medical school in 1992 and worked at the Tuen Mun Hospital. She volunteered to look after SARS patients but eventually succumbed to the disease. She became Hong Kong's heroine — the symbol of all that was noble and good in human nature.

Despite praise for Hong Kong's healthcare workers, there was one sour note. When the HKSAR Government published the 2003 honours list on 1 July 2003, the medical profession was flabbergasted at how clumsily the authorities had dealt with recognition of the health care workers who died fighting SARS. It was incomprehensible to them that while Dr. Tse Yuen-man was given a posthumous Medal for Bravery (Gold), five other public health care workers received silver medals. Two private sector doctors who died after contracting SARS from their patients received no recognition at all. In honouring the dead, it seemed unnecessary and insensitive to make any distinction between them.[18]

Beyond the frontline doctors and healthcare staff were researchers who spent many sleepless nights studying the SARS virus for data that could be used to find a cure. Professor Malik Peiris, Professor K Y Yuen and their team at the University of Hong Kong (HKU) were the first in the world to identify the coronavirus as the culprit on 21 March, while the SARS research team at CUHK, led by Dr. Dennis Lo Yuk-ming, was among the earliest in the world to complete the sequencing of the coronavirus genome. The HKU team was also instrumental in demonstrating that the SARS virus most probably jumped from the civet cat to humans.[19] Indeed, Hong Kong experts have so far accounted for half of all scientific publications related to SARS.[20] Hong Kong was suddenly aware that its resources included top class microbiologists whose work was critical to global understanding of SARS, and that the work of local experts had received international attention.

Community gratitude for the work of Hong Kong's medical professionals could be seen from the large sums donated to the *South China Morning Post*'s *Project Shield* campaign, set up to purchase protective gear for healthcare professionals after it became known that existing supplies were insufficient. More than 10,000 individuals, organisations and companies contributed to the fund throughout the ten-day campaign, which raised HK$20 million.[21]

Sadness, loss and anger

SARS claimed the lives of some 300 Hong Kong residents. The daily tally of newly infected cases and deaths from March to June was sobering for the entire community.

A poignant reminder of the unpredictable turns life can take was the case of 41-year-old Frankie Chu, who cheated death on 11 September 2001 in New York but was caught by SARS. On the morning of 11 September, he was late for a business meeting at the World Trade Centre and escaped the terrorist attack. Yet he was unlucky enough to be on Air China flight CA112 on 15 March from Hong Kong to Beijing, during which he caught SARS from a 72-year-old Beijing man — a "super-spreader" who reportedly infected 21 people.[22] Chu started to feel ill four days later and checked into hospital on 21 March, shortly after he returned to Hong Kong. When it was confirmed that he had SARS four days later, Chu was placed in isolation and never saw his wife again. On 16 April, he died alone after suffering terrible difficulties in breathing. His wife, Karen Chu, was distraught that she could not be with him. She also felt a sense of anger and frustration at not knowing whether her husband received the best care from Tseung Kwan O Hospital.[23]

There were also disturbing cases of discrimination against ex-SARS patients. The Equal Opportunities Commission (EOC) received more than 500 inquiries and complaints linked to the outbreak.[24] Doctors and the EOC noted that misunderstandings about the disease could hamper infection control if those infected felt that they would be discriminated against by the general public. According to a survey conducted by CUHK, 51.3 percent of respondents said they remain fearful of former SARS patients.[25]

Positive experiences associated with SARS were complicated by these negative memories of bitterness and suffering, which must also be recognised and acknowledged by the community. While SARS has subsided, the grief and distress of those who were directly and personally affected still need to be addressed.

Hong Kong residents took part of this responsibility upon themselves by creating funds and projects to help those in need. For example, the *Love Hong Kong, Support our SARS frontline workers* project was put together by a coalition of 28 groups to raise money for medical workers; the *Business Community Relief Fund for Victims of SARS* was launched by the Liberal Party for recovered SARS patients and the families of victims in Hong Kong and mainland China; *Project Blossom* was created by performing artists to assist SARS children in their studies; the *We Care Education Fund* was initiated by several senior civil servants to help SARS orphans; and *Teachers against SARS* aimed to offer financial assistance for families affected by SARS, including those that had experienced job losses due to the disease. On the media front, in addition to the *South China Morning Post*'s *Project Shield* campaign, *Apple Daily* set up a charitable foundation, *Ming Pao* joined in various projects and the television station TVB launched a concert to raise funds to fight SARS.[26] Numerous other private sector funds have been set up by concerned individuals and groups to offer help to SARS victims. According to a government assessment, up until the end of July 2003, a total of about HK$150 million had been raised for various funds.[27]

Hong Kong fights back

The community response to SARS was diverse and colourful, demonstrating the energy and creativity of Hong Kong people.

The earliest civic response came from CUHK alumni, who set up the *We Care Foundation* in March 2003 to support frontline medical workers and others involved in the fight against SARS. The focus was initially on workers at PWH, but was subsequently extended to the Princess Margaret Hospital and eventually to other public hospitals. The campaign raised over HK$2 million. In a gesture of personal outreach, the Foundation delivered free soup to frontline workers between 29 March and 21 May. The Cantonese have a long tradition of drinking freshly made soup according to the seasons in order to stay healthy.[28]

Another early effort was the *So Sick* website, which was put together very quickly by four young computer engineers, Edwin Chan, Bernard Chung, Nelson Kwan and John Lau. In June 2002, they registered the domain name because it sounded like the Cantonese pronunciation of Su Shi, a poet of the Northern Sung period (1037–1101). The domain was intended as a space where cyber friends could share ideas. However, during the SARS outbreak, the four friends became upset that the Hong Kong authorities were unwilling to release information on infected sites around the city. They felt the public had a right to know this information. On 24 March 2003, they decided to compile a list themselves and put it on *So Sick* as a public service. The first list was put up on 31 March. By 2 April the domain had already received 200,000 hits; by 11 April, it had over 2 million; and by 21 April, it had more than 5 million.[29] The site eventually forced the government to publish an official list of affected buildings and areas. The work of these individuals, none of whom had started out intending to track infection data or defy the government, became world famous.

As the community realised that Hong Kong would have to learn to live with SARS, people from different backgrounds and with different expertise and skills put together a number of activities. Hong Kong's universities were at the forefront of many of these efforts. One of the earliest examples was the *We Are With You* movement founded by HKU sociologists Cecilia Chan and Stephen Chau to provide support to individuals coping with SARS through the use of hotlines and provide teaching support to students when classes were suspended.[30] A large number of similar projects were created by staff and students.

The *Fearbusters* campaign germinated over lunch on 11 April when three concerned individuals met to explore what they could do to address the situation.[31] Two were in the travel and hospitality sector and the third was a seasoned community campaigner. They quickly decided that they should use their respective networks to bring together a diverse group of people to fight SARS on a community level. Many people were witnessing the collapse of their businesses while others were uncertain about what the future held. They could all benefit by discussing and exploring new ideas to help them get through SARS together as a community of concerned individuals. On 15 April, the *Fearbusters* movement was born; its role was conceived of as being like the role of a firefighter, who does his work when there is a crisis in the community but then goes back to the station when the fire is under control and waits to come out again in the future whenever necessary. On 26 April, *Fearbusters* brought together 130 people from across social and cultural sectors to brainstorm action plans.

The result was remarkable, especially as there was no budget available and most of those involved did not know each other. The participation of so many people led to a wide range of activities that was powered by their collective ingenuity, enthusiasm and commitment to Hong Kong. Some of the initiatives developed a life beyond the SARS outbreak. The earliest project was to track local and overseas data on SARS so that it could be put on a website for public access. This kind of information had been notably lacking in March when people were still trying to understand the disease and its impact on Hong Kong and the world community. Michael DeGolyer, an academic and an expert in tracking statistics, provided new numbers as they became available so that the website could be updated every other day. Other activities included a web-based survey of the level of fear within the community; the creation of a "Busketeers" team to work with overseas media in order to counteract unfair and inaccurate representations of Hong Kong's SARS experience; a series of talks given by experts from the University of Science and Technology (UST) about the scientific aspects of SARS; a new English-language website, *Hkunmasked*, that used the voices and images of residents to inform the global community about what life was really like in Hong Kong;[32] a 12-week on-line travel industry initiative to educate tour operators about travel to Hong Kong; a neighbourhood cleanup project in the Lower Ngau Tau Kok Estate, where there was a high number of SARS infections; compilation of a set of information about all the relevant laws relating to public hygiene for public reference; a campaign called *My Pledge* to engage Hong Kong residents to adopt higher personal hygiene practices than those adopted by various government entities; and the September 2003 France-Hong Kong week-long charity festival hosted by the Novotel Hotel in Wanchai.[33]

On the same day that *Fearbusters* was made public, *Operation UNITE* was also announced. Led by former Executive Councillor Rosanna Wong, the campaign's aim was to boost morale and solidarity in Hong Kong.[34] While this was not a government campaign, it involved many high profile individuals, raised substantial funding and became the community arm of the authorities' efforts to promote better hygiene. More than 100 businesses and 200 groups partnered to launch a massive territory-wide cleanup over the Easter weekend in April. Following this initiative, the campaign worked with CUHK's school of public health to launch a *Hygiene Charter* on 13 May to help various business sectors improve hygiene practices. *Fearbusters* and *Operation UNITE* shared ideas and the former also helped to promote improved hygiene practices under the latter's banner.

There were probably more government and community cleanups between April and June 2003 than anyone could recall in recent experience. SARS provided a reminder to Hong Kong of the importance of public hygiene. Apart from wearing facemasks to prevent the spread of infection, Hong Kong people were reminded that they should wash their hands well and keep their homes and offices spotless. The HKSAR Government's *Team Clean* initiative, led by the chief secretary, Donald Tsang, devised a package of measures to sustain public cleanliness post-SARS. The fine for littering, spitting and related offences was increased from HK$600 to HK$1,500 and the authorities stepped up enforcement.[35] Public housing residents were also expected to alter their behaviour to keep buildings clean through the imposition of a system under which "points" would be deducted if tenants were found to have littered or committed other acts that affected the cleanliness of the estate. Residents who exceeded the maximum number of points over two years would lose their tenancy.[36] The Housing Authority, which manages the government's public housing estates, adopted *Fearbusters' My Pledge* initiative on 13 July as one way to help residents improve hygiene practices. Subsequently, the Education Department also adopted the initiative for primary school students. These and other public-private sector collaborations helped to strengthen civil society as both sectors saw they needed to work together to change behaviour, not only through the use of fines and penalties but also through public education and persuasion.

The business sector also had an important role to play in fighting SARS by helping ease the sense of public panic as well as communicating a more accurate picture of life in the city to international colleagues and clients in order to counter the dire reports in the international media. The business community essentially called for adopting a sense of proportion and perspective:

...[The] SARS outbreak is a sobering reminder...that international travel involves risks that are different from the risks we face at home. When one travels to New York or Chicago, one is aware of the statistical risk of mugging or gunshot violence. People travel in full knowledge that tuberculosis, tetanus, typhoid, malaria, dengue fever and a host of nasty stomach viruses are endemic in many countries they visit. Perspective...is a valuable device.... We should remember that only 0.02 per cent of the Hong Kong population have become infected.[37]

Trade bodies such as the Hong Kong Trade Development Council and the various chambers of commerce also sought to help the HKSAR Government respond to SARS. For example, on 9 May the Hong Kong General Chamber of Commerce offered advice on Hong Kong economic policy through an initiative called *Re-Launch, Re-Invigorate, and Re-Build Hong Kong* that looked at what needed to be done within the next five weeks, five months and five years.[38] On 28 May, the British Chamber of Commerce provided advice to business in a document entitled, *Corporate Strategies Following the Lifting of the WHO Travel Advisory*, while the American Chamber of Commerce dedicated the May 2003 issue of its magazine to SARS-related information.[39]

Hong Kong's travel sector was particularly hard hit by SARS as international travellers stayed away, while outbound travel dropped to a minimum. Like those in the medical profession, the travel industry was hoping for some guidance and support from the authorities. However, the Hong Kong Tourism Board (HKTB) chose not to play an active role in helping guide the industry during the SARS crisis, claiming that it was waiting for the right time — once the WHO lifted the travel advisory — to do the right thing. Perhaps the unfortunate timing and unintentional irony of its Hong Kong *Take Your Breath Away* international advertising campaign, which coincided with the onset of the SARS outbreak, prevented the HKTB from reaching out to its constituencies. The travel sector realised that it had to think quickly and act swiftly to help itself.

Hong Kong's airport, voted the most efficient in the world and usually bustling with activity, became a morgue. One of its first challenges during the outbreak was to put in place body temperature screening devices in accordance with the 27 March WHO recommendation. The Hong Kong Airport Authority, which manages the airport, initiated *Operation SkyFit,* an HK$363 million (US$46.5 million) initiative to encourage airlines to reinstate cancelled flights, with discounts of up to

50 percent on landing fees, lucky draws and other extras for air travellers. Between mid-March and mid-April, Cathay Pacific Airways, which is based out of Hong Kong, lost 75 percent of its market share. Daily passenger loads fell from an average of 32,000 a day to 11,000 a day in April and just 7,000 a day in May. Cathay was forced to ground 22 aircraft in May as passenger levels dropped to a quarter of levels in May 2002. Its business planning scenarios had failed to conceive of a situation where people simply did not travel; this had not been the case during times of war or even after 11 September 2001. Despite Cathay's reassurances that it already had introduced top-end air filter, recycle and replacement systems in its aircrafts that were effective in removing airborne contaminants such as droplets, bacteria and viral particles, it was unable to convince people that it was safe to fly during the outbreak.[40] As James Hughes-Hallett, chairman of Cathay Pacific Airways, noted, irrational fears of catching SARS proved most damaging to the industry:

> The economic, rather than the medical damage done by SARS is mainly self-inflicted through panic and massive over-reaction by the public and governing institutions around the world. Human beings, both as individuals and collectively through our governing institutions, are often spectacularly bad at calculating risk. Too often we succumb to silly fears and irrational panics, too eager to join the risk of the month club. Rational risk analysis may be within our intellectual grasp, but it very seldom wins out against our basic panic instincts when confronted by unfamiliar threat.[41]

Dragonair, which provides flights from Hong Kong to mainland China and other Asian cities, also suffered. In a unique bid to restore confidence in flying toward the end of May, Dragonair invited senior people from government and the business sector to a mid-air press conference, which it called *Flightpath to Recovery*.

A Tourism Coalition established by the Board of Airline Representatives launched the *We Love Hong Kong* campaign, targeting the travel and retail sectors, in order to boost domestic consumer spending and rebuild confidence in Hong Kong as an international travel destination. Airlines, hotels, travel agencies, restaurants and taxi owners were urged to offer special packages that encouraged consumers to spend. Locals who spent a minimum of HK$700 on a local tour or hotel plus another HK$300 on retail purchases could qualify for overseas travel at very attractive rates. Between 1 May and 30 June, more than 20 airlines, over 70 hotels, hundreds of travel agents and many cinemas and taxi companies participated in the campaign, helping to stimulate spending and travel as well as convey a renewed sense of confidence in Hong Kong. Both Cathay Pacific and Dragonair offered extraordinary deals to travellers. Moreover, for the first time in its history, the Hong Kong Hotels Association managed to unite 77 of its 79 member hotels in promoting the *Be Our Guest* campaign from June through September; for the price of two nights, hotel guests could stay free for an additional night. Tour operators became more imaginative with their offerings for local tourists. Waterside areas and the countryside became popular destinations. The tours were a real eye-opener for local residents who were more familiar with Hong Kong's shopping malls than its stunning countryside and outlying islands.

Although the travel sector's primary goal was to revive business, the level of cooperation and collaboration across businesses was exceptional and invaluable. During the months of the outbreak, the frequency and intensity of networking within and between different sectors and groups was higher than at any other time in living memory. This helped to create a sense of camaraderie that went beyond mere business arrangements. People felt like they were members of a community and that they needed to look out for each other in order to survive. The community also shared the visible agony of companies that were local institutions. The pains of Cathay Pacific and the elegant Peninsula Hotel reflected everybody's pain.

Other businesses also had to cope with SARS. Large employers such as the Hongkong and Shanghai Banking Corporation (HSBC) and telephone operator PCCW had to deal with the infection of employees and customer demands for a higher level of safety in providing services. HSBC, for example, realised that one way to combat fear and panic was to provide employees with accurate and timely information about SARS through its internal communication system. The bank also immediately provided information to customers on ways that they could minimise the risk of infection, for example, by using its Internet or telephone banking services. Indeed, the biggest players in Hong Kong's financial services sector were able to put in place contingency plans for critical staff to continue to work uninterrupted from home and established "safe" offices to ensure that the city's trading and regulatory services would not be disrupted. In the case of PCCW, where a number of staff members were infected, a new home/office visiting protocol was developed to reduce the possibility of infection and maintain services for customers.

Given their strong interest in helping Hong Kong overcome SARS, members of the financial services industry also introduced several initiatives to support businesses and families affected by SARS and stimulate spending and tourism. HSBC announced a HK$100 million programme in May that included interest refunds to SARS-affected families, employees of hard-hit industries and commercial clients who had suffered a 10 percent or more drop in sales. In addition, cash refunds, coupons and gifts were offered to encourage local residents to dine out and shop throughout Hong Kong. Other local banks also announced incentive packages to help revive the territory's economy.

The city's creative community perhaps best captured the depth of emotion experienced by Hong Kong. The many photographs taken during the outbreak were displayed in public exhibitions and subsequently published in the book *Hearts in Unity*, funded by private sector sponsorship. Arts groups joined forces to help SARS victims with a series of collaborations aimed at raising money and community morale. For example, the Hong Kong Arts Centre, Goethe-Institut Hong Kong, Para/Site Art Space and Art in Hospital worked together to present the *A Time Like This* exhibition (29 May to 2 June) by inviting members of the public to submit works that conveyed their feelings during the outbreak. Musicians of all ages and backgrounds played in numerous concerts. Six of Hong Kong's major performing arts groups cooperated in putting together a special charity performance on 23 May. Hong Kong's Canto-pop stars organised the 1:99 Concert at the Hong Kong Stadium on 24 May featuring some of the biggest local names — Andy Lau Tak-wah, Aaron Kwok Fu-shing and Jacky Cheung Hok-yau. The money raised at both performances was donated to the *We Care Education Fund* for SARS orphans.

Writer-turned-painter Fong So responded to the crisis by locking himself up to let his emotions flow from brush to paper. The sense of panic within the community was captured by his use of greys and greens. At the opening of his Hong Kong 2003 exhibition on 13 July, Fong said that he had never painted so much in such a short period of time:

> When Hong Kong was hit by the epidemic, I had the feeling that the city was stifling under an airless shroud. Now the situation is getting better, but the memories of the outbreak and people's sufferings brought about by it are still fresh.... The last [painting], a bunch of flowers, is dedicated to the medical workers who did the most and sacrificed the most while fighting against the deadly disease.[42]

Hong Kong's political cartoonists, including Zunzi, Malone, Wheeler and Gavin Coates, also helped to capture the experience of SARS with their usual wit and sarcasm, particularly at moments when the authorities fumbled. The Internet provided a space for the global digital community to create SARS-inspired images. While the origin of many of the images was unknown, there was a fair representation of images from Hong Kong.[43]

Filmmakers too, put their creative abilities to good use. The coronavirus starred in thirteen productions in the summer of 2003. These included a dozen short films and *City of SARS*, a 90-minute, low-budget independent production directed by Stephen Cheung Wai-man. He shot the movie in 15 days with comedian Tsang Chi-wai playing the role of a man who wants to kill himself by trying to catch SARS. The film's scriptwriter, Edmond Wong Chi-woon noted that: "It's been intense. Such a massive, massive experience for the city. It hit everything, from Hong Kong's economy and its place in the world to the way we touch each other, it's not easy to squeeze all that into 90 minutes. I think everyone working on this film feels a tremendous sense of responsibility."[44] The movie script links three stories:

> The first part concerns a jaded doctor who catches SARS and rediscovers his vocation through the kindness of the young nurse…who treats him. The middle section deals with a teenage girl…who falls in love with a boy she meets in quarantine. It explores how SARS has tested friendships and how neighbours and family have found a new sense of community in crisis. The final story is a dark comedy that follows the owner of a chain of karaoke bars…who, having gone bust when SARS scared away his customers, tried to commit suicide by catching the virus.[45]

In addition to *City of SARS*, a number of short films were funded by the HKSAR Government as part of a collaborative artists' response to the disease.[46]

Conclusion

Hong Kong gradually managed to salvage much of its international reputation as it became clear that the city was able to deal with SARS and that some international responses had been overblown and unnecessary. There was even a measure of contrition in international attitudes towards Hong Kong. For example, two weeks after its announcement that it would bar Hong Kong youngsters from attending its summer school, the University of California at Berkeley sent a high-level team to Hong Kong to apologise for having overreacted. In larger part, this was an attempt to salvage its "SARS-ravaged reputation,"[47] particularly after the WHO rebuked US universities for placing "unnecessary" restrictions on students from Hong Kong and other affected areas.[48] Ireland eventually reversed its decision to ban athletes from SARS-affected areas from participating in the Special Olympics. Hong Kong's healthcare workers received universal praise for their courage and professionalism in fighting SARS. Their performance under extreme stress compared very well to that of their counterparts elsewhere, including Toronto, which had far fewer infections than Hong Kong.

In the final analysis, the massive slowdown in the usually hectic pace of Hong Kong life was surprisingly therapeutic. Parents spent more time with their children. Husbands and wives renewed their commitment to each other. The relocation of Amoy Gardens families to isolation camps resulted in new friendships between neighbours that would never otherwise have occurred. Busy business people realised that there was more to life than their careers. Everybody became more health conscious. People were newly conscious of the support provided by family members, friends, colleagues and even strangers. The flood of cards and flowers from members of the public to hospital workers as well as the donations to the various foundations set up for SARS workers and victims attested to the strong sense of neighbourliness and solidarity that came to the forefront during the outbreak. Usually sedentary residents took to the countryside and the seaside in large numbers and discovered Hong Kong's great outdoors — one of its best assets. Many people offered their skills and time as volunteers through programmes set up by companies, clubs and community groups. New friendships formed and networks expanded. Companies and groups that usually compete for custom or publicity collaborated with one another and found the experience energising. For the first time, competitors started communicating openly with each other. For nearly three months, Hong Kong's traditional principles of competition and profit were shelved in place of partnership and sharing of information.

Ultimately, the people of Hong Kong felt that they had passed the test presented by the SARS crisis. When push came to shove, they had not let each other down. Hong Kong people felt like members of a united community. They felt good about themselves and about their city. They realised that Hong Kong's true value could not be measured simply in terms of its economic achievements.

CHAPTER **14**

Lessons Learned

Christine Loh

S ARS provided a dramatic demonstration of the global havoc that
can ensue following the emergence of a new infectious disease.
Public health authorities, doctors, nurses, other hospital workers,
scientists and laboratory research staff around the world struggled to
cope with SARS. Public panic was widespread in many parts of the world
that were affected. Some government officials lost their jobs due to
mishandling of the situation. The short-term economic impact was severe
and painful. Hospitals, schools and many places of entertainment had
to be closed, and travel advisories were imposed that greatly limited
international travel.

Now that the outbreak has subsided, what are the lessons that need
to be learned? There are four key aspects of the 2003 SARS outbreak
that stand out, upon which all other issues hang. First, SARS was the
first severe and readily transmissible new disease to emerge in the twenty-
first century. As such, it was a reminder that while modern science has
done much to improve public health it has not conquered disease.
Second, in controlling the spread of an infectious disease, every hour
counts. Timely and effective communication among key decision-makers
is critical in crisis management; communication with the public is also
essential in keeping the community informed. Implementing
preventative and control measures requires decision action, among the
most important measures being basic, low-technology initiatives such as

235

isolation and quarantine arrangements. Third, although SARS appears to have originated in Guangdong Province as early as November 2002, because mainland China refused to acknowledge the extent and severity of the disease, Hong Kong became the de facto epicentre of the outbreak. In other words, the lead actor in the SARS story was really mainland China but Hong Kong played the key role because it was in a tiny corner of the country that had a free media and an independent medical profession, both factors that proved critical in providing information about the new disease to the nation and to the world. Last, the outbreak gave the people of Hong Kong a chance to see how their society operated under intense stress. The experience contributed to a sense of gratitude and community pride that resulted in an unexpected show of unity on 1 July 2003.

The face of the new disease

SARS' place in history is assured. It was this century's first major public health scare. The outbreak may have given the world a taste of what is yet to come, as virologists continue to worry about the possible emergence of a highly infectious disease that has the capacity to transmit efficiently from person to person. Due to modern air travel, new diseases can spread very quickly around the globe, as SARS has shown. In the case of SARS, the world was lucky that the infectivity of the virus was relatively low.

SARS reminded the world that modern medicine has yet to defeat infectious diseases, despite significant advances. Rising standards of living in many parts of the world mean that increasing numbers of people can afford better food and accommodation, leading to higher disease resistance and improved public hygiene. There have been many public health successes over the past hundred years. For example, small pox, once a major killer, can now be avoided through vaccination. Other diseases like diphtheria can be cured using antitoxins, while plagues can be brought under control by preventative measures such as isolation, quarantine and pest control. In many parts of the world, the spread of cholera has been contained by improving water supplies. Antibiotics can now be used to treat typhoid, enteric fevers, syphilis and pneumonia. The result has been a significant drop in the world's death rate, due largely to better management of infectious diseases. Yet SARS was worrying because it was a new disease that came from a virus that had the capacity to mutate, raising important questions about the future evolution of outbreaks and the development of cures.

It is easy to focus on the mechanical aspect of disease prevention and control in terms of developing better diagnostic tests and finding the right vaccine and ignore the more complex underlying concerns. Though exceptional in terms of its impact and ease of international spread, SARS is only one of around fifty internationally important outbreaks in any given year, according to the World Health Organisation (WHO).[1]

Twenty years ago, experts warned that the intensive farming of animals and the close proximity between humans and animals that is prevalent in south China provides "an ecosystem for the interaction of viruses" (see Chapter 5). Furthermore, the ways in which animals are caught or reared and slaughtered in this region are far from humane or healthy. Animal protection laws are often openly flouted. Cooped up in cages or tight spaces, animals farmed for food often develop many types of illnesses. In south China, the wild animal trade provides exotic dishes in ever-larger quantities as income levels increase. Wild animals are reservoirs for all types of viruses. The discovery of a possible linkage between the SARS-coronavirus and the civet cat and other wild animals slowed consumption of these species and led to a Chinese Government ban on the trade and transportation of wild animals in May 2003. However, by July 2003, the ban was lifted. It seems that the SARS outbreak slowed the consumption of exotic animals only temporarily.

Beyond intensive farming and hunting of wild animals for food and other uses, the degradation of the natural environment in south China, as a result of rapid development, has resulted in widespread pollution of the air, water and soil. Pollution causes ecological imbalances that have a negative impact on public health. Living in polluted environments weakens the immune system of both humans and animals, resulting in a higher incidence of sickness. Moreover, when human diseases are treated with strong drugs such as antibiotics, not only do viruses build up resistance to the drugs over time, but also the body's own defence mechanisms may become weakened.

Thus, SARS represented more than a medical challenge. Public health is intimately linked with the state of the natural environment, which goes beyond improving hygiene. No amount of superficial cleaning of streets and buildings is sufficient to reverse the kind of ecological disturbance brought on by massive development projects that clear forests, divert rivers, change the climate or poison the land and waters. To ensure a healthy future, society has to take a much more holistic approach that includes reassessing whether its development path is sustainable on a long-term basis. This is unfortunately something that authorities in Hong Kong and Guangdong have yet to consider seriously.

Every hour counts

In an infectious disease outbreak, every hour counts, "as the window of opportunity for preventing deaths and further spread closes quickly."[2] Once the disease has affected healthcare workers in significant numbers and is present in the general community, it becomes much harder to control. Governments and healthcare professionals therefore need to move quickly to contain the spread of the disease. SARS demonstrated that responding to an outbreak requires good communication among key decision-makers so that information can be amassed, analysed and acted upon. An effective response extends beyond providing medical care to patients and may continue long after the disease itself has subsided. SARS not only had a significant impact on medical treatment and practice, it also created a substantial political challenge and possibly even a legal challenge for the authorities.

In the case of Hong Kong, questions continue to be raised about the timing and effectiveness of the government's response to SARS. For example, did Hong Kong's health officials pay attention to a press statement issued by Guangdong authorities on 10 February 2003, acknowledging that there was an outbreak of atypical pneumonia across the border that had infected 305 people and caused five deaths? The report of the government-appointed SARS Expert Committee released on 2 October 2003 noted that Hong Kong's Department of Health sought information about the outbreak from Guangdong authorities on 10 February but that this request was ignored. Hong Kong then contacted the Ministry of Health in Beijing.[3] It is unclear what information Hong Kong received from Beijing but it is clear that Hong Kong officials were not provided with the expert report on atypical pneumonia in Guangdong (mentioned in Chapter 9) given to the mainland authorities on 23 January 2003. Had Hong Kong received information in early February, many lives could have been spared. While the failure to share information openly is a legacy of the mainland culture of official secrecy, it also reflects the fact that Hong Kong appears to have been totally helpless when dealing with mainland authorities.

Nevertheless, on 11 February, Hong Kong's Hospital Authority (HA) and Department of Health did take the step of setting up a joint task force, called the Working Group on Severe Community-acquired Pneumonia, to identify pneumonia cases in Hong Kong similar to those reported in Guangdong. The HA is a statutory body that manages Hong Kong's 43 public hospitals and works closely with the Department of Health. Thus, as early as February, health professionals were anticipating that the disease could easily enter Hong Kong, despite Guangdong's claim that the situation across the border was "under control." The number of daily passenger crossings between Hong Kong and Guangdong is in the region of 250,000 to 300,000 people. Describing the work of the Working Group, Director of Health Dr. Margaret Chan noted that: "…together with the Hospital Authority [the Department of Health] examined all community-acquired pneumonia admitted into hospitals. We had to find out about the origins of the infection, whether they were caused by germs, virus or flu…. At that time what concerned us most was influenza. It was the winter peak for flu."[4] Doctors participating in the task force surveillance exercise reported no unusual cases of flu or pneumonia.[5] However, between 12 and 21 February, the pre-existing influenza infection guidelines and a specially prepared information package entitled "Frequently Asked Questions" about Severe Community-acquired Pneumonia were circulated to all public hospitals in Hong Kong.

On 21 Februrary, Dr. Liu Jianlun, Hong Kong's index case patient, arrived in Hong Kong from Guangdong. Piecing together the data, researchers have concluded that Dr. Liu, "patient zero," infected 12 people, who then infected many more around the world within a matter of days. Hong Kong's Metropole Hotel also became infamous as the point of contact between Liu and other hotel guests who would subsequently become infected. By mid-May 2003, the WHO estimated that of the 8,000-plus SARS cases worldwide at that time, more than 4,000 could be traced back to Liu's two-day stay at the Metropole Hotel.

When Liu was admitted to the Kwong Wah Hospital on 22 February, he was already very sick. He told doctors and nurses that he had come in contact with patients in Guangdong suspected to have atypical pneumonia, but thought that he had recovered. As his condition was poor, he was put into intensive care in an isolation room immediately. His case was also promptly reported to the HA as well as the Department of Health. On 28 February, Liu's brother-in-law was also admitted to Kwong Wah Hospital with the same symptoms. While the Report of the Hospital Authority Review Panel on the SARS Outbreak, released on 16 October 2003, noted that the HA and the Department of Health Working Group did issue information on infection control to all hospitals, it was critical of the limited efforts by health authorities to alert other hospitals of the potential risks of the disease. For example, while information on infection control was provided to infection control officers in the form of "Frequently Asked Questions" and posted on the HA website, the Review Panel found that the content of informational materials and the way in which they were circulated "failed to get the attention of, and thus warn, staff about the risk of infection."[6] The Panel also noted the failure to assemble all available data "held by a range of people inside and outside the HA into a single picture,"[7] and recommended that in the event of an emerging unknown infectious disease, "any indications that it is infective to heathcare workers should be communicated to frontline staff immediately."[8]

According to the Review Panel, the passivity of health and hospital authorities was due to the fact that "there was no strategy or contingency plan suitable for dealing with a major disease outbreak,"[9] and no "comprehensive, multi-agency strategy for disease prevention and control that puts the health of the public first."[10] The lack of a clear overall leadership structure also raised problems.[11]

In the rush to put the new Principal Officials Accountability System (POAS) in place by 1 July 2002, the Chief Executive did not allow time to clearly demarcate the responsibilities of a number of official posts. This resulted in some overlap between the responsibilities of the Secretary for Health, Welfare and Food and the Director of Health, leaving Hong Kong without the equivalent of a surgeon general or chief medical officer.[12] In its October 2003 report, the SARS Expert Committee noted that there was an "imbalance between responsibility, authority and accountability in the health system. For example, [the Secretary] has accountability for the health system as a whole...but statutory public health powers are vested in the Director of Health."[13] More astute members of the Legislative Council (LegCo) had foreseen this type of problem in 2002 when the POAS was implemented, but the Tung administration chose to prioritise speed over clarity of the leadership structure. The confusion inherent in the way the POAS was implemented was evident following the "penny stocks" incident in 2002. At that time, a review panel noted that the specific responsibilities and powers of the relevant ministerial posts were unclear.[14]

Jurisdictional confusion within the system was compounded by the failure of administrators to anticipate the public health implications of the initial outbreak at the Prince of Wales Hospital (PWH). On 10 March, after 11 PWH staff working in Ward 8A became ill, doctors immediately closed the ward to admissions and visitors. On 11 March, hospital administrators upheld the decision to stop patient admissions to Ward 8A but began re-admitting visitors wearing protective gear because they did not want to cause anxiety among patients. Between 11 and 19 March, PWH management increased protective measures incrementally, first cordoning off the floor where Ward 8A was situated and eventually closing its accident and emergency department completely. During this ten-day period, the WHO issued two global alerts about the new disease. Despite the finding of the SARS Expert Committee that the various decisions on the management of the disease were made "collectively at meetings" attended by both administrative and senior healthcare professionals, controversy over the series of decisions that led to a gradual approach in closing PWH never subsided because of the numerous and continued objections from frontline healthcare workers and the medical faculty at the Chinese University of Hong Kong (CUHK), which uses PWH as its teaching facility.[15]

The HA Review Panel was much more critical of decision-making at PWH than the SARS Expert Committee. In its report, the Panel described the reopening of Ward 8A to visitors on 11 March as "a step down in the strict infection control measures" introduced on the previous day. Despite the fact that PWH administrators put stricter precautions for visitors in place, the decision to reopen the ward "potentially exposed [visitors], and hence the wider community to infection."[16] The Panel also noted that CUHK began calling for the closure of PWH on 12 March, "but because there was no effective mechanism for ensuring that the key stakeholders could properly consider the benefits and consequences of such a complex decision, then by default the hospital was never closed."[17] By contrast, the SARS Expert Committee merely stated that "there was a lack of clarity in the role of university staff in a hospital outbreak situation and failures of communication between HA, DH [Department of Health] and the university."[18] The price paid for this "lack of clarity" was substantial: a total of 239 people were infected during the PWH outbreak.

It should also be noted that by the end of February, virologists such as Professor Malik Peiris and his colleagues at the University of Hong Kong (HKU), had already begun to believe that they might be dealing with a new virus.[19] Indeed, on 7 March, the HA's own Working Group reported to its board (which included top government officials) that the atypical pneumonia cases might have been caused by an "unusual virus."[20] Thus, senior management at the HA and the Department of Health knew that there was a strong possibility that the disease was not just a variant of winter flu and that whatever its identity, its impact on patients was serious.

The HA Review Panel made an interesting observation on this point:

> Looking back, information about the virus and the potential havoc it could cause was scant prior to early February. Those privy to information were reluctant to share it, and what was shared often only had the status of rumour. It still remains unclear what was known, by whom and when. It was clear however, that something unusual was happening.[21]

By 15 March, the day the WHO named the new disease "severe acute respiratory syndrome" or "SARS," it was impossible for Hong Kong authorities to ignore the extent of the outbreak, which had now spread to many countries around the world and resulted in the infection of more than 150 people. Despite these facts, health authorities continued to deny the severity of the outbreak, prompting Professor Sydney Chung, Dean of the Faculty of Medicine at CUHK, to go public on 17 March to contradict statements by the Secretary of Health, Welfare and Food and the Director of Health that the disease had not spread to the general community in Hong Kong. The SARS Expert Committee partially exonerated the Secretary for this lapse by saying that his statement was technically correct at the time it was made but noting that he could have used "a more prudent phrase" — which sounds more like an apology.[22] By 21 March, virologists in Hong Kong knew that the causative agent for the disease was a coronavirus. Yet it was only on 24 March that the authorities finally created a special inter-departmental task force to coordinate the fight against SARS; only on 27 March that the government advised people to quarantine themselves for ten days if they had come into contact with SARS patients; and it was 31 March when they decided to isolate Block E of Amoy Gardens, ten days after large numbers of residents had begun to fall ill. The SARS Expert Committee acknowledged "there were significant shortcomings of system performance during the early days of the epidemic" but was not prepared to find anyone at fault.[23]

From the community's point of view, government prevarication resulted in the loss of valuable opportunities to minimise the spread of SARS. The government even mishandled the setting up of a SARS Expert Committee to review the government management of the SARS crisis. The Committee received bad press from the start, after Chief Executive Tung Chee-hwa appointed the Secretary for Health, Welfare and Food Dr. EK Yeoh as its head. His reasons for doing so seemed incomprehensible because Dr. Yeoh's own decisions and conduct during the outbreak had to be included in the review. Although the Chief Executive finally replaced Dr. Yeoh as head of the Committee on 17 July, the damage to the government's credibility had already been done. This is why the public continues to question the Committee's refusal to apportion blame to key decision-makers. Its explanation that it sought to avoid the "hazards of retrospective judgement"[24] is suspect because it would then make it hard to hold officials accountable for any issue or event they do not foresee.

In a further display of public dissatisfaction, more than half a million Hong Kong people took to the streets on 1 July 2003. While the immediate cause of the protest was the Article 23 national security legislation, it was also clear that Hong Kong people had a litany of complaints regarding the performance of the Tung administration since 1997. His insistence on appointing an implicated party to head an inquiry is only one illustration of his governing style, and raised doubts about the sincerity and value of the evaluation process. In this light, one of the local members of the SARS Expert Committee, Dr. Rosie Young, made an extraordinary statement on television on 4 October when she referred to the handling of SARS victims: "The government was very indifferent and did not have enough care for the people. I guess the whole government should learn."[25]

On 29 October 2003, LegCo voted to use the powers granted to it under the Power and Privileges Ordinance to conduct an inquiry into how the Hong Kong authorities handled SARS. Both the LegCo process and the HA Review Panel report may help to address public dissatisfaction with the SARS Expert Committee report, but clearly the preferable situation would have been for the Chief Executive to appointment an independent public inquiry team whose credentials were beyond dispute at the outset. Furthermore, the SARS crisis may give rise to many private law questions in the months to come. There are legal issues to be addressed concerning would-be plaintiffs and potential defendants.[26] The government has committed itself to a range of ex gratia payments to certain relatives of healthcare workers who died of SARS. For example, in three cases, the families of the deceased will receive HK$3 million in assistance payments.[27] Nevertheless, frontline medical staff, families of those who died from SARS, those who contracted SARS in hospitals and the residents of Amoy Gardens may still bring lawsuits against the government.

In terms of timeliness, what was truly impressive was the work of the WHO's Global Outbreak Alert Response Network (GOARN), as discussed in Chapter 9, and the network of 13 research laboratories studying the SARS virus that was convened by Dr. Klaus Stohr at the WHO's Geneva headquarters (see Chapter 4). With the help of modern telecommunications and in a spirit of collaboration that enabled professional rivalries to be put aside in the interests of the greater good, experts were able to make impressive strides in understanding the new virus in a relatively short period of time. While much more research remains to be done, the effort by international institutions to work together demonstrated the speed with which information can be transmitted worldwide, contributing to global knowledge. It was also a reminder that expertise and technology are available if the decision-makers responsible for public health understand how to use them. When it is possible to coordinate so many parties in so many parts of the world to work to their highest efficiency, it is harder to excuse poor communication and decision-making within one hospital, such as the PWH, or between two government bodies, such as the HA and the Heath, Welfare and Food Bureau.

A further aspect of timeliness is the importance of information management and dissemination in a highly wired world. Modern information technology enables the rapid dissemination of legitimate information, but it also offers a way to publicise rumours and misinformation that can lead to widespread panic. Despite clinical uncertainty about the nature and identify of the new disease at the initial stage of the outbreak in Hong Kong, an important lesson for governments and public institutions is that it is their responsibility to put out timely information on matters of public concern, otherwise they may lose the opportunity to address public confusion and fears. This became apparent on April Fool's Day when a teenager in Hong Kong used the Internet to make a false announcement that Hong Kong had been declared an "infected port" (see Chapter 13). Again, failure by the authorities to release information about the spread of SARS within the community led four information technology engineers to take matters into their own hands by setting up the website www.sosick.org to provide information to the public on affected areas and buildings. The lesson for the authorities is that failure to take the initiative can result in a "lose-lose" situation where others put out incorrect or false information or citizens end up doing their jobs for them. Either scenario creates perceptions of official ineptitude. Furthermore, Chapter 6 provides a reminder that there is still much useful information about the outbreak that the HA and the Department of Health have not released to the public. The message is clear: in fostering a true knowledge-based society, the authorities play a critical role in how they promote access to information.

Mainland China

The initial response of mainland authorities to the emergence of a new infectious disease in Guangdong was to downplay the situation and attempt to control information. The lesson for Chinese leaders is that stonewalling no longer works well in a wired world. Indeed, in the event of a future outbreak, the best strategy is to be transparent about what is happening, especially in such a vast country. National leaders in Beijing need to have timely information about local events in order to make the right decisions. At the time of the outbreak, national leaders were so preoccupied with the politics of the transition in leadership that they did not see the storm on the horizon even though, as Chapter 9 points out, it seems inconceivable that top level officials were unaware that something unusual was occurring. The Chinese Government should not lose sight of the fact that it lost a valuable opportunity to inform the nation about SARS at the National People's Congress meetings in March 2003, an occasion that could have been used to provide information to the entire country on preventative and control measures. The price

China had to pay for its oversight was substantial — many deaths and loss of credibility worldwide.

Mainland China should have been the epicentre of the SARS outbreak as the disease originated and affected the largest number of people there, not in Hong Kong. As a result of the mainland's refusal to acknowledge the extent of the outbreak in China up until mid-April 2003, Hong Kong, which has a free flow of information, became the de facto epicentre.

As a Special Administrative Region (SAR) of the People's Republic of China, Hong Kong operates under the "one country, two systems" principle. There are many aspects of life in Hong Kong that are fundamentally different from practices on the Mainland. Hong Kong residents enjoy freedom of expression and a free media, neither of which is available to Chinese citizens on the mainland. When SARS hit Hong Kong in February, the local media pursued the story relentlessly once it realised that SARS was an important issue. In fact, reports coming out of Hong Kong about the situation in south China enabled the WHO to press mainland China for more information on what was happening there. No doubt, additional pressure was supplied in the form of diplomatic messages relayed to Beijing from other nations — who were also operating on the basis of information reported by the Hong Kong media. Had it not been for Hong Kong's separate "system," it might well have taken China even longer to address SARS. At least in the case of SARS, the "one country, two systems" principle may be viewed as a blessing in disguise for both mainland China and the global community.

Another difference between Hong Kong and mainland China concerns the role of the Chinese Communist Party, which dominates the mainland government. On the mainland, the Party and therefore the government play a key leadership role in numerous aspects of Chinese life, including the conduct of healthcare professionals. Contrasting the role of Dr. Jiang Yanyong in Beijing and Professor Sydney Chung in Hong Kong, it is clear while both men felt that they must put evidence and professionalism ahead of official objectives, Dr. Jiang faced greater obstacles in finding a way to get out the message that mainland officials were not admitting to the hundreds of SARS cases in Beijing's military hospitals. Although Jiang became a folk hero for telling the truth, he was eventually silenced by the authorities. By contrast, medical professionals in Hong Kong, like Professor Chung, do not regard the government as a superior. They operate independently from the authorities in the exercise of their professional judgment. Professor Chung always chose his words carefully when speaking in public, as would be expected from a person of his standing.

The SARS crisis showed how important it is to ensure that professionals operate independently of government and can speak out to maintain standards and ensure that official statements are based on actual evidence. On the mainland, the Community Party has yet to allow truly independent groups to function. There is no shortage of competent, dedicated and courageous professionals on the mainland, but they lack the political environment that permits true independence — a basic requirement for true professionalism. It remains unclear how the Party and the Chinese Government view Dr. Jiang today. It is to be hoped that the fact that Jiang and other mainland physicians did speak out about the official cover-up during the outbreak is a sign that things could be changing for the better. There is no doubt about how Professor Chung is regarded — for Hong Kong people he is a hero.

The culture of official secrecy dies hard even at a moment when Hong Kong, Guangdong and Macau have agreed to be more transparent in sharing information. While the respective authorities have agreed to cross-border reporting on eight diseases and information exchange on all notifiable diseases in their own jurisdictions, this information is still treated as confidential and has not been made available to the public. One important concession is that medical professionals can have access to the information for research purposes, although it remains unclear how the issue will be handled in publishing research findings.

Official abhorrence of openness rubs in other ways as well. The first example is with regard to scientific research. As the Communist Party and mainland government denied the true extent of the outbreak up until 17 April, when the Politburo changed its tune by calling for accurate reporting, mainland scientists were denied the opportunity to carry out scientific studies of the new virus at the first opportunity. The official cover-up therefore also prevented mainland scientists from participating in groundbreaking research. Again, scientists in one tiny corner of the country — Hong Kong — came to the forefront in the investigation of the disease and eventually won international recognition for their work in identifying the SARS-coronavirus.

The second example is the lack of trust in official information. Chapter 9 notes that Shanghai wisely took early precautions to prevent the spread of SARS; this, coupled with some good luck, was critical in preventing an outbreak on the scale of that experienced by other cities in China and around the world. Yet doubts about the accuracy of Chinese information persist. Lastly, even though government health ministers and the mayor of Beijing were fired as a sign that Chinese leaders wanted accountability, it is doubtful that any internal review reports will be made public. It seems likely that the enquiries on Hong Kong's handling of SARS will be the only reports made publicly available in China.

A renewed sense of dignity

Hong Kong people appeared to have lost their self-confidence since 1997 as the economy softened. Perhaps even more significant in the minds of Hong Kong people has been their adjustment from subjects of a small British colony to citizens of a large country experiencing rapid modernisation. It has undoubtedly been difficult for Hong Kong to redefine itself within the context of an evolving People's Republic of China. As the mainland continues to advance economically, Hong Kong's traditional role as a gateway to China seems to have become obsolete.

Chapter 11 provides a useful perspective on Hong Kong's current economic situation. Hong Kong remains highly competitive, not necessarily in terms of cost (although costs are now more competitive than before), but certainly in terms of its social "software," which includes its management capacity, professionalism, openness and transparency, free media, personal liberties and rule of law. The SARS outbreak brought out many of these strengths, including the ability of the community to work together in the face of tough times. Hong Kong people saw how well many aspects of their society worked. Even in terms of the government, the public saw that despite poor crisis management at the early stages of the outbreak, once the severity of the situation was fully understood and acknowledged, solid advances were quickly made in many areas. For example, Hong Kong developed an impressive contact tracing system for people who had come into contact with SARS patients. Hospitals and healthcare workers revised infection control procedures. These innovations will prove very useful in case of future outbreaks, both in Hong Kong and elsewhere. The calibre of Hong Kong's response to SARS allowed the people of Hong Kong to feel good about themselves and about their community.

Between March and May 2003, Hong Kong dropped almost

everything else to focus on fighting SARS. As the outbreak waned, people began to pick up their lives again where they had left off. One pressing issue was the national security legislation proposed by the government in compliance with Article 23 of the Basic Law, Hong Kong's post-1997 constitution. The article requires Hong Kong on its own to pass laws to prohibit treason, secession, subversion, sedition, theft of state secrets and links between local and overseas political bodies. The Tung administration hoped to pass the legislation on 9 July 2003. As soon as public attention was transferred away from SARS to Article 23, objections to the content of the draft legislation mounted day by day. Non-governmental groups joined forces to organise a demonstration against the draft bill on 1 July 2003 — a public holiday to commemorate the return of Hong Kong to Chinese rule in 1997. In the week leading up to the holiday, it became clear that a large number of people were likely to join the demonstrations. Media reports suggested that there would be over 100,000 protesters.

On the day, over 500,000 people showed up to participate in a march that was entirely peaceful and yet was a powerful expression of the deep discontent of the community with the Tung administration.[28] Among the protesters were healthcare workers who wanted to vent their frustrations regarding the government handling of SARS. As noted above, the Chief Executive's subsequent decision to remove Dr. EK Yeoh as the head of the SARS Expert Committee was a response to public dissatisfaction. Furthermore, in the same way that healthcare professionals became local heroes during the SARS outbreak, Hong Kong's legal professionals played a pivotal role in taking a vocal stance against Article 23 and helping the public to understand the complexities of the legislation. This was another confirmation of the strength of Hong Kong's social software and the importance of independent commentary by professionals for the community as a whole. Post–1 July, Hong Kong's interest in politics seems to have been awakened. The call for democratic reform is unambiguous.

SARS presented an unprecedented challenge for Hong Kong. Facing and overcoming this challenge allowed Hong Kong people to feel as though they had regained their dignity. The events of 1 July also forced leaders in Beijing to reassess Hong Kong and consider the possibility that there were many aspects of its development that they did not adequately understand. The rest of the world, which was close to writing off Hong Kong as a has-been because of SARS and Hong Kong's soft economic performance against rapid advances on the mainland, began to reassess Hong Kong's importance as well. While the stakes for Hong Kong are high, it is clear that it has the capacity to push for changes that will have reverberations on the mainland. This process of change could yield positive results if the protagonists keep a cool head.

NOTES

CHAPTER 2

1. K.W. Tsang, P.L. Ho, G. Ooi, et al., A cluster of cases of severe acute respiratory syndrome in Hong Kong, *New England Journal of Medicine* 2003; 345: 1977–85; S.M. Poutanen, D.E. Low, B. Henry, et al., Identification of severe acute respiratory syndrome in Canada, *New England Journal of Medicine* 2003; 348: 1953–66; N. Lee, D. Hui, A.Wu, et al., A major outbreak of severe acute respiratory syndrome in Hong Kong, *New England Journal of Medicine* 2003; 248: 1986–94; and C.M. Booth, L.M. Matukas, G.A. Tomlinson, et al., Clinical features and short-term outcomes of 144 patients with SARS in the Greater Toronto Area, *Journal of the American Medical Association* 7 May 2003, **http://jama.ama-assn.org/cgi/content/full/289.21.JOC30885vl**.
2. The report of the Hong Kong Hospital Authority Review Panel on the SARS outbreak, released to the public on 16 October 2003, also provides a very useful summary of events and facts. See Section IV: A chronological overview of the outbreak of SARS in Hong Kong, and Section V: The detailed facts. *Report of the Hospital Authority Review Panel on the SARS Outbreak,* Hospital Authority, Hong Kong, September 2003.
3. C.C. Luk, Chief Executive, Kwong Wah Hospital, "Index patient," *South China Morning Post* 29 May 2003, Letter to the Editor.
4. N. Lee, D. Hui, A. Wu, et al., A major outbreak of severe acute respiratory syndrome in Hong Kong, *New England Journal of Medicine* 2003; 348: 1986–94.
5. SARS Expert Committee, *SARS in Hong Kong: From Experience to Action,* 2 October 2003, pp. 23–35.
6. Ella Lee, "Waging war on an unknown enemy," *South China Morning Post* 26 March 2003, p. A11.
7. See endnote 5.
8. See endnote 5.

9. World Health Organisation, First data on stability and resistance of SARS coronavirus compiled by members of WHP laboratory network, 4 May 2003, **www.who.int/csr/sars/survival_2003_05_04/en/index/html**.

10. Department of Health, HKSAR Government, Main findings of an investigation into the outbreak of Severe Acute Respiratory Syndrome at Amoy Gardens, 17 April 2003, **www.info.gov.hk/dh**.

11. See endnote 1.

12. K.T. Wong, G.E.A. Frazer, D.S.C. Hui, et al., Severe acute respiratory syndrome: Radiographic appearances and pattern of progression in 138 patients, *Radiology* August 2003, 228(2): 401–6 and N. L. Muller, G.C Ooi, P.L. Khong, N. Savvas, Severe acute respiratory syndrome: Radiographic and CT findings, *American Journal of Roentgenology* 2003 (in press).

13. K.W. Tsang, P.L. Ho, G. Ooi, et al., A cluster of cases of severe acute respiratory syndrome in Hong Kong, *New England Journal of Medicine* 2003; 345: 1977–85.

14. Hospital Authority (Hong Kong), Information on management of SARS: Case definition, 30 April 2003, **www.ha.org.hk/sars/sars_index_e.html**.

15. World Health Organisation, Case definition for surveillance of severe acute respiratory syndrome (SARS), 5 May 2003, **www.who.int/csr/sars/casedefinition/en**.

16. J.S.M. Peiris, C.M. Chu, V.C.C. Cheng, et al., Clinical progression and viral load in a community outbreak of coronavirus-associated SARS pneumonia: A prospective study, *Lancet* 2003; 361: 1767–72; and World Health Organisation, Use of laboratory methods for SARS diagnosis, 5 May 2003, **www.who.int.csr.sars.labmethods/en**.

17. World Health Organisation, Use of laboratory methods for SARS diagnosis, 5 May 2003, **www.who.int.csr.sars.labmethods/en/**; and World Health Organisation, Recommendations for laboratories testing by PCR for presence of SARS coronavirus-RNA, 13 May 2003, **www.who/int/csr/coronarecommendations/en**.

18. J.S.M. Peiris, C.M. Chu, V.C.C. Cheng, et al., Clinical progression and viral load in a community outbreak of coronavirus-associated SARS pneumonia: A prospective study, *Lancet* 2003; 361: 1767–72; and World Health Organisation, Recommendations for laboratories testing by PCR for presence of SARS coronavirus-RNA, 13 May 2003, **www.who/int/csr/coronarecommendations/en**.

19. W. Ho, Guideline on management of severe acute respiratory syndrome (SARS), *Lancet* 2003; 361: 1313–5.

20. L.K.Y. So, A.C.W. Lau , L.Y.C. Yam, et al., Development of a standard treatment protocol for severe acute respiratory syndrome, *Lancet* 2003; 361: 1615.

21. J. Gerberding, Lack of in vitro activities of Ribavirin against coronavirus, Centres for Disease Control and Prevention, Press briefing, 22 April 2003.

22. W.K. Lam, K.W. Tsang, C. Ooi, M. Ip, M. Chan-Yeung, Severe acute respiratory syndrome, in *Respiratory Disease: An Asian Perspective*, edited by M.S. Ip, M. Chan-Yeung, N.S. Zhong, W.K. Lam. Hong Kong: Hong Kong University Press 2004.

23. J.S.M. Peiris, C.M. Chu, V.C.C. Cheng, et al., Clinical progression and viral load in a community outbreak of coronavirus-associated SARS pneumonia: A prospective study, *Lancet* 2003; 361: 1767–72.

24. K.L.E. Hon, C.W. Leung, W.T.F. Cheng, et al., Clinical presentations and outcome of severe acute respiratory syndrome in children, *Lancet* 2003; 361: 1701–3.

25. C.A. Donnelly, A.C. Ghani, G.M. Leung, et al., Epidemiological determinants of spread of causal agent of severe acute respiratory syndrome in Hong Kong, *Lancet* 2003; 361: 1773–8.

26. Department of Health. Health, Welfare & Food Bureau, SARS Bulletin, 30 May 2003, **www.info.gov.hk/info/infection-c.htm**.

27. Ibid.

28. See endnote 5.

CHAPTER **4**

1. Matt Pottinger, Elena Cherney, Gautam Nail and Michael Waldholz, "How a global effort identified SARS virus in a matter of weeks," *The Wall Street Journal* 16 April 2003.

2. David Heymann, Executive Director, Communicable Diseases, World Health Organisation, from a transcript of a conference call on 8 April 2003 in CLSA Speaker Series, *SARS — Hype from Reality*, published by CLSA Emerging Markets. See also Chris Taylor, "In China, it seems the 'big one' is yet to come," *South China Morning Post* 11 May 2003, p. 4.

3. World Health Organisation, Severe acute respiratory syndrome (SARS): Status of the outbreak and lessons for the immediate future, 20 May 2003.

4. See endnote 2. The father, a 33-year-old man, and his nine-year-old son were admitted to hospital on 11 and 12 February respectively. The mother was admitted on 13 February. The father died but the son and mother recovered. The family also had a second daughter who remained asymptomatic throughout.

5. See endnotes 3 and 4.

6. See endnote 1.

7. See endnote 3.

8. See endnote 1.

9. D. Normile, Up close and personal with SARS, *Science* 2003; 300: 886–7, **www.sciencemag.org**.

10. World Health Organisation Multiple Collaborative Network for Severe Acute Respiratory Syndrome (SARS) Diagnosis, A multiple collaboration to

investigate the cause of severe acute respiratory syndrome, *Lancet* 2003; 361: 1730–3.

11. J.S.M. Peiris, S.T. Lai, L.L.M. Poon, et al., Coronavirus as a possible cause of severe acute respiratory syndrome, *Lancet* 2003; 361: 1319–25.

12. Mary Ann Benitez, The struggle to profile a killer, *South China Morning Post* 25 June 2003, p. A14.

13. T.G. Ksiazek, D. Erdman, C.S. Goldsmith, et al., A novel coronavirus associated with severe acute respiratory syndrome, *New England Journal of Medicine* 2003; 348: 1953–66; and C. Drosten, S. Gunther S, W. Preiser, et al., Identification of a novel coronavirus in patients with severe acute respiratory syndrome, *New England Journal of Medicine* 2003; 348: 1967–76.

14. See endnote 1.

15. Lawrence K Altman, "Experiments on monkeys zero in on SARS cause," *New York Times* 16 April 2003.

16. Koch's Postulates are:

    (a) The organism has to be isolated from diseased tissues of the patient.
    (b) The organism can induce the same disease in another individual or a close species.
    (c) The same organism can be isolated again from the infected individual or a close species.

17. K.V. Holmes, SARS-associated coronavirus, *New England Journal of Medicine* 2003; 348: 1848–1951.

18. See endnote 1.

19. Mary Ann Benitez, "SARS study puts civet cats back in the dock," *South China Morning Post* 5 September 2003, front page.

20. Ibid.

21. E.G. Brown and J.A. Tetro, Comparative analysis of the SARS-coronavirus genome: A good start to a long journey, *Lancet* 2003; 361: 1756–7.

22. M. Enserimk, Calling all coronavirologists, *Science* 2003; 300: 413, **www.sciencemag.org**.

23. Centers for Disease Control and Prevention, CDC Lab sequences genome of new coronavirus, 2003, **www.cdc.gov/od/oc/media/pressrel/r030414.htm**; P.A. Rota, M.S. Oberste, S.S. Monroe, et al., Characterization of a novel coronavirus associated with severe acute respiratory syndrome, *Science* 2003; 300: 1394–9; M.A. Marra, S.J.M. Jones, C.R. Astell, et al., The genome sequence of the SARS-associated coronavirus, *Science* 2003; 300: 1399–404; and Y.J. Ruan, C.L. Wei, A.I. Ee, et al., Comparative full-length genome sequence analysis of 14 SARS coronavirus isolates and common mutations associated with putative origins of infection, *Lancet* 24 May 2003; 361(9371): 1779–85.

24. See endnote 12.
25. See endnote 21.
26. See endnote 12.
27. M. Enserimk, Clues to the animal origins of SARS, *Science* 2003; 300: 1351, **www.sciencemag.org**.
28. Robert J. Saiget, SARS antibodies found in wild animal traders in Southern China, Agence France-Press, 25 May 2003.
29. Rob Stein, "Test results reveal a tough virus," *The Standard* 5 May 2003, p. B6.
30. World Health Organisation, First data on stability and resistance of SARS-coronavirus compiled by members of WHO laboratory network, **www.who.int/csr/sars/survival_2003_05_04/en/index.html**, 4 May 2003.
31. Agencies, Josephine Ma and Mary Ann Benitez, "SARS probe will focus on laboratories," *South China Morning Post* 10 September 2003, front page.
32. Staff reporters, "SARS labs tighten up after Lion City case," *The Standard* 11 September 2003, p. B4.
33. World Health Organisation Update, What happens if SARS returns? **www.who.int/csr/sars/survival_2003_06_26/en/index.html**, 26 June 2003.

CHAPTER 5

1. Vu TH, Cabau JF, Nguyen NT, Lenoir M, SARS in Northern Vietnam, *New England Journal of Medicine* 2003; 348: 2035.
2. Poutanen SM, Low DE, Henry B, et al., Identification of severe acute respiratory syndrome in Canada, *New England Journal of Medicine* 2003; 348: 1995–2005.
3. Tsang KW, Ho PL, Ooi GC, et al., A cluster of cases of severe acute respiratory syndrome in Hong Kong, *New England Journal of Medicine* 2003; 348:1 977–85.
4. Lee N, Hui D, Wu A, et al., A major outbreak of severe acute respiratory syndrome in Hong Kong, *New England Journal of Medicine* 2003; 348: 1986–94.
5. Shortridge KF, Stuart-Harris CH, An influenza epicentre? *Lancet* 1982; 2: 812–3.
6. Wickramasinghe C, Wainwright M, Narlikar J, SARS — A clue to its origins? *Lancet* 2003; 361: 1832.
7. Hospital Authority, Section II: Prologue and summary of our analysis, *Response to the report of the Hospital Authority Review Panel on the SARS outbreak,* 16 October 2003, p. 54, paragraph 2.18.
8. Donnelly CA, Ghani AC, Leung GM, et al., Epidemiological determinants of spread of causal agent of severe acute respiratory syndrome in Hong Kong, *Lancet* 2003; 361: 1761–6.

9. Riley S, Fraser C, Donnelly CA, et al., Transmission dynamics of the etiological agent of SARS in Hong Kong: Impact of public health interventions, *Science* 20 Jun 2003: 300(5627): 1961–66.

10. Ibid.

11. Lipsitch M, Cohen T, Cooper B, et al., Transmission dynamics and control of severe acute respiratory syndrome, *Science* 20 Jun 2003: 300(55627): 1966–70.

12. Anderson RM, May RM, *Infectious Diseases of Humans*. Oxford: Oxford University Press 1991, p. 70.

13. Ferguson NM, Galvani AP, Bush RM, Ecological and immunological determinants of influenza evolution, *Nature* 2003; 422: 428–33.

14. See endnote 9.

15. See endnote 9.

16. See endnote 9.

17. Galloway G, Scope of SARS outbreak understated, critics say, *The Globe and Mail* 29 May 2003, p. A1.

18. Leung GM, Hedley AJ, Ghani AC, et al., Case fatality rate in 1529 inpatients with severe acute respiratory syndrome (SARS) in Hong Kong, 2003 (under review).

19. So LKY, Lau ACW, Yam LYC, et al., Development of a standard treatment protocol for severe acute respiratory syndrome, *Lancet* 2003; 361: 1615–7.

20. Booth CM, Matukas LM, Tomlinson GA, et al., Clinical features and short-term outcomes of 144 patients with SARS in the Greater Toronto Area, *Journal of the American Medical Association* 4 Jun 2003: 289(21): 2801–9.

21. Personal communication, Dr. Allison McGeer, 30 May 2003.

22. The Harvard Team, *Improving Hong Kong's Health Care System: Why and For Whom?* Hong Kong: Government Printer 1999.

23. WD Scott and Co, *The Delivery of Medical Services in Hospitals: A Report for the Hong Kong Government*. Hong Kong: Government Printer 1985.

24. Hutzler C, Beijing missteps on virus show research failings, *Asian Wall Street Journal* 4 June 2003, p. A1.

25. Horton R, The new public health of risk and radical management, *Lancet* 1998; 352: 251–2.

26. Horton R, The new public health, *Lancet* 1998; 352: 904.

27. Reason J, Human errors: Models and management, *British Medical Journal* 2000; 320: 768–70.

CHAPTER **6**

1. Gro Harlem Brundtland, Day One Conclusion — The response so far, Speech by the Director General at the World Health Organisation global

meeting on SARS, Kuala Lumpur, 17 June 2003, **www.who.int/csr/SARS/conference/june_2003/materials/presentations/brundtland/en.**

2. World Health Organisation, SARS — Status of the outbreak and lessons for the immediate future, May 2003, **www.who.int/csr/media/SARS_wha.pdf.**

3. *People's Daily*, WHO officials study SARS situation in S. China province, 5 April 2003, **www.english.peopledaily.com.cn/200304/05/eng20030405_114618.shtml.**

4. World Health Organization, SARS epidemiology to date, 11 April 2003, **www.who.int/csr/SARS/epi2003_04_11/en.**

5. World Health Organisation, Update 49 — SARS case fatality ratio, incubation period, 7 May 2003, **www.who.int/csr/SARSarchive/2003_05_07a/en.**

6. Karen Richardson and Betsy McKay, WHO's methodology may understate SARS death rate, some officials say, *The Wall Street Journal*, 22 April 2003, **www.aegis.com/news/wsj/2003/WJ030410.html.**

7. Hong Kong SAR Government Press Release, **www.info.gov.hk/gia/general/200304/26/0426132.htm.**

8. Hong Kong SAR Government Press Release, **www.info.gov.hk/gia/general/200304/19/0419180.htm.**

9. Oliver Razum, Heiko Becher, Annette Kapaun, Thomas Junghanss, SARS, lay epidemiology, and fear, *Lancet* 17 May 2003.

10. In contrast, the change in the ICU/hospital ratio at the end is less significant as the number of patients in hospital is a lot lower.

11. S. Riley, C. Fraser, C.A. Donnelly, et al., Transmission dynamics of the etiological agent of SARS in Hong Kong: Impact of public health interventions, *Science* 23 May 2003, **www.sciencemag.org/cgi/rapidpdf/1086478v1.pdf.**

12. C. Dye and N. Gay, Modeling the SARS epidemic, *Science* 20 June 2003, **www.sciencemag.org/cgi/reprint/300/5627/1884.pdf.**

13. World Health Organisation, Cumulative number of reported probable cases of SARS, **www.who.int/csr/SARS/country/2003_07_11/en**; Data from the United States is not included, since only eight of the reported 75 SARS cases have been confirmed to be SARS by serology tests. See US Centers for Disease Control, Reported Suspect and Probable SARS Cases, by SARS-Associated Coronavirus (SARS-CoV) Serology, United States, 15 July 2003. Available at **www.cdc.gov/ncidod/SARS/casecount.htm.**

14. Ministry of Health, People's Republic of China, **www.moh.gov.cn/zhgl/yqfb/index.htm.**

15. Loretta Yam, Lecture on SARS-related issues given at Hong Kong Science Museum on 7 June 2003, **t.hk/~avwork/MyDir/Archive/Archive/OUDPA/SARS/SARS01_070603.ram.**

16. Ibid.

17. See Chapter 7.

CHAPTER 7

1. Certain sections of this chapter are reprinted with permission from Elsevier from the article entitled "Possible role of an animal vector in the SARS outbreak at Amoy Gardens" by Dr. Stephen Ng (*Lancet* 2003; 362: 570–2).

2. All chronology is based on data obtained from the Department of Health on 4 April 2003. Subsequent more up-to-date data are not available at the time of the writing of this chapter.

3. Department of Health, Hong Kong Government, *Outbreak of Severe Acute Respiratory Syndrome (SARS) at Amoy Gardens, Kowloon Bay, Hong Kong, Main Findings of the Investigation,* 2003.

4. *Ming Pao* (Hong Kong), 27 March 2003.

5. *Ming Pao* (Hong Kong), 11 April 2003.

6. *Ming Pao* (Hong Kong), 5 May 2003.

7. Ibid.

8. See endnote 3.

9. World Health Organisation Laboratory Network, First data on stability and resistance of SARS coronavirus, **www.who.int/csr/sars/survival_2003_05–04/en/**.

10. Lipsitch M, Cohen T, Cooper B, et al., Transmission dynamics and control of severe acute respiratory syndrome, *Science* 20 June 2003; 300(5627) 1966–70.

11. Ibid.

12. Due to incomplete data, the epidemic curves are constructed using 187 confirmed SARS cases instead of the 267 cases that were reported at the time.

13. Jacoby RO, Rat coronavirus, in *Viral and Mycoplasmal Infections of Laboratory Rodents: Effects on Biomedical Research,* edited by Bhatt PN, Jacoby RO, Morse AC III and New AE. Orlando: Academic Press 1986, pp. 625–38.

14. The University of Arizona Cooperative Extension, **www.cals.arizona.edu/pubs/insects/az1280.pdf**.

15. Professional Pest Management Association, **www.pestworld.org/homeowners/spotlight/roof_black_ship_rat.asp**.

16. *New York Times* (New York), 24 May 2003.

17. Peiris JSM, Chu CM, Cheng VCC, et al., Clinical progression and viral load in a community outbreak of coronavirus-associated SARS pneumonia: A prospective study, *Lancet* 2003; 361: 1767–72.

18. *Ming Pao* (Hong Kong), 8 May 2003.

19. *South China Morning Post* (Hong Kong), 28 May 2003.

20. Rota PA, Oberste MS, Monroe SS, et al., Characterization of a novel coronavirus associated with severe acute respiratory syndrome, *Science* 2003; 300: 1394–9.

21. Marra MA, Jones SJM, Astell CR, et al., The genome sequence of the SARS-associated coronavirus, *Science* 2003; 300: 1399–404.

22. Haijema BJ, Volders H, and Rottier PJM, Switching species tropism: An effective way to manipulate the feline coronavirus genome, *Journal of Virology* April 2003; 77: 4528–38.

23. Researchers from the US National Institute of Allergy and Infectious Disease have just reported that they had successfully inoculated mice with the SARS coronavirus (*Science* vol. 302, 10 October 2003). Mice showed no symptoms of disease despite active replication of virus in their bodies.

CHAPTER **8**

1. Yash Ghai, *Hong Kong's New Constitutional Order* (Hong Kong: Hong Kong University Press 1997), pp. 113–184 discusses extensively the legal and constitutional theory of autonomy in Chinese law. However, in practice, the Central Peoples Government kept Hong Kong practically sealed off from access by the rest of the country, allowing limited tourism, and then only in authorised, vetted groups. Business trips had to be approved by central authorities, with the Hong Kong and Macau Affairs Office and the Central People's Government Liaison Office jealously guarding their respective authorising powers over Hong Kong-mainland exchanges. Contacts between Hong Kong and Shenzhen and Guangdong authorities were largely ceremonial, highly bureaucratic or unofficial, except for those focused mainly on cross-boundary policing issues. Contours of the Hong Kong-mainland relations between mid-1997 and mid-2003 are best discerned from the initiatives registered in the "One Country, Two Systems Research Institute" (see the list of research projects at **www.octs.org.hk/e_page_research.htm**), which urged various changes in the relationship. Compare to the Hong Kong government website under the listing "mainland of China and Hong Kong" (see for example "infrastructure coordination with the mainland" at **info.gov.hk/topic_f.htm**). The rigid lines of official communication and the negotiated dates and agenda of formal meetings highly restrained cooperation and coordination in the case of emergencies such as SARS. See endnote 5.

2. Keith Bradsher, "Hong Kong doctor's ordeal as SARS patient," *New York Times*, 25 April 2003; and Mary Ann Benitez's interview of Dr. Tom Buckley, acting director of the PWH intensive care unit from 12 to 22 March who alerted physicians worldwide to the severity of the atypical pneumonia outbreak while Hong Kong officials were denying its seriousness, in "Doctor overwhelmed after launching e-mail campaign," *South China Morning Post* 31 March 2003.

3. See Chapter 4; and Cannix Yau, "Too little, too late in battle to stop killer," *The Standard* 15 April 2003.

4. Patsy Moy and Marcal Joanitho, "Pneumonia prompts WHO health alert," *Sunday Morning Post* 16 March 2003, lead story. Also see next endnote for repeated calls for calm.

5. Mary Ann Benitez and Leu Siew Ying, in "WHO accused of spreading panic as pneumonia numbers hit 83," *South China Morning Post* 18 March 2003, p. 1, quote Guangdong Health Bureau official Feng Shaoming as saying "We will monitor the situation in Hong Kong very closely but as for any exchange or cooperation, we need to get approval (from the central government)."

6. See below for details of the Article 23 controversy.

7. The 2003–04 Budget Address, see especially pages 75–93, "Raising Revenue," available at the Hong Kong Government website: **www.budget.gov.hk/2003/eng/index.htm**.

8. See statement of the Financial Secretary to the press on his reprimand. Available on the Hong Kong Government website at: **www.info.gov.hk/gia/general/200303/15/0315217.htm**. See also Margaret Ng, "The case against Antony Leung," *South China Morning Post* 28 March 2003.

9. See *China Daily* 17 July 2003 where Ip is highly praised while Leung receives very different treatment. Available at: **www1.chinadaily.com.cn/en/doc/2003-07/17/content_245828.htm**. Contrast this dry recital with the AP report at: **www.twincities.com/mld/twincities/news/world/6313397.htm** and especially the *Shenzhen Daily's* account at: **www.szed.com/szdaily/20030718/ca437983.htm**.

10. John Pomfret, "Chinese authorities ordered doctors in Beijing to hide SARS patients," *Washington Post* 20 April 2003. Warnings by mainland officials not to assess the mainland government's handling of SARS were reported in July, on the day following the gigantic protest over Article 23 legislation, which included proposed new restraints on media reportage of state secrets in Hong Kong. "Media and academics 'gagged by officials' over SARS," *South China Morning Post* 2 July 2003.

11. Bates Gill and Andrew Thompson, "Why China's health matters to the world," *South China Morning Post* 16 April 2003.

12. Charges that the Hong Kong Government also tried to hide aspects of SARS or kept information away from the public appeared throughout the period. See, for example, Chow Chung-yan, "Police told not to cause panic by using masks," *South China Morning Post* 31 March 2003; Matthew Lee, "Officials 'played down' killer virus," *The Standard* 14 April 2003; and Philip Bowring, "What the outbreak reveals: Hong Kong at its worst," *South China Morning Post* 7 May 2003. Bowring complained about the Hong Kong Government's secrecy with basic data, and attributed it, in part, to the political structure that empowered cliques with information denied to the rest.

13. The first call for a 100,000 person turnout was reported 20 June in the *South China Morning Post* (Jimmy Cheung, "Rally against security law promoted

via postcards"). By 25 June, 100,000 were expected to attend (Ambrose Leung and Stella Lee, "Democrats prepare to begin 100-hour hunger strike," *South China Morning Post*). The next day, after Tsang Yok-sing, Executive Councillor and head of the DAB, stated that "even if 200,000 attended the rally the government would not withdraw the bill." This prompted Lee Cheuk-yan to call for 300,000 to 400,000 to attend, but no one predicted such a turnout. See "Cannix Yau, Massive protest urged on Article 23," *The Standard* 26 June 2003. The highest forecast number appeared in Christine Loh, "Welcome to an unhappy Hong Kong, Premier Wen," *South China Morning Post* 30 June 2003. Loh noted that "Estimates (for the turnout) range from 100,000 to even 250,000 people." The title of Loh's op-ed piece refers to the TBWA report, *Marketing Premium Brands in Asia,* that found Hong Kong people to be "the unhappiest in the region by a wide margin — and that was before the added depression brought on by SARS." Victoria Button, "Hong Kong people saddest in region," *South China Morning Post* 29 June 2003.

14. For accounts of the unrest in the 1920s see Chan Lau Kit-ching, *From Nothing to Nothing, The Chinese Communist Movement and Hong Kong 1921–1936* (Hong Kong: Hong Kong University Press 1999) pp. 53–77. Compare to Norman Miners, *Hong Kong Under Imperial Rule, 1912–1941* (Hong Kong: Oxford University Press, 1987), pp. 12–20. See Ian Scott, *Political Change and the Crisis of Legitimacy in Hong Kong* (Hong Kong: Oxford University Press, 1989), pp. 81–126, for an account and analysis of the 1966–67 disturbances.

15. Elaine Wu, "No arrests throughout orderly protest," *South China Morning Post* 2 July 2003.

16. "Over-focus on politics to harm HK's interests," *China Daily, Hong Kong ed.* 16 July 2003, **www.1.chinadaily.com.cn/en/doc/2003-07/16/content_245665.htm**. Also, "Miscalculation of public opinion," *China Daily, Hong Kong ed.* 10 July 2003, **www1.chinadaily.com.cn/en/doc/2003-07/10/content_244251.htm**.

17. Polly Hui, Linda Yeung and Gary Cheung, "100 schools decide to shut their doors, but the education minister remains adamant that there is no need for blanket closures," *South China Morning Post* 27 March 2003.

18. The connection between the Aw case and Leung was made repeatedly in the press. For example, Stella Lee and Ravina Shamdasani, "Whether to prosecute is my business, says Elsie Leung," *South China Morning Post* 17 July 2003; the lead editorial in the *South China Morning Post* 19 July 2003, "The prosecution test that must be passed"; and an op-ed piece in the same newspaper by Christine Loh, "A crisis we could have avoided," 18 July 2003. For an account of the Aw case, see Albert H.Y. Chen, "Continuity and change in the legal system," in *The Other Hong Kong Report 1998*, edited by Larry Chuen-ho Chow and Yiu-kwan Fan, Hong Kong: Chinese University Press 1998, pp. 46–47.

19. See the Hong Kong Fearbusters website for ages of everyone who died in Hong Kong at **www.fearbuster.org.hk**. Only one person under the age of 30 died: a 28-year-old.

20. The best account of these events was written by John Pomfret of the *Washington Post* from Beijing. See "China orders end to SARS coverup, officials begin belated campaign against disease" (19 April 2003); "Coverup spurs shakeup in Beijing" (21 April 2003); "China's crisis has a political edge" (27 April 2003); "Outbreak gave China's Hu an opening, president responded to pressure inside and outside country on SARS" (13 May 2003).

21. The Health Minister Zhang Wenkang and Beijing mayor Meng Xuehong were sacked on 20 April. By 26 April, Robert Chung's POP polls were reporting that trust in the Hong Kong government had dropped while that for the mainland had soared. See "Beijing firings win our trust," *The Standard* 26 April 2003. Fong Tak-ho, "Leaders get tough with local officials," *South China Morning Post* 9 May 2003, reported 120 mainland officials had been sacked for bad performance during the SARS emergency.

22. Indications that the Article 23 legislation was in trouble in LegCo could be seen on 4 July 2003 on the front page of the *South China Morning Post*. The Post, running a headline "On Tuesday, 500,000 people marched against Article 23. Today, we ask our 60 legislators how they will vote . . . and whether events of the past week have affected their decision." The article took up the whole front page with colour photos of each LegCo member and indications of how they stood on the vote slated to take place 9 July. On 6 July 2003 the *Sunday Morning Post* front page announced "Tung makes Article 23 concessions" but this was not enough to stop criticism, and not enough to satisfy Tien, who resigned late that night. See Fanny Fung, "Tung shelves bill," *The Standard* 7 July 2003.

23. Under-employment is an economic term used to indicate that workers are working part-time but desire full time employment.

24. A study by the University of Hong Kong's Centre for Suicide Research and Prevention, reported by Patsy Moy, "Depression fears as suicides soar," *South China Morning Post* 8 September 2003.

25. Tung's character traits and the trouble they caused for governance could be clearly seen within the first year of his regime. See Michael DeGolyer, "Civil Service" in *The Other Hong Kong Report 1998*, edited by Larry Chuen-ho Chow and Yiu-kwan Fan, Hong Kong: Chinese University Press 1998, pp. 73–114. These troubles were comprehensively analysed in the joint Civic Exchange-National Democratic Institute publication reviewing the accountability system, "Accountability without Democracy," (September 2002) available at **www.civic-exchange.org/n_pub_cont_j02.htm#january2002**. See also the author's "The First Five Years" (June 2002) a Hong Kong Transition Project report, and "Accountability and Article 23" (December 2002) at **www.hkbu.edu.hk/~hktp/**.

26. See endnote above. See also Michael DeGolyer, "Broken rules," *The Standard* 4 September 2003, and the Hong Kong Government "organisation chart" (which breaks all the rules) at **www.info.gov.hk/govcht_e.htm** (see notes on this website especially).

27. Michael DeGolyer, "Legitimacy and leadership: Public attitudes in post-British Hong Kong," in *Hong Kong in Transition*, edited by Robert Ash et al, London: RoutledgeCurzon 2003, pp. 125–146; Lo Shiu-hing, *Governing Hong Kong*, New York: Nova Science Publishers 2001; Ian Scott, "The disarticulation of Hong Kong's post-handover politicial system," in *Hong Kong Government and Politics*, edited by Sing Ming, Hong Kong: Oxford University Press 2003, pp. 663–94.

28. This self-observation has been reported in the press numerous times and also by interviewees of the author who prefer anonymity. These interviewees have interacted with the Chief Executive, some many times, during both formal and informal exchanges.

29. The Government's Department of Health and the quasi-independent Hospital Authority have two separate inquiries underway.

30. This strategy is described by Lau Siu-kai, now head of Tung's Central Policy Unit, in "Government and political change in the Hong Kong Special Administrative Region," in *Hong Kong the Super Paradox*, edited by James C. Hsiung, New York: St. Martin's Press 2000, pp. 35–57.

31. As evidenced by the more than 30 interventions in the property market, including Michael Suen's famous nine steps actions in late 2002. Tung has also indicated many times he considers high wage levels part of why he considers Hong Kong "uncompetitive." See, for example, his remarks in December 2002 at the Hong Kong General Chamber of Commerce annual business summit, at **www.info.gov.hk/ce/speech/cesp.htm**. Also see the Chief Executive Office website in general for copious examples of these views.

32. Joseph Lo and Jimmy Cheung, "Li Ka-shing proud of protesters," *South China Morning Post* 22 August 2003.

33. Chris Patten's memoir, *East and West* (London: Macmillan 1998) discusses these events in passing, but Jonathan Dimbleby, *The Last Governor* (London: Little, Brown, and Co. 1997) gives a blow by blow account.

CHAPTER **9**

1. David Heymann, Executive Director, Communicable Diseases, WHO, from transcript of a conference call on 8 April 2003, CLSA Speaker Series, "SARS – Hype from reality," published by *CLSA Emerging Markets*. See also Chris Taylor, "In China, it seems the 'big one' is yet to come," *South China Morning Post* 11 May 2003, p. 4.

2. Henk Bekedam, WHO's China Representative in Beijing, from transcript

of a conference call on 29 April 2003, CLSA Speaker Series, "SARS in China — Where to from here?" published by *CLSA Emerging Markets*.

3. Carrie Chan and Mary Ann Benitez, "Mid-June hint on travel advisory," *South China Morning Post* 22 May 2003, p. A1.

4. HKSAR Government Press Release, **www.info.gov.hk/gia/general/200304/02/0402260.htm**.

5. An "affected area" is defined by the WHO as a region at the first administrative level where the country is reporting local transmission of SARS, **www.who.int/csr/sars/areas/2003_03_16/en**.

6. The criterion for 20 continuous days of no new cases being detected automatically determines when a place is SARS-free. The criterion is based on two incubation periods of ten days each.

7. HKSAR Government Press Release, **www.info.gov.hk/gia/general/200305/03/0503138.htm**

8. SARS Bulletin, Health, Welfare & Food Bureau, 7 May 2003, **www.info.gov.hk/dh/diseases/ap/eng/bulletin0507.pdf**. The criterion for the number of active cases not to exceed 60 was derived from the experience in Hanoi, where the number of cases topped at 63, according to the WHO's David Heymann at a press conference in Hong Kong at the Foreign Correspondents' Club on 19 June 2003.

9. HKSAR Government Press Release, **www.info.gov.hk/gia/general/200305/20/0520250.htm**.

10. The father, a 33-year-old man, and his nine-year-old son were admitted to hospital on 11 and 12 February respectively. The father died on 17 February while the son recovered. The mother of the family was admitted to hospital on 13 February and also recovered. The family had a second daughter who remained asymptomatic throughout.

11. A doctor from the Hanoi French Hospital, which received the SARS patient, contacted the WHO's Dr. Carlo Urbani to look at the case because it appeared highly unusual. Urbani doubted it was a case of influenza and was alarmed by the case. Together with other WHO officials, they persuaded the Vietnam Government to take action to prevent the spread of the strange disease.

12. WHO's global alert about SARS, **www.who.int/csr/sars/archive/2003_03_12/en**.

13. Matt Pottinger, Elena Cherney, Gautam Nail and Michael Waldholz, "How a global effort identified SARS virus in a matter of weeks," *The Wall Street Journal* 17 April 2003.

14. WHO's emergency travel advisory, **www.who.int/csr/sars/archive/2003_03_15/en**.

15. Chris Taylor, "In China, it seems the 'big one' is yet to come," *South China Morning Post* 11 May 2003, p. 4.

16. Rob Stein, "On the pulse: SARS has revealed the skills and limitations of the WHO disease hunters," *The Standard* 3 June 2003, p. A19.

17. Hui Li, "Atypical pneumonia: SARS in China," *CLSA Emerging Markets* 17 April 2003, p. 7.

18. WHO SARS Update: **www.who.int/csr/sars/archives/2003_04_02/en/**.

19. David Heymann, WHO, see endnote 1 for full reference.

20. Michael Backman, "SARS: A WHO-induced panic?" Commentary, *Far Eastern Economic Review*, 22 May 2003. Backman was in fact mistaken in stating that the WHO had issued a travel advisory for Vietnam and Hanoi, although the WHO did include Hanoi on its SARS "affected area" list on 16 March 2003.

21. The WHO, *The World Health Report 2000*, 21 June 2000. The rankings had been set aside after vigorous objections from a number of UN member states.

22. Yeoh Siew Hoon, "Who did the right thing by SARS and travel", interview with Dr. Max Hardiman, *TravelWeekly*, 23 May 2003, p. 16.

23. WHO SARS Update: **www.who.int/csr/sars/archive/2003_04_29/en/**.

24. WHO SARS Update: **www.who.int/csr/sars/archive/2003_05_14/en/**.

25. Thomas Crampton, "WHO assails China for faltering on SARS," *International Herald Tribune*, 3 June 2003.

26. WHO SARS Update: **www.who.int/csr/don/2003_05_23/en/** and **www.who.int/csr.don/2003_05_24/en/**.

27. WHO SARS Update: **www.who.int/csr/don/2003_05_26/en/**.

28. WHO SARS Update: **www.who.int/csr/don/2003_06_04/en/**.

29. WHO SARS Update: **www.who.int/csr/don/2003_06_13/en/**.

30. Health Canada, *Learning from SARS: Renewal of Public Health in Canada*, October 2003, p. 40.

31. Jonathan Mirsky, "Containing SARS: The scandal over Taiwan," *International Herald Tribune*, 12 May 2003.

32. Ibid.

33. "Who will stand up for Taiwan?" *Taipei Times*, 17 May 2003, p. 9. Taiwan was invited to attend a technical briefing on SARS however and was allocated time to make a short report on the development of SARS in Taiwan, see Melody Chen and Wang Ping-yu, Taiwan makes progress at WHO, *Taipei Times* 19 May 2003, p. 1.

34. Lin Chieh-yu, "WHO campaign stays on track," *Taipei Times*, 19 May 2003, p. 2.

35. Melody Chen, "Invitation from WHO reeks of politics," *Taipei Times*, 14 June 2003, p. 1.

36. Editorial, *Asian Wall Street Journal*, 31 March 2003. Long's statement was made on 27 March 2003.

37. Henk Bekedam, WHO, see endnote 2 for full reference.

38. Statement from the Standing Committee of the Politburo read on Chinese TV on 17 April 2003.

39. Meng Xuenong was appointed as the Deputy Director of the North-South Water Diversion Office on 1 October 2003.

40. John Aglionby, "China opens door to world help with its SARS crisis," *The Guardian*, **www.guardian.co.uk/sars/story/0,13036,946201,00.html**, 30 April 2003.

41. Staff reporter, "Deadly 'cover-up'," *The Standard* 19 June 2003, p. B20.

42. John Pomfret, "China's slow reaction to fast-moving illness fearing loss of control, Beijing stonewalled," *Washington Post Foreign Service* 3 April 2003.

43. *People's Daily*, **english.peopledaily.com.cn/200304/05/print20030405_114618.html**. What is unclear from available reports is whether the Guangdong Department of Health sent Xiao's report or merely some information based on the report. Further, there are also discrepancies from published information as to when Guangdong issued the guidelines to hospitals informing them about the new disease. The *People's Daily* reported the 23 January, whilst according to John Pomfret's report (endnote 42), it could only have been after the 27 January since Xiao's report was not supposed to have been read till then. The exact dates are perhaps unimportant since the fact is systemic secrecy within the Chinese system caused information to not be acted upon to China's own detriment.

44. Ibid.

45. Josephine Ma and Staff Reporters, "Guangdong 'reported on the outbreak in February'," *South China Morning Post* 21 May 2003, p. A3.

46. Henk Bekedam, WHO, see endnote 2 for full reference, p. 3.

47. WHO SARS Update: **www.who.int/csr/sars/archive/2003_04_09/en/**.

48. *People's Daily*, **english.peopledaily.com.cn/200304/05/print20030405_114618.html**

49. Bekedam, WHO, see endnote 2 for full reference.

50. Jonathan Mirsky, "How the Chinese spread SARS," *The New York Review of Books* 29 May 2003, p. 42.

51. Matthew Lee, "Only Beijing to blame: Yeoh," *The Standard* 14 June 2003, p. B5.

52. SARS Expert Committee report, *SARS in Hong Kong: From Experience to Action*, 2 October 2003, available online at **www.sars-expertcom.gov.hk**.

53. While protective gear was sent, no medical workers were dispatched. See HKSAR Government's Press Release, **www.info.gov.hk/gia/general/200305/08/0508110.htm**

54. Christine Loh, "Love thy neighbour," Hong Kong Strategy, *CLSA Emerging Markets*, March 2003, **www.civic-exchange.org** under publications 2003.

55. Bekedam, WHO, see endnote 2 for full reference.

56. The author is grateful to Su Liu of Wirthlin Worldwide for the use of her research on Shanghai.

57. Bekedam, WHO, see endnote 2 for full reference.
58. Jonathan Mirsky noted in "How the Chinese spread SARS," *The New York Review of Books* 29 May 2003, page 42, that there was a 1996 law that classified "highest level infectious diseases" as "highly secret" with the secrecy extending from the first occurrence of the disease until the day it is announced. However, in checking the status of that law, Jerry Li of the United Nations Development Project's (UNDP) office in Beijing advised that the Ministry of Health's Legal Section told the UNDP that there was a Regulation on the Specific Scope of Secrecy of its Classification in Public Health Work but it had been invalidated in 2001, personal communication, 15 July 2003.
59. *Nanfang Ribao* 20 February 2003.
60. John Pomfret, "China's crisis has a political edge," *Washington Post Foreign Service* 27 April 2003, p. A33.
61. Ibid.
62. Matthew Forney, "China stops the presses, again," *Time*, Asia Edition 30 June 2003.
63. HKSAR Government Press Release, **www.info.gov.hk/gia/general/200307/07/0707200.htm**, 7 July 2003.

CHAPTER **10**

1. "China's Chernobyl," *The Economist*, 26 April 2003, pp. 9–10.
2. James C F Wang, *Contemporary Chinese Politics: An Introduction*, 7th Edition, Upper Saddle River, N. J.: Prentice Hall, 2002, p. 70.
3. The Central Secretariat has seven major departments: propaganda, organization, united front work, liaison office with overseas Chinese bodies, publication office of the *People's Daily*, policy research, and the office of the party school.
4. Kenneth Lieberthal, *Governing China: From Revolution Through Reform*, New York: W.W. Norton & Company Inc, 1995, pp. 169–170.
5. Ibid, pp. 170–171.
6. Ellen Lee, "Officials from HK to Visit Hospitals in Guangdong," *South China Morning Post* 1 April 2003, p. A2.
7. "Whose security? — "State security" in China's new criminal code, *Human Rights in China and Human Rights Watch/Asia*, Vol. 9, No. 4, April 1997, pp. 21–25.
8. "China wakes up," *The Economist* 26 April 2003, p. 19.
9. See Chapter 9 for more details.
10. WHO Updates, **www.who.int/csr/sars/archives/2003_03_26a/en/**, 26 March 2003. For this chapter, we have used the WHO figures rather than those of China's Ministry of Health or those reported by the media as there are discrepancies.

11. WHO Updates, **www.who.int/csr/sars/archives/2003_03_27b/en/**, 27 March 2003.

12. WHO Updates, **www.who.int/csr/sars/archives/2003_03_28/en/**, 28 March 2003; and Hugo Restall, "Examining Asian: Keep Up the Pressure on China," *Asian Wall Street Journal* 4 April 2003.

13. WHO Updates, **www.who.int/csr/sars/archives/2003_03_31/en/**, 31 March 2003.

14. WHO Updates, **www.who.int/csr/sars/archives/2003_02_02b/en/**, 2 April 2003.

15. WHO Updates, **www.who.int/csr/sars/archives/2003_04_03/en/**, 3 April 2003.

16. WHO Updates, **www.who.int/csr/sars/archives/2003_04_04/en/**, 4 April 2003.

17. WHO Updates, **www.who.int/csr/sars/archives/2003_04_07/en/**, 7 April 2003.

18. For details see Chapters 9 and 14.

19. Henk Bekedam, "SARS in China: Where to from here?," Transcript of a conference call from Beijing, CLSA Speaker Series, 29 April 2003, *CLSA Emerging Markets*.

20. Siew-ying Leu and Bill Savadove, "Who says mainland officials continue to hinder investigation," *South China Morning Post* 1 April 2003, p. A1; and Peter Wonacott and Susan V Lawrence and Matt Pottinger, "Health officials express doubt about China's SARS figures," *Wall Street Journal* 17 April 2003.

21. "Worldwide criticism of outbreak cover-up," *South China Morning Post* 18 April 2003, p. A3.

22. "Taiwanese urged to avoid mainland as 13th case is revealed," *South China Morning Post* 31 March, 2003, p. A5.

23. WHO Updates, **www.who.int/crs/sars/archives/2003_04_18/en/**, 18 April 2003.

24. Various news reports indicated that 100–200 officials have been fired throughout the country. Private communication indicated that as many as 500 have been dismissed.

25. WHO Updates, **www.who.int/crs/sars/archives/2003_04_21/en/**, 21 April 2003.

26. "The fund will be used to finance the treatment of farmers and poor urban residents infected by SARS and to upgrade country-level hospitals and purchase SARS-related medical facilities in Central and Western China and for research programmes on the virus," China Creates SARS Task Force, Special Fund, Ministry of Foreign Affairs of the People's Republic of China, 24 April 2003, **www.frnprc.gov.en/eng/47496.html**. News reports indicated that some areas did not follow the central authorities' order that poor people would be given free medical care; see John Pomfret, "SARS Spread in Rural China Raises Concerns," *Washington Post Foreign Service* 7 May 2003.

27. Ibid.

28. "Jun Yi Jin Zhu Xiaotangshan" (Military surgeons stationed in Xiaotangshan Hospital), *Ming Pao* 1 May 2003, p. A18.

29. Fred Hu, "Will SARS derail China's economy?," *China Insight*, Goldman Sachs, 25 April 2003.

30. National Bureau of Statistics of China, **www.stats.gov.cn/tjfx/jdfx/ 1200307170031.htm**, 17 July 2003.

31. "WHO experts praise SARS hospital on Beijing's outskirt," *Xinhuanet* 4 June 2003.

32. Brad Adams, "China's other health cover-up," *Asian Wall Street Journal* 12 June 2003

33. "Jie Zhong Guo Yin Man yi Qing Yi Sheng Jiang Yan Yong Zao Jian Kong" (Dr. Jiang Yanyong, who revealed SARS cover-up was under surveillance), *Asia Times Online*, **http://asiatimes-chinese.com/514chsars.htm** 14 May 2003.

34. Eric Sautede, "The snares of modernity: Internet, information and the SARS crisis in China," *China Perspectives,* No. 47, May-June 2003, p. 25.

35. Xia Liping, "China: A responsible great power," *Journal of Contemporary China* 2001, p. 17.

36. Joint State of the Special ASEAN-China Leaders Meeting on SARS, Ministry of Foreign Affairs of the People's Republic of China, 29 April 2003. In respect of the pledge, it was interesting that none of the ASEAN nation pledged money to the fund. It indicated that ASEAN did not think money was the issue.

37. CNN.com/World, "China promises openness on SARS," **www.edition.cnn.com/2003/WOOLD/asiapcf/06/28/sars.apec/reut/index.html**, 28 June 2003.

38. Judith Banister, "Population, public health and the environment in China," in *Managing The Chinese Environment,* edited by Richard Louis Edmonds, Oxford: Oxford University Press, 1998, pp. 262–91.

39. "China: 'One in 3 Chinese kids suffers from lead poisoning'," *Straits Times,* 8 April 2003.

40. Dexter Roberts, "Breakdown: How China's decentralized health care is failing," *Business Week* 28 April 2003, pp. 22–23.

41. Ibid.

42. Chris Taylor, "In China, It seems the 'Big One' is yet to come," *South China Morning Post* 11 May 2003, p. A4.

43. Christopher Bodeen, "China bans wildlife cuisine on SARS fears," *Associated Press* 31 May 2003.

44. Dexter Roberts, "Breakdown: How China's decentralized health care is failing," *Business Week* 28 April 2003, p. 22.

45. Ibid.

46. "Foreign direct investment increased steadily. In 2002, the contracted foreign capitals through foreign direct ivestment stood at 82.8 billion US dollars, up 19.6 percent, and the foreign capitals actually utilized were 52.7 billion US dollars, up 12.5 percent," "Statistical Communique 2002," National Bureau of Statistics, People's Republic of China, **www.stat.gov.cn/english/ newrelease/statisticalreports/1200303120088.htm,**28 February 2003.

47. Minxin Pei, "China's governance crisis," *Foreign Affairs*, September/October 2002, p. 97.

48. Joseph Kahn, "Beijing effectively beats SARS: WHO declares," *New York Times* 26 June 2003.

49. "No watchdog," *Asian Wall Street Journal* 9 August 2001, p. 6.

50. Wu Zhong and agencies, "70 dead in China's 'first sub accident'," *South China Morning Post*, p. A1.

CHAPTER **11**

1. Trade Shipping Industries Fisheries Agriculture Land, Hong Kong Administrative Report 1910.

2. Hong Kong Administrative Report 1934.

3. Hansard: The Financial Secretary, The Appropriation Bill, 1 March 1972.

4. Ibid.

5. Ibid.

6. World Trade Organization Agreement 1994.

7. The Federation of Hong Kong Industries and The Hong Kong Centre for Economic Research, *Made in PRD*, June 2003.

8. Ibid.

9. Ibid.

10. Gross Domestic Product 2002, HKSAR Government.

11. Corporation of the City of London, *The London/New York Study*, June 2000.

12. Corporation of the City of London, *The London/New York Study*, June 2000; US Census Bureau, 2000; and Census 2000; and HKSAR Government.

13. Annual Digest of Statistics 1990, HKSAR Government.

14. Gross Domestic Product 2002, HKSAR Government.

15. Corporation of City of London, *The London/New York Study*, June 2002.

16. Gross Domestic Product 2002, HKSAR Government.

17. Greater London Authority Housing in London, 2003; Rating and Valuation Department Report, Hong Kong 2003; New York City Rent Guidelines Board 2003 report; and New York Housing Supply Report 2003.

18. Grubb and Ellis, *New York Special Report 2001*; and Corporation of City of London, *London/New York Study*, June 2000.

19. ACI Traffic Data: World airports ranking by total cargo – 2002. Memphis, the major US domestic hub, is the world's busiest cargo airport having lifted almost 3.4 million metric tonnes of freight in 2002. Hong Kong is the world's second largest air cargo hub, carrying 2.5 million metric tonnes in 2002. Hong Kong, however, only carries freight internationally.

20. The Mayor's of London Report 2003, *Visit London*; and NYC & Co., the official body promoting tourism in New York City information available at: **www.nycvisit.com/home/index.cfm**

21. NYC & Co; and London Tourist Board and Convention Bureau, information available at: **www.londontouristboard.co.uk**.
22. Ibid.
23. Ibid.
24. World Travel and Tourism Council, *SARS has a Massive Impact on Travel & Tourism in Affected Destinations,* 15 March 2003.
25. The Hong Kong Government relies for approximately 40% of its income from various real estate-related sources, principally from selling development rights as it continues to own all the land in Hong Kong. The decline in property prices dramatically reduced revenue at the same time that it was appropriate to run expansionary fiscal policies. This has resulted in a budget deficit that is about 5% in the year 2003/04. However, the total reserves of the HKSAR is probably of the order of US$100 billion (HK$776.8 billion), excluding reserves dedicated to supporting the linked exchange rate mechanism, which total US$80 billion (HK$621.4 billion).
26. Page 2, of the Preface to the Annual General Report for 1925 prepared by the Governor.

CHAPTER **12**

1. The Hospital Authority's "probable SARS case" definition requires an X-ray with evidence of pneumonia, a fever and two of the following four symptoms: chills, cough, myalgia and/or exposure to a SARS patient. The WHO's "probable SARS case" definition requires a fever, cough or breathing difficulty and contact with SARS patient, or travel to or residence in a SARS-affected area.
2. WHO SARS Update, **www.who.int.csr/sars/archives/2003_05_12/en/**, 12 May 2003.
3. Danylo Hawaleshka, "Is this your best defense?" *Maclean's* 14 April 2003.
4. WHO Press Release, Malaria is alive and well and killing more than 3,000 African children, **www.who.int/mediacentre/releases/2003/pr33/en/**, 25 April 2003.
5. Carolina Uribe and Victor Rodriguez, "Pues Yo Me Vuelvo a Hong Kong" [Well, I'm returning to Hong Kong]," *El Mundo Cronica*, **www.el-mundo.es/cronica/2003/393/1051447606.html**, 27 April 2003.
6. Warren Kinsella, "The racist face of SARS," *Maclean's* 14 April 2003; see also Jan Wong, "How SARS has become the latest yellow peril," *The Globe and Mail*, **www.globeandmail.com/servlet/story/RTGAM.20030411.cowong0411/BNStory**, 11 April 2003.
7. David Baltimore, "Take a balanced approach to SARS," *Asian Wall Street Journal*, 29 April 2003.
8. WHO SARS Updates, **www.who.int/csr/sars/archive/2003_03_24/en/**, 24

March 2003 and **www.who.int/csr/sars/archive/2003_03_25/en/**, 25 March 2004.

9. The many stories of business lost by Hong Kong companies, particularly in the travel and tourism sectors, led to accusations that the WHO was insensitive to the economic consequences of its travel recommendations. To show that the WHO had overreacted, business people pointed to other illnesses, including the common flu, that every year kill more people than SARS. Public health professionals around the world, on the other hand, stressed the necessity of travel advisories from a public health perspective, especially given the novelty of the SARS virus, its unknown potential and the fact that it was spreading quickly via air travel. The travel advisories, although designed to warn people travelling to Hong Kong or Guangdong, also affected Hong Kong business overseas because people from SARS-affected areas were seen as potential carriers of the virus. Two major US and Swiss luxury goods trade fairs banned Hong Kong business people from participating for this reason. Immediately prior to the commencement of the Basel World Watch and Jewellery Show, Swiss officials told Hong Kong representatives that they could not participate in the Fair as exhibitors but could still be admitted as visitors. HKSAR Government officials intervened without success. A similar event occurred involving a jewellery show in Las Vegas, but intervention there did help to reverse the decision.

10. Leslie Chang, "China's petri dish to the world," *Asian Wall Street Journal* 2 April 2003.

11. Sarah Schafer and Fred Guterl, "How to make a virus," *Newsweek* 21 April 2003.

12. Elisabeth Rosenthal, "SARS forces Beijing to fight an old but unsanitary habit," *New York Times* 28 May 2003.

13. One direct consequence of the outbreak was the massive clean-ups in Hong Kong and in mainland Chinese cities.

14. Arnaud Bédat, "Dans la Cité de Tous les Dangers [In the city of all danger]," *L'illustré*, **www.illustre.ch/2003/18/pro_1.html**, 30 April 2003.

15. Alan Fung, "How Singapore outmanaged the others," *Asia Times*, **www.atimes.com/atimes/China/ED09Ad03.html**, 9 April 2003.

16. Keith Bradsher of the *New York Times* raised the point at the Panel Discussion: "Rebuilding Asia's World City" at the Hong Kong Foreign Correspondents' Club, 20 June 2003.

17. "Pro-government camp criticises the Government's PR handling of SARS," *Ming Pao* 5 May 2003.

18. HKSAR Government Press Release, **www.info.gov.hk/gia/general/200304/13/0413193.htm**, 12 April 2003.

19. Maggie Fox, "HK health-care system on the verge of collapse," *Indian Express*, **www.expressindia.com/fullstory.php?newsid=2-471#compstory**, 11 April 2003.

20. James Kong of the Hospital Authority's Health Informatics and Information Technology team developed "eSARS," Personal Communication, 21 July 2003. See also WHO SARS Update, **www.who.int/csr/sarsarchive/2003_05_06/en/**, 6 May 2003.

21. "Fearless and professional reporters in quarantine camps and SARS hotspots," *Ta Kung Pao* 14 June 2003, p. A09.

22. "SARS and the media," *Sing Tao Daily* 15 May 2003, p. E06.

23. *Media Digest*, "Conclusions of the Hong Kong media's handling of the SARS crisis," Radio Television Hong Kong, **www.rthk.org.hk/mediadigest/20030515_76_79208.html**, May 2003.

24. Sensational reporting prevailed in the early days of the crisis. See for example, "Killer pneumonia set panic in Hong Kong," *Oriental Daily* news headline 11 February 2003; and "Fatal pneumonia is spreading and is airborne," *Apple Daily* 11 February 2003 (front page headline). See also "Mutant flu outbreak – Truth behind fatal pneumonia," *Next Magazine* 13 February 2003, which portrayed the disease as one that affected less educated mainlanders.

25. Many Hong Kong newspapers and magazines frequently show nude pictures as well as enlarged images of victims who have died gory deaths. Detailed narratives in sex-related news stories are also quite common. The Hong Kong media is often under attack for the deterioration of social conduct and values. For more criticism of specific newspapers and magazines, see Yu Fu Kwok, "The 21st century network of sinners: A study of cases of violations committed by the local press," *The Candle Network*, The Society for Truth and Light, Issue 31 Vol. 6 No. 4, July 2003. For more on the local media's effect on Hong Kong society, see Yu Wing On, "The anti-intellectualism of the Hong Kong Media," Media Digest, RTHK, **www.rthk.org.hk/mediadigest/20020315_76_17701.html**, March 2002.

26. "Social responsibility," *Hong Kong Economic Times* 1 April 2003, p. C13.

27. The discussion took place on 26 April 2003 at the Fearbusters Workshop, see meeting record at **www.fearbuster.org.hk**.

28. "School of medicine dean: About 10 SARS infections in the community untold by officials; the Government was hiding infections, the Chinese University Shows," *Sing Tao Daily* 18 March 2003, p. A02.

29. "What have we learned from SARS?" *Ta Kung Pao* 26 June 2003, p. A26.

30. "Singapore closes all schools, but Hong Kong Government insists it is not for HK," *Apple Daily* 27 March 2003, headline.

31. Cheung Kwai-yeung, "The media has become the protector in the fight against SARS," *Wen Wei Pao* 28 May 2003, p. A11. The mainland-controlled media in Hong Kong adopted a more rigorous monitoring role after 17 April when fighting SARS and truthful reporting were identified as explicit priorities of China's national policy on SARS. *Tai Kung Pao* quoted Chinese

president Hu Jintao, premier Wen Jiabao and state councillor Tang Jiaxuan in saying that the media's monitoring role and push for transparency improved many government policies on many occasions. See "Fearless and professional reporters in quarantine camps and SARS hotspots," *Ta Kung Pao* 14 June 2003, p. A09.

32. Richard Cullen, "The media and society in Hong Kong," in *Building Democracy: Creating Good Governance for Hong Kong*, edited by Christine Loh and Civic Exchange; Hong Kong: Hong Kong University Press 2003.

33. See "SARS and the media," *Sing Tao Daily* 15 May 2003, p. E06.

34. *Media Digest*, see endnote 23 for full reference.

35. Albert Cheng took leave from 16 to 27 June 2003 after the Broadcasting Authority warned him for calling a government official "doglike" and criticising a Hospital Authority official without giving him enough time to defend himself on air. For further discussion on the influence of radio talk shows in Hong Kong politics, see Hannah Beech, "Making waves," *Time* 14 July 2003.

36. The show was highly acclaimed for its role in protecting pregnant medical workers, a group which was particularly vulnerable to SARS.

37. Critics focused on the Expert Committee's refusal to identify any maladministration, lack of diligence or negligence on the part of individual officials in handling the SARS epidemic. The SARS Expert Committee report, entitled *SARS in Hong Kong: From Experience to Action*, is available online at **www.sars-expertcom.gov.hk**.

38. Bryan Walsh, "System failure," *Time Asia* 28 April 2003.

39. Timeline, **www.sosick.org/timeline.html**, last update 16 June 2003.

40. "Fearless and professional reporters in quarantine camps and SARS hotspots," *Ta Kung Pao* 14 June 2003, p. A09. See also "Sydney Chung praises the media for effectively monitoring the Government and encouraging medical workers," *Ming Pao* 15 May 2003, p. A08.

41. Mary Lee Wing Ming, "The role and influence of the media in the SARS crisis," *Hong Kong Economic Journal* 12 June 2003, p. 25.

42. Chris Sorensen, "Toronto safe to visit: Lastman assures CNN audience," *Toronto Star* 25 April 2003.

43. On 29 April, after heavy lobbying by Canadian political heavyweights, the WHO lifted the travel advisory for Toronto, after which local media interest in SARS waned somewhat until the number of infections rose again and a second advisory had to be imposed on 26 May. Chapter 9 provides a fuller account of the politics involved in the WHO's unfortunate flip flop policy in the case of Toronto.

44. Jan Wong of the *Globe and Mail*, personal communication, 18 July 2003.

45. Anecdotal evidence indicated that Westerners living in Hong Kong had a lower incidence of wearing facemasks than their Chinese counterparts.

46. By contrast, Toronto's population density is 800 per square kilometre. See Population Density by Area, **www.info.gov.hk/censtat/hkinf/population/pop5_index.html**, Census & Statistics Department, 2003; and Population of 30 Metropolitan Areas in Canada, **www.canadainfolink.ca/cities.htm**, March 2003.

47. "Central Government fully supports SARS control efforts in HK: Hu Jintao," *People's Daily*, **english.peopledaily.com.cn/200304/14/eng20030414_115104.shtml**, 14 April 2003.

48. "HK's new SARS patients number under one digit per day," *People's Daily*, **english.peopledaily.com.cn/200305/13/eng20030513_116587.shtml**, 13 May 2003. However, as mainland controls on what the domestic media could report were relaxed slightly, there were many stories about the Amoy Gardens outbreak and the experience of residents. The suffering of the residents was recognised nationally when Premier Wen Jiabao took time to visit Amoy Gardens during a trip to Hong Kong on 30 June 2003. Wen also paid a visit to Kwok Sin-hung and his two young children at the neighbouring Lower Ngau Tau Kok Estate. Kwok lost his wife to SARS. Elaine Wu and Ambrose Leung, "For a devastated family, words of comfort," *South China Morning Post* 1 July 2003, front page.

49. The information was originally found at **www.chinacdc.net.cn/feiyan/default.asp** but the authors have not been able to access the information again subsequently.

50. "Transparency widespread, China opening wider," *People's Daily*, **english.peopledaily.com.cn/200306/28/eng20030628_119023.shtml**, 28 June 2003.

51. John Pomfret, "Doctor says Health Ministry lied about disease," *Washington Post Foreign Service* 10 April 2003; and Eric Sautede, "The snares of modernity: Internet, information and the SARS crisis in China," *China Perspectives*, Number 47, May-June 2003, p. 26.

52. Benjamin Kang Lim, "Chinese doctor gagged over SARS cover-up," Yahoo! News UK & Ireland, **uk.news.yahoo.com/030522/80/e0lbm.html**, 22 May 2003.

53. Staff Reporter, "Media and academics 'gagged by officials' over SARS," *South China Morning Post* 2 July, 2003.

54. See for example, Andrew Brown, *Killer Pneumonia*, CNN, aired 27 March 2003.

55. Indira Lakshmanan, "Exploring China's silence on SARS: New details surfaces on initial cover-up," *Boston Globe* 25 May 2003.

56. In May 2002, 10.3 million people crossed the Hong Kong-China border — an average of 343,000 people per day. In May 2003, the number dropped to 7.5 million people, an average of 250,000 per day.

57. "Chinese university professor: Pneumonia outbreak in Guangzhou did not cease," *Ming Pao* 24 March 2003.

58. Jesse Wong, "SARS shows dangers posed by Article 23," *Asian Wall Street Journal* 11 June 2003.

59. Joseph Man Chan, "Extending news monitoring to the mainland: Starting with SARS coverage," *Media Digest,* Radio Television Hong Kong, **www.rthk.org.hk/mediadigest/20030616_76_84871.html**, June 2003.

60. Michael Yahuda, *Hong Kong: China's Challenge,* London: Routledge 1996, p. 130.

61. Chris Yeung, "Separation and integration: Hong Kong-mainland relations in a flux," in *The First Tung Chee-hwa Administration — The First Five Years of the Hong Kong Administrative Region,* edited by Lau Kiu-kai. Hong Kong: Chinese University Press 2002, pp. 249–251.

62. Carrie Chan, "Encephalitis exposes system flaws," *South China Morning Post* 19 June 2003, p. A4.

63. *Media Watch*, Radio Television Hong Kong, aired 31 May 2003. The survey found that 88.8% of respondents thought they received sufficient information; 67.9% did not think they received too much information; 63.9% thought the coverage or information was accurate; 37.4% thought the coverage tended to be on the positive side while 30.5% thought it was on the negative side; and 63.8% thought the media had done a good job monitoring the government.

64. Ibid. Also see "The atypical military reporter," *Hong Kong Economic Journal* 28 March 2003, p. 13.

65. The HKSAR Government announced on 7 July that it would defer the legislation after the Liberal Party chairman resigned from the Executive Council the day before, which meant that the government would not carry the vote in the Legislative Council if it pushed ahead on the 9 July.

66. Chris Yeung, "The media and politics: A balancing act," *Sunday Morning Post* 13 July 2003, p. 10.

CHAPTER **13**

1. SARS Expert Committee, *SARS in Hong Kong: From Experience to Action,* pp. 71–74, available online at **www.sars-expertcom.gov.hk**.

2. Keith Bradsher, "A deadly virus on its mind, Hong Kong covers its face," *New York Times* 31 March 2003.

3. Joe Havely, *Mystery Bug Sets Tongues Wagging,* CNN, aired 1 April 2003.

4. Throughout April and the first week of May 2003, the US Business Travel Coalition conducted four surveys of major buyers of commercial air transportation, Fortune 500 Corporations and other companies. On 1 April, 27% of those surveyed barred corporate travel to Asia; by the time of the 7 April survey, it had increased to 58%, on 16 April to 61% and on 6 May to 59%. As of 6 May, the largest restrictions were 96% to mainland China, 93%

to Hong Kong, 81% to Singapore and 33% to Toronto. 96% of the respondents feared catching SARS; 59% said employees returning from Asia had to go through long period of quarantine; and 100% said they would only travel to Asia again after the WHO lifted the travel advisory.

5. David Pang of the Hong Kong Airport Authority, Personal Communication, 12 June 2003.

6. Joseph Tung of the Travel Industry Council, Personal Communication, 24 May 2003.

7. Alison Langley, "Fear of respiratory disease stymies Swiss jewelry fair," as printed in the *International Herald Tribune* 10 April 2003, p. 15.

8. Pupils Sent Into Quarantine, BBC News, **www.news.bbc.co.uk/1/hi/education/ 2957951.stm**, 18 April 2003.

9. Ella Lee, Michael Gibb and Agencies, "WHO rebukes US universities for SARS ban," *South China Morning Post* 10 May 2003, p. A1.

10. Harry Doran and Tim Maitland, "Athletes Face Special Olympics Ban," *South China Morning Post*, 17 May 2003, p. A3.

11. James Lu of the Hong Kong Hotels Association, Personal Communication, 24 May 2003.

12. Steve Friess, "In Hong Kong, SARS fears infect hearts and minds," *USA Today* 15 April 2003, p. D06.

13. Ella Lee, "Waging war on an unknown enemy," *South China Morning Post* 26 March 2003, p. A11.

14. The Chinese University of Hong Kong, *Fighting SARS: We Care, We Serve*, **www.cuhk.edu.hk/sars/**, June 2003.

15. Dr. York Chow, "What's going on, and what shall we do?" Internal Memo for Medical Colleagues, 13 April 2003.

16. The Chinese University of Hong Kong, *Fighting SARS: We Care, We Serve*, **www.cuhk.edu,hk/sars/**, June 2003.

17. See endnote 15.

18. Mary Ann Benitez, "SARS heroes denied top honour," *South China Morning Post* 1 July 2003, page C16.

19. Shaoni Bhattacharya and Debora MacKenzie, "Exotic animals likely source of SARS," *New Scientist*, **www.newscientist.com/hottopics/sars/ article.jsp?id=99993763&sub=News%20update**, 23 May 2003.

20. Hong Kong Government Press Release, **www.info.gov.hk/gia/general/200307/ 19/0719079/htm**, 19 July 2003.

21. **www.register.scmp.com/projectshield/acknowledgements.html**

22. Indira A R Lakshmanan, "Exploring China's silence on SARS: New details surface on initial cover-up," *Boston Globe* 25 May 2003.

23. Anna Healy Fenton, "My husband should not have died like this," *South China Morning Post* 10 June 2003, p. A16.

24. Teddy Ng, "SARS job complaints swamp watchdog," *The Standard* 29 July 2003, p. B3.

25. Patsy Moy, "SARS stigma puts control of disease at risk," *South China Morning Post* 29 July 2003, p. C1.

26. Niki Law, "Generous spirit thrives in a time of great need," *South China Morning Post* 19 May 2003.

27. Hong Kong Government Press Release, **www.info.gov.hk/gia/general/200307/19/0719079/htm**, 19 July 2003.

28. See **www.alumni.cuhk.edu.hk/eng/wecare**.

29. See **www.sosick.org**.

30. **www.hku.hk.gened/withu/Frame3_contents.htm**.

31. The lunch was attended by the two authors for this chapter and another person in the hotel sector.

32. **www.hongkongunmasked.com** is a collaboration between Civic Exchange and Lemon, both members of Fearbusters. Another site created as a response to SARS was BrightenHK **www.brightenhk.org.hk**, which as a collaboration between The Outstanding Young Persons' Association, Internet Professional Association, Better Hong Kong Foundation and World Trade Centres Association.

33. The various Fearbusters campaigns are described in their Newsletters, **www.fearbuster.org.hk**. This book is also a direct result of the campaign.

34. See **www.operateunite.hkcss.org.hk**.

35. See **www.teamclean.gov.hk**.

36. See **www.info.gov.hk/gia/general/200305/29/0529228.htm**.

37. See **www.vision2047.org.hk**. The Vision 2047 group's mission is to strengthen understanding of Hong Kong international role. They wrote a letter in April 2003 which was sent to all the members' contacts all around the world. Other business groups also posted the letter on their websites.

38. See **www.hkgcc.org.hk/hkcomesback**.

39. See **www.britcham.com** and **www.amcham.org.hk**.

40. Jonathan Sharp, "SARS wars: Cathay fight back," *Hong Kong Business* July 2003, pp. 64–66.

41. James Hughes-Hallett, Chairman of Cathay Pacific Airways, *Flying Through Turbulent Skies*, speech to the Aerospace Forum Asia Industry Luncheon, 21 May 2003.

42. Hong Kong 2003, exhibition catalogue, Fong & Yeung Studio, 2003.

43. See **www.sarsart.org**.

44. Tom Hiditch, "The mask of sorrow," Post Magazine, *South China Morning Post* 8 June 2003, p. 10 & p. 12.

45. Ibid, p.12.

46. Ibid.

47. Katherine Forestier, "Academics in a spin to contain the SARS fallout," *South China Morning Post* 24 May 2003, p. W3.
48. Ella Lee, Michael Gibb and Agencies, "WHO rebukes US universities for SARS ban," *South China Morning Post* 10 May 2003, front page.

CHAPTER **14**

1. World Health Organization (WHO), *Severe acute respiratory syndrome (SARS): Status of the outbreak and lessons for the immediate future*, 20 May 2003.
2. Ibid.
3. SARS Expert Committee, *SARS in Hong Kong: From Experience to Action*, 2 October 2003, pp. 68–70, available online at **www.sars-expertcom.gov.hk**.
4. Mary Anne Benitez, "Taskforce was on alert pre-SARS," *South China Morning Post* 6 June 2003, p. C6.
5. See endnote 3, p. 17, Figure 3.3.
6. Report of the Hospital Authority Review Panel on the SARS Outbreak, released by the Hospital Authority on 16 October 2003, pp. 17–18, paragraph 2.13.
7. Ibid, p. 17, paragraph 2.12.
8. Ibid, pp. 145–147, paragraphs 6.96, 6.97 and 6.102.
9. Ibid, p. 16, paragraph 2.8.
10. Ibid, p. 30, paragraph 3.8.
11. See endnote 3, pp. 87–90.
12. Ibid, pp. 87–88.
13. Ibid, p. 88.
14. Civic Exchange and the National Democratic Institute for International Affairs (NDI), *Accountability Without Democracy*, September 2002, p. 29 paragraph 7.6.
15. Ella Lee, "Hospital vetoed SARS ward closure," *South China Morning Post* 31 July 2003, p. 1. The SARS Expert Committee noted that "the absence of a pre-determined hospital outbreak control plan and the inadequate involvement of [Department of Health] staff in critical decisions about outbreak control measures at PWH were not conducive to the management of the outbreak," see *SARS in Hong Kong: From Experience to Action*, p. 71.
16. See endnote 6, p. 18, paragraphs 2.15–2.16.
17. Ibid, p.19, paragraph 2.20.
18. See endnote 3, p. 72.
19. Mary Ann Benitez, "The struggle to profile a killer," *South China Morning Post* 25 June 2003, p. A14.
20. Ibid
21. See endnote 6, p. 16, paragraph 2.9.
22. See endnote 3, p. 74.

23. Ibid, p. 67.

24. Ibid.

25. Patsy Moy, "Leaders showed indifference towards outbreak, says panelist," *South China Morning Post* 5 October 2003, front page.

26. For a useful discussion of the possible legal issues, see D K Srivastava and Richard Cullen, "SARS in the HKSAR: Some Important Legal Issues," *Hong Kong Lawyer* July 2003, pp. 71–83.

27. Ravina Shamdasani, "Payout to 3 more medics' families," *South China Morning Post* 30 June 2003, p. C14.

28. The University of Hong Kong's Public Opinion Programme conducted many surveys before and after 1 July 2003 that provide useful information on how members of the Hong Kong public felt about how they were being governed. See **http://hkupop.hku.hk**.

CONTRIBUTORS

Stephen Brown has lived in Hong Kong for twenty years. He is married with two teenage children. He is head of regional research at Kim Eng Securities, a leading Asian securities firm. He is particularly interested in the economics of public policy decisions and has become increasingly interested in the history of public policy development in Hong Kong. He is a regular columnist with *The Standard* newspaper in Hong Kong, appears regularly on both television and radio and is a director of Civic Exchange, Hong Kong's independent public policy think tank.

Moira Chan-Yeung is on leave as a Professor of Medicine at the University of British Columbia (UBC) and is currently Chair Professor of Respiratory Medicine at the University of Hong Kong. She has headed the Occupational and Environmental Lung Diseases Unit at UBC since 1989. She has also served as the Chairperson of the Assembly of Environmental and Occupational Health for the American Thoracic Society; as a member of the Pulmonary Disease Advisory Committee, National Heart, Lung, and Blood Institute, part of the US National Institutes of Health; and as Chairperson of the Respiratory Diseases Section for the International Union Against Tuberculosis and Lung Disease. Professor Chan-Yeung's research interests include occupational asthma and lung disease, environmental and genetic risk factors in asthma and lung cancer, and the epidemiology and control of tuberculosis.

Gregory Cheng was born in Hong Kong and completed secondary school at St. Joseph's College. In 1971 he studied in Canada and obtained MD and PhD degrees at the University of Toronto, specialising in Haematology, Transfusion Medicine and Oncology. Dr. Cheng returned to work in Hong Kong in 1992, first at the Queen Mary Hospital and then at the Prince of Wales Hospital, where he has been since 1997. He is now a fellow of the Hong Kong Academy of Medicine, and Professor at the Faculty of Medicine, Chinese University of Hong Kong.

William Chiu received his Bachelor of Science in Business from the University of Minnesota, USA, in 1997. Upon returning to his hometown of Hong Kong, he took up business planning and support roles on the trading floors of JP Morgan and Citibank and also assisted in the founding of an internet start-up business. Chiu has been a Researcher for Civic Exchange since April 2003 and is currently an MBA student at the Hong Kong University of Science and Technology.

Michael E DeGolyer has been Director of the Hong Kong Transition Project since 1993. He obtained his PhD in 1985 from Claremont Graduate University, USA, in comparative and historical political economy and is Associate Professor of Government and International Studies at Hong Kong Baptist University. He has co-authored two books and is the author of more than 70 research papers/reports and over 60 published research articles and book chapters. DeGolyer has also been a weekly columnist for *The Standard* (a China-region business daily) since May 2000 and an invited columnist for the *South China Morning Post*, *Apple Daily*, *Hong Kong Economic Times*, and the *Asian Wall Street Journal*. He is a contributor to the Economist Intelligence Unit quarterly *Country Reports on Hong Kong* (1995-1998, 2000-present). Since 1989, he has made over 2,500 briefings to local and international media, businesses, consulates and other officials of more than 50 countries, Hong Kong Government departments, and academics on Hong Kong and China affairs.

Veronica Galbraith obtained her BA in Psychology from Huron University College at the University of Western Ontario, Canada. From 1998-2001 she managed tutors and students with Frontier College, a Canadian literacy organisation, as part of its London (Ontario) executive. She also worked at the Canadian Consulate in Hong Kong between 1999 and

2003. Galbraith joined Civic Exchange in March 2003 as a Researcher. As such, she has worked on a wide range of projects including a report on corporate social responsibility, the Fearbusters campaign, and the publication *Building Democracy: Creating Good Government for Hong Kong.*

Anthony J Hedley has been Chair Professor of Community Medicine in the University of Hong Kong since 1988. He was formerly professor of public health in the University of Glasgow. His main research and public health advocacy interests in recent years have been in the field of environmental health, including outdoor and indoor air pollution, and the prevention of disease caused by tobacco. An important goal of the University of Hong Kong's Department of Community Medicine is to translate epidemiological research findings into public health policy.

Tai-Hing Lam graduated from the Faculty of Medicine of the University of Hong Kong in 1975 and obtained his MD degree there in 1988. He has been Chair Professor and Head of the Department of Community Medicine of the University of Hong Kong since 2000. His research spans the areas of epidemiology, occupational and environmental health, tobacco control, lifestyle factors, sexual and adolescent health, and molecular epidemiology.

Alexis Lau is an environmental scientist and Associate Director of the Center for Coastal and Atmospheric Research of the Hong Kong University of Science and Technology. A native of Hong Kong, Alexis graduated from the Chinese University of Hong Kong in 1984, got his PhD in Atmospheric and Oceanic Sciences from Princeton University in 1991, and returned to Hong Kong just before 1997. His specialty is in modelling and statistical data analysis for environmental and atmospheric sciences, with particular focus on air quality issues over Hong Kong and the Pearl River Delta. A true believer in the importance of explaining science to the public, he also works actively to promote science education in primary schools.

Edith MC Lau is a Professor in the Department of Community and Family Medicine in the Chinese University of Hong Kong. She is also the Deputy Director of the School of Public Health and the Director of the Jockey Club Center for Osteoporosis Care and Control in the Chinese University of Hong Kong. She is currently the President of the Hong Kong College of Community Medicine. She is an expert in the field of epidemiology, and has conducted much research in women's health, osteoporosis and other chronic diseases. She has contributed to original epidemiology research and the development of public health policy in the recent SARS outbreak. She has published more than 100 papers in international medical journals.

Gabriel M Leung is currently Clinical Assistant Professor at the Department of Community Medicine of the University of Hong Kong. He is a key member of the SARS Epidemiology and Public Health Research Group, a collaboration between the University of Hong Kong and Imperial College, London. His research spans the areas of epidemiology, health services research, and health policy and economics. As a Fulbright Scholar, he graduated from Harvard University School of Public Health and received his undergraduate and postgraduate medical education at the Universities of Western Ontario and Toronto.

Christine Loh is Chief Executive Officer of Civic Exchange, an independent public policy think-tank. She holds a law degree from England and a Masters Degree in Chinese and Comparative Law from City University, Hong Kong. She also has been awarded the degree of Doctor of Law, *honoris causa*, from her alma mater, the University of Hull, England. In 1992, she was appointed to the Legislative Council. She gave up her business career in 1994 to become a full-time legislator and ran successfully in the 1995 and 1998 elections. She chose not to stand for re-election in 2000 to start Civic Exchange. Her work in public policy and promoting environmental protection and equal opportunity is well known. Loh writes extensively for local and international publications.

Stephen K.C. Ng graduated from the Faculty of Medicine, University of Hong Kong in 1972. He subsequently went to the United States and became a board-certified paediatrician in 1979. He obtained his Doctor of Public Health (Epidemiology) from the School of Public Health, Columbia University in 1986. Dr. Ng was a lecturer of Community Medicine at the University of Hong Kong between 1974-76. He was Professor of Paediatrics and Epidemiology at Columbia University between 1986-93 doing research in perinatal and cancer epidemiology before returning to Hong Kong in 1993. He is now Adjunct Associate Professor of Community Medicine at the Chinese University of Hong Kong as well as Special Lecturer in Epidemiology at Columbia University.

Alexandra A Seno is a freelance journalist and the Hong Kong correspondent for *Newsweek* magazine. As the granddaughter, daughter and sister of medical doctors, the SARS outbreak was a story that was personally important to her. Alexandra has covered Asian economics, politics, health and pop culture for over a decade, including seven and a half years at *Asiaweek* Magazine (a Time Inc. weekly publication based in Hong Kong). After receiving her Bachelor of Science undergraduate business law degree from the Ateneo de Manila University in the Philippines, she attended Xiamen University in Fujian for a year on a Chinese Education Ministry scholarship. Alexandra's work has also appeared in the *Washington Post* and the *International Herald Tribune*. She has lived in Hong Kong since 1994.

Jennifer Welker is editor of *TravelWeekly* China, a travel trade magazine published by a division of Reed Elsevier PLC. She also contributes to *TravelWeekly*'s sister publications for the Asia-Pacific region based in Hong Kong. Born in El Paso, Texas, she moved on soon after, and travelling became a very natural part of her life. At the age of 11, she moved to Hong Kong for two years and witnessed China just as it opened to the outside world in the early 1980s. She then realized Asia is where she wanted to spend the rest of her life. Upon graduation from the University of Missouri-Columbia's School of Journalism in 1993, she flew directly to Beijing where she spent three years in intensive Mandarin-language courses at the Beijing Capital Teacher's University. She has remained in Asia ever since.

YIP Yan-yan is a Researcher at Civic Exchange. She has assisted in Civic Exchange's various projects such as the Clean Environment Campaign and research on the Principal Officials Accountability System. She also took part in research for the HKSAR Government's Central Policy Unit on the Third Sector development in Hong Kong in 2002. She is now co-ordinating the Enhancing Democratic Participation Project at Civic Exchange and a project on how to sustain a cleaner environment at the Lower Ngau Tau Kok Estate post-SARS. Yip received her MSc in International Relations from the London School of Economics, UK.